University of Tehran Science and Humanities Series

Series Editor
Central Acquisitions Office, University of Tehran, Tehran, Iran

The *University of Tehran Science and Humanities Series* seeks to publish a broad portfolio of scientific books, basically aiming at scientists, researchers, students and professionals. The series includes peer-reviewed monographs, edited volumes, textbooks, and conference proceedings. It covers a wide range of scientific disciplines including, but not limited to Humanities, Social Sciences and Natural Sciences.

More information about this series at http://www.springer.com/series/14538

Ali Akbar Moosavi-Movahedi
Editor

Rationality and Scientific Lifestyle for Health

 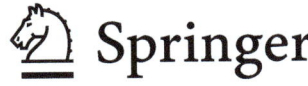

Editor
Ali Akbar Moosavi-Movahedi
Institute of Biochemistry
and Biophysics (IBB)
University of Tehran
Tehran, Iran

ISSN 2367-1092   ISSN 2367-1106   (electronic)
University of Tehran Science and Humanities Series
ISBN 978-3-030-74325-3   ISBN 978-3-030-74326-0   (eBook)
https://doi.org/10.1007/978-3-030-74326-0

© The Editor(s) (if applicable) and The Author(s), under exclusive license to Springer Nature Switzerland AG 2021

This work is subject to copyright. All rights are solely and exclusively licensed by the Publisher, whether the whole or part of the material is concerned, specifically the rights of translation, reprinting, reuse of illustrations, recitation, broadcasting, reproduction on microfilms or in any other physical way, and transmission or information storage and retrieval, electronic adaptation, computer software, or by similar or dissimilar methodology now known or hereafter developed.

The use of general descriptive names, registered names, trademarks, service marks, etc. in this publication does not imply, even in the absence of a specific statement, that such names are exempt from the relevant protective laws and regulations and therefore free for general use.

The publisher, the authors and the editors are safe to assume that the advice and information in this book are believed to be true and accurate at the date of publication. Neither the publisher nor the authors or the editors give a warranty, expressed or implied, with respect to the material contained herein or for any errors or omissions that may have been made. The publisher remains neutral with regard to jurisdictional claims in published maps and institutional affiliations.

This Springer imprint is published by the registered company Springer Nature Switzerland AG
The registered company address is: Gewerbestrasse 11, 6330 Cham, Switzerland

This book is dedicated to all the people of the world who sincere to knowledge, reason, science and ethics.

Human beings are members of a whole

In creation of one essence and soul

If one member is afflicted with pain

Other members uneasy will remain

If you've no sympathy for human pain

The name of human you cannot retain

Saadi Shirazi

Preface

Probably the few books have been written in the field of rationality, science and lifestyle. In this book, an attempt has been made to link science with reason and lifestyle so that the anomalies of technology branching out from science are under the control of rationality.

In the past, scientists discovered and developed science with good intentions for humanity, but today most abnormal technologies are created to generate large incomes without considering sustainable development, that caused industrial diseases, mental disorders, lack of peace for humanity.

This book raises the issues that science is supported by rationality and lifestyle and science is imbued with ethics to promote the effectiveness of science for human society.

This book not only introduces science and technique but also introduces knowledge as a combination of transcendental sciences, peripheral sciences (not just systems), human experience, conscience, strong imagination and inspiration, networking of data and information. In fact, science is the existence of enriched human (really science = scientist) being who can make the best use of better data and information to make the right decision. Based on the maturity, thinking and wisdom of the scientist, science yields and develop. Science is a correct analysis that can identify any phenomenon and provide solutions to problems. Science is different from research, but research has a narrow position that creates points, but science is integrated and connects points to reveal the true meaning. The important thing in the realm of science is that man can make the right analysis and make the right decision.

This book is written for the health and well-being of people to lead everyone to true prosperity. This states that man for his/her health should be in love with nature and be balanced with them as much as possible. The guidance is: if do not unbalance the nature so that its own balance is not disturbed. The best and healthiest for human beings is to have a balance in life and nature. Here introduces what is useful nutritious, functional foods, nutraceuticals, antioxidants and how natural molecules, which are from the generosity of nature, can be the best medicine for human beings.

In this book, the molecular meaning of stress is defined by the presence of unbalanced free radicals in the body. Most diseases, especially type 2 diabetes, which makes up most diabetics, come from this pathway. Our scientific evidence shows that diabetes type 2 is not just a disease of sugar but it is a disease of stress. In this book expresses about healthier lifestyle by considering psycho-emotional dimension of wellness. And finally this book states that good sleep is the principle of health and happiness for humanity and how it removes stress from mankind and how unbalanced free radicals in good sleep are expelled from human beings.

We hope that the contents of this book will be useful and make tranquility for the readers, especially during the outbreak of COVID-19 that man needs inner quietness, and we hope that the mores suggested in this book will show a new path to a better life.

Trhran, Iran   Ali Akbar Moosavi-Movahedi

Acknowledgments The support of University of Tehran, Iran National Science Foundation (INSF), Iran National Elites Foundation, UNESCO Chair on Interdisciplinary Research in Diabetes affiliated at University of Tehran, Center of Excellence in Biothermodynamics affiliated at University of Tehran, Iran Society of Biophysical Chemistry, Chemistry & Chemical Engineering Research Center of Iran (CCERCI), Standard Research Institute, Functional Food Research Core (FRC) at University of Tehran are gratefully acknowledged.

About This Book

This book will guide you how to find knowledge, how to get acquainted with nature, how rationality helps to promote science, and how a good lifestyle makes a person healthy and happy.

Contents

Philosophy Virtue of Nature, Mankind and Natural Health 1
Ali Akbar Moosavi-Movahedi

Bioinspiration and Biomimicry in Lifestyle 9
Sedigheh Abedanzadeh, Maryam Nourisefat,
and Zainab Moosavi-Movahedi

Nature's Generosity in Protecting Human Health 31
Nazanin Seighal Delshad, Bahareh Soleimanpour,
and Peyman Salehi

**Biodiversity and Drug Discovery Approach to Natural
Medicine**.. 61
Mansooreh Mazaheri and Ali Akbar Moosavi-Movahedi

Nutraceuticals and Superfoods............................. 75
Mehdi Mohammadian, Maryam Salami, Maryam Moghadam,
Zahra Emam-Djomeh, and Ali Akbar Moosavi-Movahedi

Spices as Traditional Remedies: Scientifically Proven Benefits ... 91
Mona Miran, Maryam Salami, and Zahra Emam-Djomeh

Halal Products and Healthy Lifestyle 115
Elnaz Hosseini, Mahdie Rahban, and Ali Akbar Moosavi-Movahedi

Lifestyle in the Regulation of Diabetic Disorders 129
Fereshteh Taghavi, Mahdie Rahban,
and Ali Akbar Moosavi-Movahedi

**Healthier Lifestyle by Considering Psychoemotional Dimension
of Wellness**.. 155
Monireh-Sadat Mousavi and Gholamhossein Riazi

Good Sleep as an Important Pillar for a Healthy Life 167
Faezeh Moosavi-Movahedi and Reza Yousefi

Index 197

Editor and Contributors

About the Editor

Ali Akbar Moosavi-Movahedi is currently Professor of Biophysical Chemistry at Institute of Biochemistry and Biophysics (IBB), University of Tehran. Born in Shiraz, Iran, in 1953, graduated from National University of Iran (NUI) with a B.Sc. in Chemistry, 1975, from Eastern Michigan University (EMU), USA, with a M.Sc. in Chemistry (Bioanalytical Chemistry), 1979 and from University of Manchester, UK, with a Ph.D. in Biophysical Chemistry, 1986. He is the author of 20 books written in Persian and numerous research full papers published in mostly international research journals mainly in the area of structural elucidation of protein, enzyme and DNA. He is a Fellow of the World Academy of Sciences (TWAS) and Fellow of the Islamic Academy of Sciences (IAS) and the member of a few of related international scientific societies and is currently the president of Iran Society of Biophysical Chemistry. He is the Editor-in-Chief of *Science Cultivation* (Journal) that is the journal of popularization and enculturation of science. The banner of this journal is: the plant is cultivated in the soil but science in the mind.

For more information: ibb.ut.ac.ir/∼moosavi

Contributors

Sedigheh Abedanzadeh Faculty of Chemistry, Kharazmi University, Tehran, Iran;
Institute of Biochemistry and Biophysics (IBB), University of Tehran, Tehran, Iran

Zahra Emam-Djomeh Department of Food Science and Engineering, University College of Agriculture & Natural Resources, University of Tehran, Karaj, Iran

Elnaz Hosseini Institute of Biochemistry and Biophysics (IBB), University of Tehran, Tehran, Iran

Mansooreh Mazaheri Standard Research Institute, Research Center of Food Technology and Agricultural Products, Karaj, Iran

Mona Miran Department of Food Science and Engineering, University College of Agriculture & Natural Resources, University of Tehran, Karaj, Iran

Maryam Moghadam Department of Food Science and Engineering, University College of Agriculture & Natural Resources, University of Tehran, Karaj, Iran

Mehdi Mohammadian Department of Food Science and Engineering, University College of Agriculture & Natural Resources, University of Tehran, Karaj, Iran

Ali Akbar Moosavi-Movahedi Institute of Biochemistry and Biophysics (IBB), University of Tehran, Tehran, Iran

Faezeh Moosavi-Movahedi Institute of Biochemistry and Biophysics (IBB), University of Tehran, Tehran, Iran

Zainab Moosavi-Movahedi Chemistry and Chemical Engineering Research Center of Iran, Tehran, Iran

Monireh-Sadat Mousavi Laboratory of Neuro-Organic Chemistry, Institute of Biochemistry and Biophysics (IBB), University of Tehran, Tehran, Iran

Maryam Nourisefat Institute of Biochemistry and Biophysics (IBB), University of Tehran, Tehran, Iran

Mahdie Rahban Institute of Biochemistry and Biophysics (IBB), University of Tehran, Tehran, Iran

Gholamhossein Riazi Laboratory of Neuro-Organic Chemistry, Institute of Biochemistry and Biophysics (IBB), University of Tehran, Tehran, Iran

Maryam Salami Department of Food Science and Engineering, University College of Agriculture & Natural Resources, University of Tehran, Karaj, Iran

Peyman Salehi Department of Phytochemistry, Medicinal Plants and Drugs Research Institute, Shahid Beheshti University, Tehran, Iran

Nazanin Seighal Delshad Department of Phytochemistry, Medicinal Plants and Drugs Research Institute, Shahid Beheshti University, Tehran, Iran

Bahareh Soleimanpour Department of Phytochemistry, Medicinal Plants and Drugs Research Institute, Shahid Beheshti University, Tehran, Iran

Fereshteh Taghavi Faculty of Biological Science, Tarbiat Modares University, Tehran, Iran

Reza Yousefi Protein Chemistry Laboratory (PCL), Department of Biology, College of Sciences, Shiraz University, Shiraz, Iran

Philosophy Virtue of Nature, Mankind and Natural Health

Ali Akbar Moosavi-Movahedi

Abstract

The universe is high in spirituality, and the abstract of the universe is also a human being who owns all the wonders of being. Thus, human health is formed by a balance between external nature and human inner nature. Whatever man departs from his nature, approach to unbalanced diseases and make a balance, which is the principle of human health. Self-knowledge is thus the foundation of human health and happiness. Human beings need comprehensive knowledge to know themselves, so they can appreciate themselves and not self-harm. If one realizes that it does not harm itself, it certainly does not harm others. Humankind has created technologies based on inferior knowledge, whereas it needs vast knowledge to produce healthy technologies. Today, a large part of man-made technologies is anomalous and create pollutants that produce unbalanced free radicals for humans and other creatures. Unbalanced free radicals created by pollutants that caused human disease and damage to the planet and the environment. Technologies must be linked to ethics, sustainable environment, bio-model, biomimetic and bioinspiration and health.

Keywords

Nature · Human · Natural health · Bio-model · Biomimetic · Ethics · Free radicals · Diseases

1 Introduction

Man is the abstract of the whole universe, and his health must be in balance with nature outside the body. A moderate man with nature has guaranteed his health and happiness. The secret of moderation in humans is the knowledge from the self and nature outside the body. Self-scrutiny is the base of human health and fortune. A man has two beings: the human body who needs water, food, air, clothes, and the human reality (soul) needs a healthy spirit. The healthy soul and spirit is also the capital of a healthy body. A healthy spirit is achieved by spirituality and a healthy body with a balance with nature. So, the logic of life teaches us to increase and practice our knowledge for a healthy soul and body. Be capable of being wise. Man needs knowledge-based on wisdom to understand himself and creation. Wisdom or wise knowledge means the attainment of the truth of knowledge, science, and reason, and is a solid issue in which there is no false. The meaning of wise knowledge is the set of knowledge, interdisciplinary sciences and understanding of the experience that leads man to the truth so that there is no doubt. Science is

A. A. Moosavi-Movahedi (✉)
Institute of Biochemistry and Biophysics (IBB), University of Tehran, Tehran, Iran
e-mail: moosavi@ut.ac.ir
URL: https://ibb.ut.ac.ir/~moosavi

© The Author(s), under exclusive license to Springer Nature Switzerland AG 2021
A. A. Moosavi-Movahedi (ed.), *Rationality and Scientific Lifestyle for Health*,
University of Tehran Science and Humanities Series,
https://doi.org/10.1007/978-3-030-74326-0_1

discovering realities as it is the scientist does not create anything but knows what is created. However, wise knowledge is the discovery of facts that certain people have access to. The world is a representation of knowledge, cognition and wisdom.

In this world we live in, everything is created for us, and according to the first law of thermodynamics, man cannot create even a small new thing in existence just can change the material and energy (Edsall and Gutfreund 1983). So must know and model the world, design and produce natural and healthy technologies based on it, and present it to mankind. The most optimal technologies come from biomimetics (Bar-Cohen 2011). It is appropriate to model the being in which we live. The purpose of being is not just the earth, but all the universe. Thinkers have extraterrestrial thinking. They know that they live on earth, but their livelihood comes from heaven.

All Earth's reactions originate from heat, and Earth's heat comes from the sun and other fiery spheres. So, we have to know that everything is not just on Earth. The planet is where we live, but it is ruled by invisible forces from the sky. Therefore, to understand the fundamental of terrestrial creatures, we must know the celestial creatures and secret forces, so we need to think and think extraterrestrial. Modeling the phenomena of being and living to create natural, man-made nature is the key to success in developing healthy and sustainable technologies. So, modeling nature, life and creature is the right way. To follow the right path is called wisdom. The purpose of this article is to pay attention to wisdom and creation that can be identified by nature's modeling, knowledge and innovation, and then to obtain the technology of reality and the product of biostructure based on the knowledge of reality.

Today, much of the technology is anomalous, producing pollutants that produce unbalanced free radicals in humans and other organisms.

Unbalanced free radicals created by pollutants cause disease to humans and damage to the planet and the environment. The creation of technologies must be linked to ethics, a sustainable environment, and health, not just economic benefits. In today's world, where technology growth is more economical and less about the ethics of technology, one needs to define and adopt a healthy lifestyle to deal with anomalies. Stress avoidance is one of the most important criteria of a good lifestyle, and one of the highest wealth in the world today is relaxation. The new definition of a developed country seems to be that the people and society of that country are at peace and tranquility. So, we need to know how to avoid stressful relationships. Molecular stress generates a variety of unbalanced free radicals from which many diseases originate (Özben 1998). One of the diseases of today's society that is shaped by stress and unbalanced free radicals and has many effects on the body is diabetes. Statistics show that 90% of diabetes is type 2 and known as an industrial disease. Diabetes complicates other types of diseases; that is why it is called "diabetes and its complications." Our research shows that type 2 diabetes is not just come from sugars but comes from stress (Taghavi and Moosavi-Movahedi 2019). In order to prevent stress in the body and reduce the development of diabetes, the right lifestyle should be chosen to diminish stress and diabetes. The following are some of the most important lifestyle modes of stress and diabetes management.

2 Exercise

Exercise is known to reduce stress in the body, free radicals and eventually to reduce or delay diseases in the body. Exercise enhances longevity and vitality. Aerobic exercise in the open environment and nature, its effect is a hundred times more. Exercise and mobility rebuilding the physical organs, also provide mental, intellectual, psychological ability. Of course, sports are various, and each can have a unique effect on the human condition. Scientific sources have always emphasized is the effect of physical activity in the prevention of diseases such as diabetes. The effects of exercise on health can be explained in terms of physiological, psychological, biochemical, metabolic capacity, and improvement of blood nutrient function. Type 2 diabetes is associated with overweight in adult and non-active lifestyles. However, physical inactivity alone can increase the risk of diabetes. Communities with good physical activity have a lower incidence of diabetes (Fentem 1994).

Numerous studies have shown that exercise, especially its regular form, affects metabolic processes by increasing insulin sensitivity, improving glucose tolerance and weight loss, and having an exact effect on cardiovascular health by decreasing blood pressure (Helmrich et al. 1991). Exercise alone can prevent many of the complications of diabetes, but, surprisingly, this treatment has been uniquely suited to people, but it is not much attention to this issue (Tanasescu et al. 2003).

The importance of sport has been so far that a new branch of medicine has emerged since the late twentieth century as sports medicine as one of the most important ways of preventing and treating many diseases. Indeed, Sports Medicine is a branch of medical knowledge that focuses on physical fitness, treatment, and disease prevention (Fentem 1994). On the other hand, meditation practices have been replaced by the scientific perspectives for clear effects in the treatment of diseases and its beneficial effects have been emphasized on insulin resistance, glucose tolerance, insulin sensitivity, lipid-lipoprotein levels, blood pressure, oxidative stress, and blood coagulation factors (Alexander et al. 2008). However, the critical point is that exercise in the open air and the use of nature's air is vital to human health and well-being. Exercise activities in the polluted air have the opposite effect and should be treated with caution.

3 Nutrition and Diet

The type and quality of food consumed are directly related to people's health, so determined a proper diet will be necessary. It is so essential that it is said, "You say what you eat, and I say who you are." Part of human transcendence comes from the quality consumption and quantity of food. If you look at the quantity and quality of your food, you will not need any medication. One should not even take medication as much as possible, but his food should be his/her medicine "to eat food as medicine." This type of food is called super or functional food. Eating a healthy diet, maintaining an ideal weight, normal blood sugar, providing enough energy in diabetes conditions, and keeping blood fats at optimum levels. Nutrition of fresh foods containing vegetables and fruits due to the antioxidant that reduces free radicals removes toxins from the body and improves the body's immune system. But consuming industrial foods that contain oxidant preservatives can cause stress and increase unbalanced free radicals. If industrial food is eaten several times a week, it must be eaten fresh several times to reduce or counteract the effect (Wheeler et al. 2012).

Foods are considering their effects on diabetes or glycemic index; it is crucial to consider how they are used in diabetic patients. Modern lifestyles and changes in conventional eating habits have led to high consumption of fast foods and ready meals, fat intake and reduced consumption of vegetables and fruits. These factors have led to an increase in the prevalence of diseases. Research suggests that the use of preservatives and antimicrobial agents in a variety of food industries has led to the development of diabetes and other diseases (Meyer et al. 2001). Proper diets, regular exercise and weight control have the potential to control diseases, primarily type 2 diabetes. In ancient societies, traditional methods of using nutrients, processed foods and herbal therapies effectively prevent and treat many diseases, including stress and diabetes. Wholesome foods have created another crucial natural pathway for disease prevention and treatment. Many of these processed foods have antioxidant and anti-inflammatory properties (Boaz et al. 2011). The ancient healing method has a tremendous impact on the application of differentiated or combination methods and approaches to plants, animals, minerals-based medicines, spiritual therapies in preventing and treating diseases, and maintaining health. In industrial societies, tradition, medicine has been termed complementary or alternative medicine. Traditional medicine can benefit from the achievements of modern medicine, and modern medicine can benefit from the experience and achievements of traditional medicine. The integration of traditional medicine and modern medicine will be one of the most critical decisions in the medical field. It should be developed databases, software in the combination of modern medicine and traditional medicine to benefit medical doctors and patients' treatment. Both methods bring science and experience, and wisdom to humankind. Traditional medicine is a comprehensive term that refers to traditional Chinese medicine, Indian Orodha, Greek medicine, Iranian medicine, and various natural medicine forms. Traditional medicine includes herbal remedies, medications with an animal or mineral section, and non-pharmacological treatments, including acupuncture, manual treatments, and spiritual therapies (Zhang and Organization 2002). Of course, it is noteworthy if a person can do to heal his soul can have a counteraction in the health of his body.

4 Spiritual Beliefs

The biochemistry of the human body derives from consciousness and belief. Consciously reinforced beliefs become one's biochemistry. Certainly, even the smallest cell in the human body is fully aware of one's thoughts, feelings, and beliefs. Recent research has substantiated much of the biological science behind beliefs. The human belief system is actually formed by refining all the experiences learned through personality (Bogousslavsky and Inglin 2007; Abdoli et al. 2011).

In the meantime, culture and spirituality can play an essential role in empowering people to live a better life and cope with the disease. Empowerment is a positive and dynamic phenomenon that is increasingly playing a role in modulating diseases, especially those with stress. Feeling responsible for maintaining the body as a divine blessing is full-fledged management of health and well-being. A human being with a morality cares for, safeguards and protects his health. In fact, this is one of the empowerment solutions (Lipton 2016).

A man with good deeds can use the law of reaction and bring goodness back into his/her life. If anyone does a good deed, he/she will return several times more. You do good and open up to the goddess who gives you God in the desert.

5 Reduce Stress and Anxiety

Urbanization, especially in big cities, and its consequences, such as chemical pollution, traffic congestion, street traffic, and mental disorders, are major causes of stress and anxiety in today's world. Recent research has well established that diverse stresses eventually play an essential role in the pathogenesis of diabetes and its associated vascular complications by causing oxidative stress and systemic inflammation (Davì et al. 2010).

Oxidative stress is an acute state of imbalance between the production of oxidative agents and the antioxidant defense mechanism that leads to poor tissue function and destruction. This stress is part of the disease-causing processes of reactive oxygen species (ROS) that plays a role in insulin resistance (Betteridge 2000). The mentioned species are also the hallmarks of type-2 diabetes. On the other hand, elevated blood glucose causes spontaneous oxidation of glucose, glycation of proteins (producing radical and non-radical active species, especially ROS) and activation of some metabolic pathways. These changes themselves accelerate the production of ROS and cause chemical and oxidative changes of lipids, DNA and proteins in various tissues (Davì et al. 2010). The production of a chain of new free radical-generating interactions will lead to more exposure to macromolecules and the formation of toxic compounds (Betteridge 2000). Oxidative stress also plays a key role in the development of diabetes complications such as cataracts, kidney and nerve damage due to the production of toxic products (Davì et al. 2010). The occurrence of stress will have many effects on the body's metabolism through its mechanism action (Brindley and Rolland 1989; Engström et al. 2003).

The presence of inflammatory markers is a signal of the onset of obesity. Overweight is directly proportional to the concentration of these inflammatory markers. Recent research has shown that the use of potassium sorbate as a widely used preservative in the food, pharmaceutical, health, and cosmetic industries can have damaging effects. These substances also have a direct and acute interactive effect on the development or exacerbation of diabetes mellitus. They mediate the production and intensification of a variety of oxidative toxic species, and in particular, a role in guiding the structure of human serum albumin to fibrillogenesis (Taghavi et al. 2013, 2014), due to the harmful effects of preservatives in altering the structure of proteins and producing toxic intermediate structures and interfering roles. They emphasize the process of forming and exacerbating diabetes, eliminating or restricting the use of these substances in the industries mentioned above, and emphasize that consumers modulate these substances.

Of course, it is worth noting that if antioxidants are discovered as antimicrobial and antibacterial, they may be used as antioxidant preservatives in industrial foods in the near future. Our research team reported the first report of antimicrobial and antibacterial peptides of camel milk proteins (Salami et al. 2010, 2017; Moslehishad et al. 2013, 2014; Moosavi-Movahedi 2013; Rahimi et al. 2016; Khalesi et al. 2017), then reported the antibacterial peptides of walnut proteins (Jahanbani et al. 2016, 2018).

6 Sleep

Scientific research shows that sleep detoxifies the body and removes waste from the brain. Sleep is healing and restorative, and one of the best antioxidants called melatonin is produced in healthy sleep and relieves stress. During waking up, the body experiences a variety of stresses, and sleep is a remedy. It is worth noting that sleep is different from the rest and that healthy sleep is defined at night when the sun is not present. In today's urban and urbanization, people overuse virtualized social media, changing their sleeping hours and usually getting up late. Even as they fall asleep, they wake up to the unnatural noise of the city, and insomnia just starts for them and may fall asleep at non-biological hours instead. This story does not detoxify well the body and causes a lot of stress that is induced by a variety of disasters and anomalies for the individual and society. In this state of the body and brain infraction, human learning also comes down. Insomnia causes people to spend the whole day constantly sleeping and waking, which drastically reduces focus and accuracy. Also, in these situations, people are not able to perform precise and sensitive tasks that depend on high alertness and concentration (Heijden et al. 2005). Therefore, it is necessary for a healthy lifestyle for the people and society to control the anomalies. A good lifestyle is a collection of old and new knowledge that must be collected from all cultures of the nations and applied in today's life (Foley et al. 2004; Spiegel et al. 1999).

Understanding the body's biological clock is very important. The theme of "Body Biology Clock" won the 2017 Nobel Prize in Medicine and Physiology. The Nobel Committee jointly awarded the prize to three scientists because of the tremendous impact of this finding on health. The body clock or biological rhythm is a 24-h cycle that regulates the activity of the organs as it rotates around the Earth and passes day by night and vice versa. It plays an important role in regulating body temperature, hormone secretion, and metabolism. This is the hour that makes us sleep at night and wake up in the morning. Disruption of the biological clock can have a profound effect on health, such as working in shifts or the phenomenon of long-haul flights, where the destination and origin time differences are high and cause the body clock to adapt to a 24-h rhythm. In the short term, it opposes effects on memory, concentration and alertness, and other cognitive abilities, but over the long term, it increases the risk of developing type 2 diabetes and other diseases (Allada et al. 1998;

Dembinska et al. 1997; Emery et al. 1998). They identified a portion of DNA called the periodic gene that plays a role in this twenty-four-hour cycle (Frisch et al. 1994). The recurrent gene contains a specific protein synthesis (Hege et al. 1997). This protein increases during the night, and we fall asleep and get lower in the day and wake up and stay awake.

Insomnia increases and disrupts metabolism, resulting in insulin resistance and the development of type-2 diabetes, as insomnia decreases during night time sleep. Previous research suggests that insulin resistance in diabetic patients with insomnia (poor sleep quality) is 82% higher than those with normal sleep (Ananthakrishnan et al. 2013). In fact, prolonged periods of inadequate sleep can increase the level of fatty acid in the blood, disrupting the metabolism of fats and impairing insulin's ability to properly regulate blood sugar. In the long run, these destructive phenomena can cause people to develop diabetes. Fatty acids levels typically fluctuate throughout the day but usually follow a pattern that rises in the afternoon and decreases at midnight. Studies have shown that nocturnal insomnia increases the level of fatty acids at night. According to research conducted in adolescents, increased night time sleep by reducing metabolic regulation of fatty acids reduces the risk of diabetes (Vgontzas et al. 2009). Nocturnal insomnia speeds up the erosion of nerve cells in the brain and exacerbates diseases such as Alzheimer's and Parkinson's. This is why a lack of sleep can lead to the formation of amyloid plaques because the brain's cleaning system will be active during sleep, and this cleaning may defeat due to insomnia (Dauvilliers 2007).

6.1 Optimize Melatonin Levels in the Body

Two common environmental factors that can disrupt the sleep process are light and heat pollution. Therefore, they should not watch TV or use the computer for at least one hour before bedtime. These devices emit blue light itself, which makes the brain mistakenly imagine that it is still day. The brain normally begins to release the melatonin between 9 and 10 PM, and light emitted by these devices may stop the process. Regular exposure to sunlight helps to produce the melatonin pineal gland in the absolute darkness of the night. So, the bed should be a completely dark environment. Even a slight amount of light entering the bedroom can disturb the bio-clock and affect melatonin production. It is recommended to use yellow, orange or red low light bulbs if need a light source for night time in the bedroom. Light with such bandwidth may not disrupt melatonin production as much as blue and white lights. For this purpose, salt lamps can also be used. Bedroom temperature should not exceed 21 °C. Studies show that the proper room temperature for sleeping is between 15 and 20 °C (Haim and Zubidat 2015). Sunbathing in the morning will help the body's biological clock, which needs a little bit of daylight to reset. The scientific research results show that 10–15 min of morning sun exposure send a precise message to the body's internal clock and announces the start of the day. This phenomenon makes the body have a distinct and complete definition of the day and does not confuse it with night time artificial light (Krauchi et al. 1997).

Therefore, insomnia is one of the biggest problems of mankind, and given its widespread implications that encompass various aspects of personal and social life, there is a need for education and awareness of the body about the biological clock. It is also imperative that precise and rapid planning be put on the program of life that plans to improve the sleep patterns of society, especially youth of life.

7 Activate Happiness Hormones

Hormones are chemicals produced by various glands in the body (Farhud et al. 2014). They travel through the bloodstream, act as messengers, and are involved in many body processes and help regulate mood. Some hormones help boost positive emotions, including happiness and pleasure. The "happy hormones" are:

Dopamine is known as the "feel-good" hormone and is a neurotransmitter. Dopamine is associated with pleasant emotions associated with learning, memory, motor function and more.

Serotonin is a neurotransmitter that helps regulate mood as well as sleep, appetite, digestion, learning ability and memory.

Oxytocin, often referred to as the "love hormone." It can also help boost trust, empathy, and bond in relationships.

Endorphins are analgesics that the body responds to stress and reduces discomfort.

8 Conclusion

Today, stress invades the human body in many ways, inside and outside the body. The more people move away from their natural life; the more stress they have on them. In today's life, human beings are more exposed to offensive technologies and their adverse effects. A good lifestyle modulates the anomalous effects of industrial pollutants that move humans away from their natural paths. We have reported the subject of stress inhibition manners (Taghavi and Moosavi-Movahedi 2019). It seems that having a good lifestyle requires a lot of experience and knowledge that should be available from the old to the new era. The software needs to be developed to rationalize the old knowledge and new knowledge-based mostly on technical science to compile and optimize it. The most important thing a human being should seek is certainly a "tranquility and peace" that is not achieved by living in modern cities with great wealth and money. Tranquility and relaxation come from the blessing of others, living with nature, living with contentment, sleeping and being well-nourished, gaining knowledge and wisdom, and receiving inspiration from the pure self.

References

Abdoli S, Ashktorab T, Ahmadi F, Parvizy S, Dunning T (2011) Religion, faith and the empowerment process: stories of Iranian people with diabetes. Int J Nurs Pract 17(3):289–298

Alexander GK, Taylor AG, Innes KE, Kulbok P, Selfe TK (2008) Contextualizing the effects of yoga therapy on diabetes management: a review of the social determinants of physical activity. Fam Community Health 31(3):228–239

Allada R, White NE, So WV, Hall JC, Rosbash M (1998) A mutant drosophila homolog of mammalian clock disrupts circadian rhythms and transcription of period and timeless. Cell 93(5):791–804

Ananthakrishnan AN, Long MD, Martin CF, Sandler RS, Kappelman MD (2013) Sleep disturbance and risk of active disease in patients with crohn's disease and ulcerative colitis. Clin Gastroenterol Hepatol 11(8):965–971

Bar-Cohen Y (2011) Biomimetics: nature-based innovation. CRC press

Betteridge DJ (2000) What is oxidative stress? Metab Clin Exp 49(2):3–8

Boaz M, Leibovitz E, Dayan YB, Wainstein J (2011) Functional foods in the treatment of type 2 diabetes: olive leaf extract, turmeric and fenugreek, a qualitative review. Funct Foods Health Dis 1(11):472–481

Bogousslavsky J, Inglin M (2007) Beliefs and the brain. Eur Neurol 58(3):129–132

Brindley DN, Rolland Y (1989) Possible connections between stress, diabetes, obesity, hypertension and altered lipoprotein metabolism that may result in atherosclerosis. Clin Sci 77(5):453–461

Dauvilliers Y (2007) Insomnia in patients with neurodegenerative conditions. Sleep Med 8(Suppl 4):S27-34

Davì G, Santilli F, Patrono C (2010) Nutraceuticals in diabetes and metabolic syndrome. Cardiovasc Ther 28(4):216–226

Dembinska M, Stanewsky R, Hall J, Rosbash M (1997) Circadian cycling of a period-lacz fusion protein in drosophila: evidence for an instability cycling element in per. J Biol Rhythms 12:157–172

Edsall JT, Gutfreund H (1983) Biothermodynamics: the study of biochemical processes at equilibrium. Wiley, New York

Emery P, So WV, Kaneko M, Hall JC, Rosbash M (1998) Cry, a drosophila clock and light-regulated cryptochrome, is a major contributor to circadian rhythm resetting and photosensitivity. Cell 95(5):669–679

Engström G, Hedblad B, Stavenow L, Lind P, Janzon L, Lindgärde F (2003) Inflammation-sensitive plasma proteins are associated with future weight gain. Diabetes 52(8):2097–2101

Farhud D, Malmir M, Khanahmadi M (2014) Happiness and health: the biological factors-systematic review article. Iran J Public Health 43(11):1468

Fentem PH (1994) Benefits of exercise in health and disease. BMJ 308(6939):1291–1295

Foley D, Ancoli-Israel S, Britz P, Walsh J (2004) Sleep disturbances and chronic disease in older adults: results of the 2003 national sleep foundation sleep in America survey. J Psychosom Res 56(5):497–502

Frisch B, Hardin PE, Hamblen-Coyle MJ, Rosbash M, Hall JC (1994) A promoterless period gene mediates behavioral rhythmicity and cyclical per expression in a restricted subset of the drosophila nervous system. Neuron 12(3):555–570

Haim A, Zubidat AE (2015) Artificial light at night: melatonin as a mediator between the environment and epigenome. Philos Trans Royal Soc B Biol Sci 370 (1667):20140121

Hege DM, Stanewsky R, Hall JC, Giebultowicz JM (1997) Rhythmic expression of a per-reporter in the Malpighian tubules of decapitated drosophila: evidence for a brain-independent circadian clock. J Biol Rhythms 12(4):300–308

Helmrich SP, Ragland DR, Leung RW, Paffenbarger RS Jr (1991) Physical activity and reduced occurrence of non-insulin-dependent diabetes mellitus. N Engl J Med 325(3):147–152

Jahanbani R, Ghaffari SM, Salami M, Vahdati K, Sepehri H, Sarvestani NN, Sheibani N, Moosavi-Movahedi AA (2016) Antioxidant and anticancer activities of walnut (Juglans Regia L.) Protein hydrolysates using different proteases. Plant Foods Hum Nutr 71(4):402–409

Jahanbani R, Ghaffari M, Vahdati K, Salami M, Khalesi M, Sheibani N, Moosavi-Movahedi AA (2018) Kinetics study of protein hydrolysis and inhibition of angiotensin converting enzyme by peptides hydrolysate extracted from walnut. Int J Pept Res Ther 24(1):77–85

Khalesi M, Salami M, Moslehishad M, Winterburn J, Moosavi-Movahedi AA (2017) Biomolecular content of camel milk: a traditional superfood towards future healthcare industry. Trends Food Sci Technol 62:49–58

Krauchi K, Cajochen C, Wirz-Justice A (1997) A relationship between heat loss and sleepiness: effects of postural change and melatonin administration. J Appl Physiol 83(1):134–139

Lipton BH (2016) The biology of belief: unleashing the power of consciousness, matter & miracles. Hay House

Meyer KA, Kushi LH, Jacobs DR, Folsom AR (2001) Dietary fat and incidence of type 2 diabetes in older Iowa women. Diab Care 24(9):1528–1535

Moosavi-Movahedi AA (2013) Milk and its bioactive peptides: phenomenal nutraceutical food of the century. Pertanika J Sc Technol 21. University of Putra Malaysia Press Serdang, Selangor, Malaysia

Moslehishad M, Ehsani MR, Salami M, Mirdamadi S, Ezzatpanah H, Naslaji AN, Moosavi-Movahedi AA (2013) The comparative assessment of ace-inhibitory and antioxidant activities of peptide fractions obtained from fermented camel and bovine milk by lactobacillus rhamnosus PTCC 1637. Int Dairy J 29(2):82–87

Moslehishad M, Salami M, Mirdamadi S, Ehsani MR, Moosavi-Movahedi AA (2014) Production of fermented camel milk containing antioxidant and antihypertensive peptides. Iran 29857 Patent

Özben T (1998) Free radicals, oxidative stress, and antioxidants. 1 edn. Springer, Berlin

Rahimi M, Ghaffari SM, Salami M, Mousavy SJ, Niasari-Naslaji A, Jahanbani R, Yousefinejad S, Khalesi M, Moosavi-Movahedi AA (2016) ACE-inhibitory and radical scavenging activities of bioactive peptides obtained from camel milk casein hydrolysis with proteinase K. Dairy Sci Technol 96(4):489–499

Salami M, Moosavi-Movahedi AA, Ehsani MR, Yousefi R, Haertle T, Chobert J-M, Razavi SH, Henrich R, Balalaie S, Ebadi SA (2010) Improvement of the antimicrobial and antioxidant activities of camel and bovine whey proteins by limited proteolysis. J Agric Food Chem 58(6):3297–3302

Salami M, Niasari-Naslaji A, Moosavi-Movahedi AA (2017) Recollection: camel milk proteins, bioactive peptides and casein micelles. J Camel Pract Res 24(2):181–182

Spiegel K, Leproult R, Van Cauter E (1999) Impact of sleep debt on metabolic and endocrine function. The Lancet 354(9188):1435–1439

Taghavi F, Moosavi-Movahedi AA, Bohlooli M, Alijanvand HH, Salami M, Maghami P, Saboury A, Farhadi M, Yousefi R, Habibi-Rezaei M (2013) Potassium sorbate as an age activator for human serum albumin in the presence and absence of glucose. Int J Biol Macromol 62:146–154

Taghavi F, Moosavi-Movahedi A, Bohlooli M, Habibi-Rezaei M, Hadi Alijanvand H, Amanlou M, Sheibani N, Saboury A, Ahmad F (2014) Energetic domains and conformational analysis of human serum albumin upon co-incubation with sodium benzoate and glucose. J Biomol Struct Dyn 32(3):438–447

Taghavi F, Moosavi-Movahedi AA (2019) Free radicals, diabetes, and its complexities. In: Plant and human health, vol 2. Springer, Berlin, pp 1–41

Tanasescu M, Leitzmann MF, Rimm EB, Hu FB (2003) Physical activity in relation to cardiovascular disease and total mortality among men with type 2 diabetes. Circulation 107(19):2435–2439

Van der Heijden KB, Smits MG, Someren EJV, Boudewijn Gunning W (2005) Idiopathic chronic sleep onset insomnia in attention-deficit/hyperactivity disorder: a circadian rhythm sleep disorder. Chronobiol Int 22 (3):559–570

Vgontzas AN, Liao D, Pejovic S, Calhoun S, Karataraki M, Bixler EO (2009) Insomnia with objective short sleep duration is associated with type 2 diabetes: a population-based study. Diab Care 32 (11):1980–1985

Wheeler M, Dunbar S, Jaacks L, Karmally W, Mayer-Davis E, Wylie-Rosett J, Yancy W (2012) Macronutrients, food groups, and eating patterns in the management of diabetes: a systematic review of the literature. Diab Care 35(6):434–445

Zhang X, Organization WH (2002) Traditional medicine strategy 2002–2005. Geneva, p 74

Bioinspiration and Biomimicry in Lifestyle

Sedigheh Abedanzadeh, Maryam Nourisefat, and Zainab Moosavi-Movahedi

Abstract

Biomimetics is a new language that enables man to have effective communication with nature. Every human being encounters biomimetic products in normal daily lives, but they are not often recognized as such issues! From a biomimetic point of view, every phenomenon in nature is a source of inspiration to improve human life quality. The human lifestyle undergoes fundamental changes arising from the influence of biomimicry and bioinspiration in technology, health, art, and education. Nature seems to have the best solutions for everything. Every aspect of human life would be seriously affected by the emergence of new bioinspired tools, methods and capabilities at every scale from nano to macro and beyond. Biomimetics is a leading paradigm for the development of new technologies that potentially facilitate human lives. Expanding medical investigation to new bioinspired approaches accelerates innovations in healthcare. Art, education and architecture also gain considerable benefits from the revolution that biomimicry introduces into the human lifestyle. Nature knows best; by learning from its powerful lessons, we can model innovative strategies to successfull and fulfilling personal life.

Keywords

Biomimetic · Bioinspiration · Technology · Medicine · Art · Education

1 Introduction

Bioinspiration and biomimicry are praiseworthy strategies that help us address the challenges that affect human life. Looking to nature to find out the right answers to our intractable problems is undoubtedly as old as humanity. Nature is and will continue to be the best considered powerful model, mentor, and measure for the right way of life. Systematic studies about the biological rules, concepts and principles of nature is required toward better understanding of features and capabilities. Humans have always made efforts to inspire nature to solve problems and innovate new, improved structures, systems, or processes. As a great blessing from the Lord, nature can direct mankind to the right and correct way. How best to imitate nature certainly leads to improve every facet of human living, especially in art, technology, and health. An essential share of modern science innovation mainly relies on multidisciplinary approaches across different thinking and a broad spectrum of interest fields. Nature holds treasure and brings knowledge and truth to mankind if he/she carefully listens to its voice (Whitesides 2015; Bar-Cohen 2016; Liu 2012).

Biomimicry (Bio = life, Mimicry = imitation/mimesis) is an interdisciplinary scientific subject that formally involves a direct replication from nature as a rich and readily accessible source of new concepts. Biomimetic processes imitated nature straightforwardly and study the structure and function of natural substances or materials and biological mechanisms to synthesize similar products through artificial approaches. Biomimetics and biomimicry are new branches of science and engineering expressing about the emulation of living creatures' structure and behavior. However, bioinspiration involves a more indirect pathway and tends to inspire design concepts. Bioinspiration is mostly concerned with applying the principles of natural processes in non-biological systems. The unique creation plays an enormous resource of inspiration for mankind to develop new technologies. The successful inspirations from nature lead to conceive materials, structures, and strategies to facilitate daily human life. For creating new biomimetic materials, the formation, structure, and function of natural systems are essential characteristics that should be considered. The fundamental challenge of man-made technologies focuses on the development of artificial entities with the high performance of biological functions as well as the biological structures (Mano 2013; Dicks 2016; Bensaude-Vincent 2011). Figure 1 shows the interdisciplinary scientific and technological benefited from nature.

Nature is full of secrets. Everything around us is the result of a perfect creation. The superior design of every living creature in the world is the work of a powerful creator possessed of reason and knowledge. Who, better than nature, can design a smart complex system in such a way that it can build the ideal structure–function relationship. We must learn from nature and catch the opportunities to extract meaningful strategies to have security, comfort, and a brighter future. Nature-inspired technologies are now an integral part of our everyday life (Cohen and Reich 2016; Jelinek 2013; Singh et al. 2009).

Scientists always may attempt to describe the laws of nature. They are interested in stating the scientific

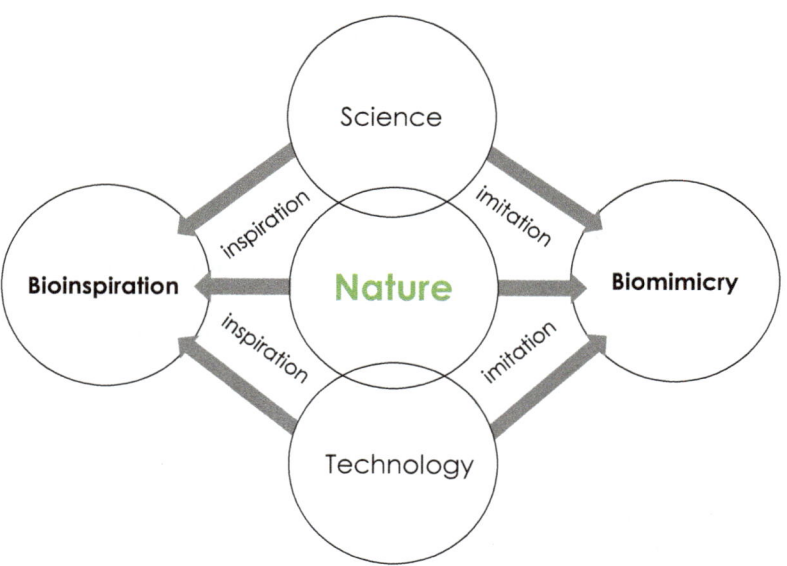

Fig. 1 The scientific and technological interactions benefited from nature

explanations for the natural parts of the universe's structure and mechanistic function. Avicenna, Copernicus, Newton, Kepler, Galileo, and other early scientists believed in the 'rational/logical' coherence of the universe. They studied the universe precisely to discover the principles and mysteries. Kepler and Newton developed gravitational theory descriptions by studying the connection and interactions between the sun and the planets. Faraday and Maxwell, two brilliant nineteenth-century scientists, revolutionized physics by discovering electromagnetism. An astonishing number of breakthroughs and remarkable scientific progress has been made through biomimetic methods, following nature's super-intelligent rules (Hwang et al. 2015; Bar-Cohen 2006).

Nature has experiences of billion years, and humans can learn and imitate this great bank of ideas and equip with its designs and strategies. Biomimetics and bioinspiration help us create an economy that follows natural evolution with more biodegradable and biocompatible products. This pathway should be a lifestyle for a better life. In this chapter, we plan to take a look at the impacts and potentials of bioinspiration and biomimicry in upgrading the living standards. The primary purpose is to reveal the enormous breadth and applications of biomimetics as a powerful scientific method in developing human knowledge of life science and the significant reflects of nature on a wide variety of human society aspects. This chapter reviews the general important bioinspired topics and highlights the key areas that humans have mimicked nature, focusing on science, technology, health, energy, art, and design. Biomimetic/bioinspired sensors, materials, medicines, locomotion models, medical implants, and architectures are the prominent successful examples that show the great power of nature to change the human lifestyle. Biologically inspired innovations and inventions have a critical role in our life to help surviving generations and provide a sustainable future for humankind.

In summary, this chapter deals with the capabilities, potential, and challenges of nature-based technologies in our lifestyle. Nature is singing a song of praising! It is up to us how to hear nature poems.

2 Nature-Based Technologies

Producing technology is a complicated business involving the combination of information, materials, and facilities. Most of the human inventions already exist in nature. Every living organism possesses perfect design and flawless creation. Among the million millions of technological marvels in nature that remain undiscovered, only a small fraction has been explored by mankind.

Some kinds of plants have light sensors in their bodies. In the absence of light, petals became closed up through an inner electrical circuit. Similar sensors were applied in lamps to go on in the dark situation and be turned off at day.

Arctic birds were never freezing in the coldest climates! This is due to the existence of strange blood circulatory systems that reduce heat loss to a minimum. While they stand on ice or their feet meet cold water, warm blood flows downward in different blood vessels running close together. In this way, the shock of cold blood circulating upwards from the feet became reduced. Whenever two fluids (liquid or gas) with different temperatures move in the opposite directions in two separate contiguous channels, heat travels from the warm fluid to the cold one. The idea of designing heat transfer machines has been emerged based on the natural heat exchange mechanism. See Fig. 2.

All of the nerve cell axons throughout the whole human body are surrounded by the special lipid-rich protective material known as myelin. Myelin is formed in the center of the nervous, either the peripheral nervous system. Each myelin sheath insulates the nervous system's wire by wrapping around the axon, facilitating the conduction of electrically encoded information, increasing the transmission rate of electrical impulses, and preventing tissue damage. Understanding the "insulating" function of the myelin plasma membrane would spark inspiration for scientists to design biomimetic multifunctional coatings for electrical systems.

The spider web has quite an incredibly strong structure, able to carry a large number of objects.

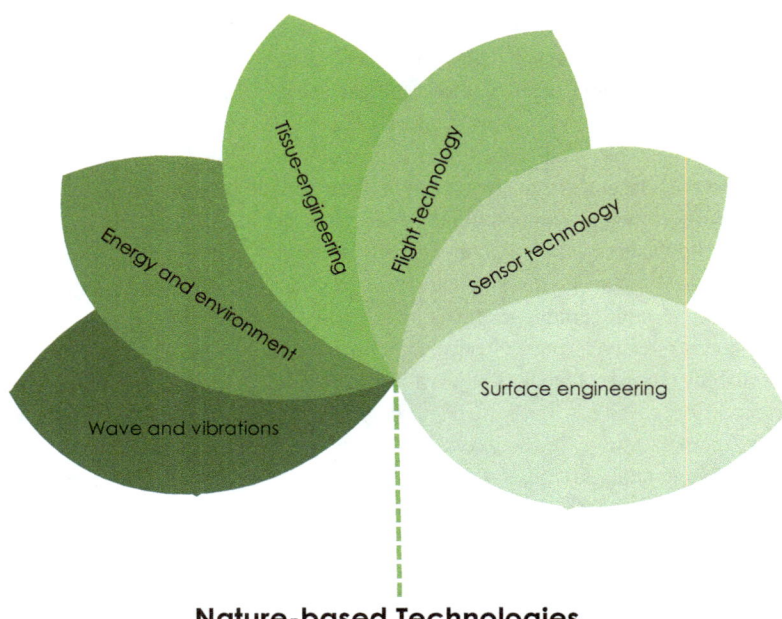

Fig. 2 Examples for nature-based technologies

The radial thread tensile strength is higher than the steel of a similar weight. According to the spider type, the distance between the fibers varies from several centimeters to a fraction of a millimeter. The wires are made from digested bugs, produced via a biologically generated chemical at room temperature and ambient atmospheric pressure. While the web is biodegradable, it can tolerate the relatively harsh conditions of various temperatures, wind, rain, and sunlight. The spider web network is a source of inspiration for humankind to make tools such as bags, wires, ropes, nets, sieves, protective covers, screens, woven fabrics, protective covers, bandage, and strainers. However, microelectromechanical systems technology developed techniques to produce fine, uniform, and continuous fibers with enormous strength.

2.1 Surface Engineering

Biomimetic surface engineering has been introduced to modify the surface structure, composition, and molecular organization and improve functional performance. With the aim of mimicking nature to modulate surfaces with desired properties, a better understanding of the fundamental aspects of chemistry and physics occurring at the surfaces and interfaces is critical. The nanostructured surface of a moth's eye, the grooved pattern of a shark's skin, and the lamellar structure of a gecko's feet confer specific functionalities to them while they would be served as promising natural sources of inspiration.

The discovery of extreme water repellency in the outer surfaces of Lotus leaves became an area of very intensive research in recent years. Surfaces coverage with natural specific coatings protects the plants against external incidents. The lotus leaves are capable of repelling contaminants and automatically clean themselves whenever they meet the smallest particle of dust to wash them away. The super hydrophobic property of lotus-like surfaces known as the term of "Lotus effect," endows self-cleaning function to the surface. Fabrication of artificial super hydrophobic surfaces with controllable surface energy and wettability is an area of active fundamental research for many practical applications, including self-cleaning coatings, oil spill cleanup, laboratory-on-a-chip devices, the functional interface for cell and tissue engineering, and water-capture devices. Thermodynamic methods have a crucial role in developing a novel class of bioinspired materials capable of self-organization (Liu 2012; Nosonovsky and Rohatgi 2011).

The surface is one of the most vulnerable parts of a biological system. Most living organisms show self-healing property through complex mechanisms in order to repair the external damages of their tissues. Based on recent advances in science and technology, now it is becoming possible to have engineered self-repairing materials of hierarchical structures at various scale levels made up of polymeric materials, concrete, and ceramics. A better understanding of the structure–property relationships in living nature serves as a guide to design and create modern smart biomimetic materials with specific properties (Nosonovsky and Rohatgi 2011).

2.2 Sensor Technology

Sight, hearing, touch, smell, and taste are five great advanced sensing systems that help the human body to receive information from the outside world. Nature serves as a wonderful model to create new sensor techniques. Sensor technology tries to create new devices and techniques as artificial receptors with high sensitivity, stability, and selectivity to simulate the ability of the five types of sense seen in humans. The biomimetic approach in sensor development relies based on reception and recognition mechanisms found in the biological systems. Biosensors and artificial senses are two essential concepts in biomimetic sensor technology (Stroble et al. 2009; Toko 2000).

In principle, a biosensor is a chemical sensor made by immobilizing a biologically active material to a sensing membrane combined with an electrochemical device as well as recording equipment. While the chemical reaction takes place on the receptor membrane, a transducer transforms the concentration of chemical substances into an electric signal, and subsequently, the output will be recorded. Biosensors are classified into the enzyme, microbial, immuno-, organelle and tissue sensors depending on the type of biomaterial used (Bogue 2009; Johnson et al. 2009).

An artificial sensor, such as so-called electronic sensing organs (eye, ear, skin, nose and tongue), plays the role of reproducing the human's five senses. The senses of sight, hearing, and touch is classified as the physical senses induced by receiving light (photon), sound wave, and pressure (or temperature), respectively, as one physical quantity. However, the sensing mechanism of smell and taste occurs through the chemoreception process, and subsequently, the organs playing these roles are called chemical sensors. The comprehensive explanation of taste and smell promotes the term "flavour" in food chemistry. The mental and physical condition of the individual, as well as the food culture of a country, affects deliciousness. HCl, NaCl, sucrose and quinine are the basic taste substances for sour, salty, sweet, and bitter tastes, respectively. Amino acids show a complex mixed taste. For example, L-valine elicits sweet and bitter taste simultaneously. By changing the R group in amino acid, the taste will be changed. Lipid/polymer membranes have revealed great potentials as biomimetic devices to reproduce a sense of taste in the human gustatory systems. An electronic tongue is a multifunctional sensor used to transform taste information into electrical signals (Johnson et al. 2009).

Artificial sensors can also enable humans to surpass the ability of their natural senses. Human beings cannot experience severe conditions, i.e., high temperature and pressure. In addition, limiting the sensory range of humankind prevents him from recognizing every kind of quantities, i.e., the supersonic sound generated by a bat. Man-made sensors are designed to have the ability to overcome humankind's sensing limitations. They can achieve demanding conditions and perceive every kind of quantity.

2.3 Wave and Vibrations

Sound is a mechanical wave that travels through a medium from one point to another. The vibrations contain a great deal of information about the distance, size, direction and speed of the motion. Millions of years before humans, living beings spread waves around to announce their positions and detect their way. The radar technology and detection system to locate targets by means of waves and vibrations are inspired by living beings; however, nature still does it in a much more sensitive and functional way. Dolphins, bats, fish and moths spread the sound waves around, known as sonar, to communicate effectively with their environments. They are able to transmit the waves toward their desired directions. The waves strike an object, be reflected, and turn back to the initial source. A great deal of accurate information about the distance, speed, and size of the target is obtained and processed through sonar technology.

The bioinspired man-made sonar system enables ships and submarines, identify targets and distinguish directions. Utilizing a small sonar system onto the pair of glasses, visually handicapped people became able to do certain activities. Accordingly, researchers have invented a similar biomimetic system with smart acoustic sensors based on the echolocation mechanism, which found use in vehicles for detecting obstacles. Vehicle parking sensors are also equipped with an ultrasonic sensing system for distance measurement in automotive applications. Ultrasonic sensor technology makes drivers aware of necessary outside features to ensure safe driving. Therefore, the natural world always surprises us with unlimited technological solutions and strategies to improve human life quality.

2.4 Tissue-Engineering

Within the human body, there is a unique complex architecture arranged in three-dimensional space exhibiting strong anisotropies. Tissue's structure and functionality may be related to the morphology, nutrition, and genetic effects. In the case of disease or defects, artificial tissues are the ultimate successful treatments. The functions of damaged, diseased, or missing organs would be replaced by medical implants fabricated through biomimetic design principles (Ingber et al. 2006).

Tissue-engineering is a relatively new, growing research field in modern medical technologies. Biomimetic inspired scaffolds were first being used in bone tissue engineering (Witte et al. 2018). Bone and dentin are biological composites consist of a well-ordered set of large amounts of organic/inorganic material structure from molecular to the macroscopic scale. Diffraction techniques are better suited to study the structure of hard tissues. Soft tissues are essential constituents of the human body, possessing robust anisotropic morphology. An emerging field of tissue engineering holds great promise for the regeneration of soft tissues. Poor healing of skin wounds in cases of severe burns or diabetic ulcers, the health problem is a common soft tissue problem.

To better understand the structure–function relationship in natural systems, new living cellular constructs with the tissue-like organization of cells and matrices have been generated. The anatomy and function of the target organ have to be analyzed in detail. Then, the most suitable material and implant design have to be selected. Molecular self-assembly introduces attractive strategies to build appropriate materials for any replacement or regeneration of hard tissues (e.g., bone, teeth, cartilage) as well as soft ones (e.g., skin, muscles, tendons). In vitro and in vivo experiments have to be studied. The achievement of medical implants strongly depends on the clinical task often described by the medical expert. Artificial tissues would be beneficial for patients whenever the mechanical properties of the implants are adapted to the surrounding body tissues. Biocompatibility, biofunctionality and stiffness of implant material have also been quantified to design effective medical implants.

2.5 Flight Technology

Birds are the most advanced aircraft and the greatest flying machines ever. They are able to fly for a long period of time during their seasonal migration, maneuvering with a fantastic performance, even catching prey during their flight. To achieve the impossible dream of flying, attempts were fixed to make this machine with all of its aerodynamic features and motions by emulating natural fliers' flight. As one of the earliest pioneers of flight technology, Leonardo Da Vinci believed that birds are complicated advanced instruments working according to the mathematical laws (Ang et al. 2009).

The flawless creation of hollow bones, a rigid skeleton, an enlarged breastbone for flight muscle attachment, lightweight and smooth feathers, a beak that exists instead of heavy and bony jaws and teeth, aerodynamic wings, powerful muscles, a metabolism that provides high energy needs, all these features enable them to have extraordinary abilities in the air. The four forces of weight, lift, drag and thrust, directly affect the flight of birds. Their bodies have been designed in such a way that during flight, air circulation plays as advanced cooling system. The marvelous shape of birds' wings has a determining effect on their ability to fly. Long, narrow and pointed wings enable the birds to fly fast. They are applied as the perfect models for flight engineers. The structure of the wings keeps them capable of flying in every condition. Birds played as the great experts on the subject for guidance. Natural flight machines can provide technological solutions to have more effective flights. Over thousands of years, evolutionary events were occurred to have more effective flights. Further developments in aerodynamic technologies led to a dramatic improvement in the performance of aircraft (Biomimetics 2005; Vincent 2003; Kato and Kamimura 2008).

2.6 Energy and Environment

The energy crisis and global environmental challenges are the greatest problems facing humanity. Burning oil and coal in order to produce energy has led to a considerable increase in greenhouse gases and climate changes, and extensive pollution arising from industrialization. Biomimicry aims to learn from nature in order to design a bright future. A Billion years of life on earth, nature has been harvesting and storing energy through a highly sophisticated process. As the world population grows, demand for renewable supplies of energy grows. Exploring nature to observe how natural living systems deal with the same issues helps humanity achieve sustainable materials and renewable energy resources to address the challenges. In order to ensure environmental protection, we need to achieve alternative energy sources. A particular focus has been devoted to energy generation from the solar power system as a reliable and long-lasting energy source.

Plants are a great source of inspiration for human livings. During millions of years, green leaves play as natural solar panels turning sunlight to energy during a complicated natural technology named "photosynthesis". Understanding and mimicking the mysterious mechanism of photosynthesis may enable scientists to produce artificial solar cells that may easily change the whole world. Natural photosynthesis takes place in the presence of sunlight, carbon dioxide, and water. When the chlorophyll molecules absorb light, electrons can go into an excitation state, causing the production of molecular oxygen, carbohydrates, and other carbon-rich products. Photosynthesis provides a number of critical vital reactions by light-induced multi electron-transfer processes (Kalyanasundaram and Graetzel 2010). Photochemical conversion and solar energy storage occur through two major pathways: conversion of solar energy to the electricity/generation of high energy fuels from water. Artificial photosynthesis aims to imitate the natural faction in a simplified manner to be able to convert and store abundant free solar radiation. However, adopting suitable architectures to imitate the chlorophyll function plays a key role in building the artificial system.

The integration of science helps to provide new strategies to save energy and find the best solutions to the world's energy crisis. A large percentage of total energy is consumed through the heating and cooling systems of buildings. The biomimetic architecture looks forward to designing solutions by understanding the rules of natural structures in order to solve human problems. Sustainable architecture would be expected to design buildings actively contributing to ecosystems, rather than causing significant future disruption to human society.

3 Biomimetic Drug Delivery

During the past four decades, nature as the primary source of compounds for therapeutic goals; besides providing natural organic chemical compounds, it is the source of inspiration for novel chemical structures for drug discovery and design of new drugs. Natural active products and their derivatives, which have been identified from plants, animals, and marine microorganisms, have long been an important source of pharmaceuticals compared to compounds that are synthesized by combinatorial chemistry (Newman and Cragg 2007).

Totally the natural sources are limited, so it is vital to develop the different strategies that can produce enough material for broad biological screening and applicability. Chemical modifications to develop therapeutic action, complete syntheses, and semi-syntheses, allow overcoming that barrier. Various drugs from synthetic sources retain the natural scaffolds and have more or less rich chemical functions to perform advantageous manufacture of a new drug with better biologic action. Drug discovery is designing the small molecules via high throughput screening, and computer-assisted ligands created alternatives to traditional drug discovery paradigms (Lourenco et al. 2012).

Many types of research have been indicated that natural compounds are "privileged structures" and play a significant role in the drug discovery and development process. As part of the biomimetics field, scientists are looking for rules, concepts, mechanisms, and biology principles to mimic novel engineering possibilities, containing manufacturing, mechanisms, materials, processes, and algorithms.

For example, Salicylic acid (SA) was initially originated from willow bark and has since been recognized in many species. First, the medicinal properties of this compound were applied in pain and fever management. Aspirin is one of the most common drugs which is derived from salicylates. Aspirin (acetylsalicylic acid) has been sold as a drug since 1899, but the pain-relieving effects of plant extracts have been appreciated since ancient times. Also, the antimalarial properties of the bark of the cinchona tree were known long before the use of quinine. To date, the breast cancer drug eribulin (Halaven) is simplified, albeit still rather complex, a synthetic analog of halichondrin B, which is produced by the marine sponge Halichondria okadai. So, it is important to take inspiration from different aspects of natural-product biosynthesis to recognize new bioactive molecules and create "natural product-bioinspired" libraries.

The use of biomimicry in medicine is an effective way to treat incurable diseases such as cancer. Therefore, scientists have attempted to perceive biological systems and processes such as the structure of proteins and their biological functions at the cellular levels in order to inspire these natural methods for biomedical usage (Venkatesh et al. 2005).

In this regard, one of the main goals of the researches is to find a targeted drug-delivery system to amend the effectiveness and safety of therapeutic agents. It is important to discover a carrier-system that carries the drug of interest with better biocompatibility, controlled drug release, reduced side effects, and no harmful toxic results for healthy tissues or organs.

A carrier system in addition to carrying the drug should: (a) enable high drug loading, (b) effectively prevents drug breakdown, (c) releases the drug under specific stimuli at the site of operation, and (d) Immunity (Batrakova et al. 2011). The immobilized drug must remain stable for a sufficient period of time, especially while crossing various biological barriers.

Nanotechnology has taken many steps in drug delivery, including the possibility of encapsulating drugs into nanocarriers. Nanoparticles, due to their small particle size, are less likely to be eliminated by the liver and kidneys of the body, so they have a longer shelf life, and the small size of nanoparticles also activates them for intercellular diffusion (Vauthier and Labarre 2008). Besides these advantages, the impact of nanoparticles for drug delivery to tumor cells has been a significant difficulty. Binding of plasma proteins such as immunoglobulin G (IgG) onto the surface of therapeutic nanoparticles causes the reticuloendothelial system (RES) to kill these particles as external invasive particles. So plenty of hydrophilic polymers such as polyethylene glycol (PEGylation) have been used as a prominent strategy to protect nanoparticles from the immune system by surface coating on nanoparticles (Sheikhpour et al. 2017). However, because of the unfavorable interactions between PEG and target cells, the loaded drugs were degraded (Amoozgar and Yeo 2012; Mishra et al. 2016). Biomimetics created intrinsic capabilities in biomimetic drug nanocarriers via the surface functionalization of PEGylated particles with specific biological ligands such as Proteins, vitamins, peptides, antibodies and aptamers, or moieties similar to the combination and functionality of external cell membrane (Gong and Winnik 2012; Meyer et al. 2015). These ligands are highly selective for binding to the receptor-mediated on the target cells and are selected because of the properties of target cells, such as the overexpression level of specific receptors on tumor cells (Hatakeyama et al. 2013; Choi et al. 2003).

Enhancing the half-life of drug carriers, inhibiting immune stimulation, releasing drugs through the process of cellular internalization in target cells, and reducing the effects of toxicity on the function of other healthy living cells are among the things that scientists are working on (Venkatesh et al. 2005; Gong and Winnik 2012; Balmert and Little 2012; Peppas 2004). So, the core materials, size, and the shape of drug carriers are so vital in a way that they are capable of imitating natural cells for cellular internalization. In the last few years, the design and production of the most promising groups of bio-inspired materials as drug-delivery systems have been explored. According to these, various nano-platforms in drug delivery systems have been introduced as bio-inspired and biomimetic materials for these applications. These may be broadly categorized as organic carriers (lipid nanoparticle, Polymeric nanoparticles) such as solid lipid nanoparticles, liposomes, dendrimers, hydrogel, micelles, and inorganic carriers, including carbon nanoparticles (such as fullerene and nanotubes), magnetic nanoparticles, metal nanoparticles, and nanoceramics (Sheikhpour et al. 2017; Rodrigues and Mota 2016). In the following, the most prominent biomimetic nanoparticles that are used in drug delivery as drug carriers are listed below.

3.1 Bioinspired Nanostructures

Therapeutic nanoparticles are multifunctional systems with a size range between 10 and 1000, similar to macromolecular structures such as proteins and DNA, enabling them to take advantage of the acting as carriers in drug delivery (Carmona-Ribeiro 2010; Alvarez-Lorenzo and Concheiro 2013).

Nanotubes and nanofibers, when properly designed, are so biodegradable, biocompatible, with the desired feature such as better stability, (bio) distribution, and pharmacokinetics (Bianco et al. 2005; Kimura 2008). Also, other appropriate inorganic nanoparticles based on some materials such as gold, silica, fullerene, and graphene are applied as drug carriers (Cordon et al. 2013).

3.2 Liposomes

Liposomes are spherical vesicles that can be produced from cholesterol and natural phospholipids via the self-assembly process in an aqueous medium. Liposomes are composites which its similarity with the cell membrane of the human body or animals makes them the most exploited types of drug nanocarriers. In liposomes, the phospholipid bilayer surrounded an aqueous core, and because of these properties, they have hydrophobic as well as hydrophilic characteristics and, due to these, most of the time, liposomes are considered as bioinspired products. Besides these, they are non-toxic, biocompatible, biodegradable, and biological inert, making them suitable for many clinical applications as the most well-established nano-platform. Liposomes can be prepared via several methods, such as mimicking the biological properties of cells using biomimetic methods. Biomimetic liposomes can provide intracellular delivery of drugs and also could release the loaded drug in a controlled way (Chandrawati and Caruso 2012; Allen and Cullis 2013).

Furthermore, the biomimetic modification of liposome surface, besides the biomimetic methods of liposome fabrication, increases the abilities of therapeutic liposomes in drug delivery and also increases the fluidity of the liposomal membrane, which can enhance the transport through cellular barriers.

3.3 Biomimetic Polymeric Carriers

One of the most applicable carriers for drug delivery applications are polymeric carriers due to their specific properties such as reliable methods of nanoscale production, the ability of drug loading in large quantities, providing drug release in a controlled manner, and the ability of the modification of the surface due to having active functional groups (Jang et al. 2012). These novel bioinspired polymers can mimic cellular interactions mechanism with the environment, transfer drugs through cellular barriers to the target cells, and reduce the undefined interactions on surface cells and elicit the desired cellular response causes reaching its target (Drotleff et al. 2004). Optimizing the chemical properties of synthetic polymers (to reduce cell-mediated immune responses), designing the biomimetic structure of the polymeric drug carriers, and modifying the surface of them by specific ligands or moieties, are essential for achieving a specific drug release pathway without undesirable effects on the function of healthy cells (Lima et al. 2013).

3.4 Dendrimers

Dendritic structures, the synthetic polymers, which are developed through a series of reactions, are considered as important innovative nanocarriers in nanomedicine. Dendritic architectures are the result of significant advances and innovations in organic chemistry and polymer science and are emerging from a novel type of highly branched polymers "cascade molecules," which are exhibiting significant improved physicochemical properties. The word dendrimer arises from the Greek dendron ("tree" or "branch") and meros ("part"). Dendrimers are composed of three parts; a central core with two or more reactive groups repeated units that are covalently attached to the central core and organized in layers called "generations" (G) and many terminal functional groups on their surface. They are first synthesized by Voegtle et al. in 1978 (Buhleier et al. 1978).

Dendrimers as highly branched three-dimensional macromolecules in a tree shape emanate from a focal core (Garg et al. 2011). This kind of structure provides more water solubility bioavailability and biocompatibility for drug molecules (Cheng et al. 2008). Dendrimers have many reactive terminal groups on their surface, making them appropriate drug carriers that can encapsulate the drugs inside its dendritic structure physically, or drugs can conjugate to the surface of the dendritic structure via electrostatic or covalent bonds. Also, the abundance of terminal functional groups enables binding different ligands or drugs in a specific and controllable manner and performs multivalent capacities in various biological systems. In addition, dendrimers can load a favorite molecule via forms of nanosized structures stabilized by noncovalent interactions. The unique structural properties of dendrimers, such as a globular, well-defined, and very branched structure, as well as monodisperse and controllable nanosize, made them very special for biomedical applications.

4 Bioinspired Materials for Medical Applications

Generally, any substance or mixture of substances with synthetic or natural sources that are compatible and also is designed to interact with biological systems for a medical, therapeutic, or diagnostic purpose is referred to as biological material. Biomaterials, as a fifty-year-old science, encompasses elements of medicine, biology, chemistry, tissue engineering, and materials science. In other words, biomaterials are a substance with an artificial or natural source, which is applied to improve, treat, heal, or replace living organisms (Recum and Laberge 1995). Although the first medical implants were hardly successful because of lack of information related to infection control and the biocompatibility of the materials, in the eighteenth and nineteenth centuries, Researchers began to understand that one of the essential characteristics of biomaterials compared to other materials is their biocompatibility (Ruys 2013). The concept of biocompatibility refers to the capability of a material to be used in a particular application accompanied by an appropriate response from the host that it has a main role in the success of using materials in the biological system (Ratner and Bryant 2004). In the past few decades, the use of nanostructured biomaterials in a variety of applications, including antimicrobial supplementation of medical and hygienic textiles, wound dressings, cosmetic textiles, body implants, drug release systems and, medical scaffolds, have been taken into consideration.

Generally, choosing the right material for medical applications in the human body is one of the most sensitive and complicated operations. There are several scientific and social characteristics considered in the development of biomaterials and associated medical products. Biomaterials should be chemically neutral, have no adverse effect on adjacent tissues, have a long lifespan, and have no detrimental effect on the body's free metabolism processes. These factors are called "biocompatibility factors" (Schmalz and Arenholt-Bindslev 2009; Vert et al. 2012). Also, toxicology, biocompatibility, healing, mechanical and performance requirements, and manufacturability skills are important parameters. Biomaterials are also applied daily in dental uses, surgery, and drug delivery. Also, it can be used in the design of medical implants, medical equipment, and also, they have several applications in nuclear medicine and basic medical sciences.

4.1 Types of Biomaterials

Biomaterials can be achieved from nature or produced artificially by using several chemical procedures. They generally include several types (Kulinets 2015). Nature-derived biomaterials (such as plant-derived and tissue-derived) are composed of different types of biopolymers, Semi-synthetic biomaterials, or hybrid and Synthetic biomaterials. Most typical classes of biomaterials that are applied individually or in the mixture to form many of the implantation devices are separated into the following groups: metals, polymers, ceramics, and composites as follows:

4.1.1 Metals

As a class of materials, Metallic biomaterials are exclusively used for some applications, such as hip and knee prostheses (artificial joints), fracture fixation wires, plates, and screws. Also, metallic implants are applicable in cardiovascular surgery and as dental implants. Besides pure metals, alloys provide improvement in material properties. However, the most commonly employed biomaterial for implants devices is stainless steels, titanium and titanium alloys, and cobalt-base alloys (Bombač et al. 2007; Kuroda et al. 2000; Sumita et al. 2004).

4.1.2 Ceramics

Ceramics are polycrystalline compounds that are generally bioinert, biocompatible, and biodegradable. The essential characteristics of ceramic materials are their hardness, having high resistance to corrosion with the ability of compression with low electrical and thermal conductivities (Parida et al. 2012). Ceramics should be non-toxic, non-carcinogenic, non-allergic, and non-inflammatory. Ceramic biomaterials are used in several different fields based on their bioactivities, such as orthopedic implants, dental applications (Binyamin et al. 2006), and different medical applications (Sáenz et al. 1999). Ceramics, as one of the important classes of biomaterials, contain three basic categories: bioinert, bioactive, bioresorbable ceramics (Dubok 2000). Alumina (Al_2O_3), Zirconia (ZrO_2), and pyrolytic carbon are labeled bioinert. Bioglass and glass ceramics are bioactive. Calcium phosphate ceramics are classified as bioresorbable ceramics. Bioinert refers to substances that keep their structure in the body after implantation and do not produce any host immune response (Siraparapu et al. 2013).

4.1.3 Biopolymers

Polymers as organic materials are widely used in biomedical applications. Also, polymers with natural origin have been applied as biomaterials in several reports (Langer and Kohn 1996). Synthetic Polymeric biomaterials are applicable in many usages in various aspects, for example, facial prostheses, drug delivery systems, tissue engineering, and dental implants (Binyamin et al. 2006). Besides that, some of the required characteristics of polymeric biomaterials such as biocompatibility, biodegradability, lightweight, flexibility, stability, adequate mechanical, physical properties, and manufacturability which make them unique in medical applications (Kumar 2007; Hanker and Giammara 1988), the advantages of the polymeric biomaterials over other biomaterials are ease of fabrication of several forms (latex, film, sheet, fibresfibers, etc.), ease of secondary processing, sensible cost, and availability of preferred mechanical and physical features. Totally, many polymeric materials have been applied as implants such as Polyvinylchloride (PVC), Polyethylene (PE), Polypropylene (PP), Polymethylmetacrylate (PMMA), Polystyrene (PS), Polytetrafluoroethylene (PTFE), Polyurethane (PU), Polyamide, Polyethylenterephthalate (PET), Polyethersulfone (PES) and Polyetherimide (PEI).

4.1.4 Composites

The term "composite" refers to the relatively new class of synthetic biomaterials that consist of distinct phases, and the combined properties of its components are significantly different from a homogeneous material. Development and applications of this class of biomaterials have been attracting considerable interest because of their environmental benefit, their combination of low density/weight, high strength, and biocompatibility. Due to a large number of benefits, there are some uses of composites in biomaterial applications such as using for filling teeth, orthopedic implants, bone cement, drug/gene delivery, tissue engineering, and cosmetic orthodontics applications.

4.2 Application Areas and Practices

One of the most prominent biomaterials applications, which were described earlier, is to apply them in physical replacements of soft or hard tissues that have lost their function because of a fracture, infection, or cancer (Davis 2003).

4.2.1 Orthopedics

Since there are millions of people who are suffering from bone-related disease, as the most prominent solutions, biomaterial compatible with bones are applied for orthopedic implant devices, and because of that, several methodologies have been applied to design bone replacement materials. Some diseases such as osteoarthritis and rheumatoid arthritis, can do harm in freely movable (synovial) joints, such as shoulder, ankle, elbow, and weight-bearing joints like hip and knee (Davis 2003). For example, hip replacement is one of the major procurements in orthopedic surgery that ceramics and metallic polymer implants applied to upper femur bone, pelvis areas replacement (Dowson 1992). Also, the lower femur, tibia, and knee cap, i.e., patella, are replaced with metal and polymeric compounds in knee replacement. Several biomaterials have been used to produce implantable scaffolds for bone tissue, such as bioceramics, biopolymers, and metals (Amini et al. 2012). Bioceramics, especially hydroxyapatite (HA) as the main bone mineral component, and bioglasses can be considered as a suitable matrix because of their effectiveness. Also, biocomposite scaffolds based on natural polymers (mainly alginate, chitosan, collagen, hyaluronic acid (HyA), and silk) have been well investigated in bone regenerative approaches (Pina et al. 2015). Titanium (Ti)-, zirconium (Zr)-, and magnesium (Mg) -based material is used in bone regeneration, as an important group of metals, because of their mechanical features and biocompatibility. Ceramics, as one of the best-studied synthetic bone substitute materials, are applied in many uses in orthopedic and craniofacial surgery (Bohner 2010) due to their chemical and structural properties such as biocompatibility, osteoconductivity, and bioactivity. Ceramic-based products contain materials, such as calcium phosphate (CaP), calcium sulfate (CaS), and bioactive glass (BG), used alone or in mixture with other grafts that among these materials, those based on CaP are the most considerable (Rodrigues and Mota 2016; Heini and Berlemann 2001; Vaccaro and Madigan 2002).

4.2.2 Cardiovascular Disease (CVD)

Cardiovascular disease is a class of diseases that cause losing heart functions and can lead to death. However, detection and treatments of CVD are limited; most of the heart problems related to heart valves and arteries, which can be successfully treated with implants.

Besides heart transplant, regenerative medicine offers a wide variety of treatment methods such as septal wall for ventricles and valves and the use of biomaterials and scaffolds to promote cardiac regeneration (Rodrigues and Mota 2016). Among different cardiovascular implants, polymer-based biomaterial implants are essential constituents for vascular prostheses. Also, multifunctional shape-memory polymers are high relevance due to their biocompatibility and self-expansion ability for cardiovascular applications

such as stent technology, which is a very tiny mesh of metals introduced into the dilated arterial site. Polyurethane/polycaprolactone (PU/PCL) blend is an example of shape-memory stents. Treatment of myocardial infarction is usually done by using injectable biomaterials with hydrogel origin because of their biocompatibility. This kind of biomaterial involves alginate, fibrin, chitosan, collagen or matrix gel (Khan et al. 2014).

4.2.3 Wound Healing

Skin is the soft outer tissue that plays a crucial role in protecting the body from toxins and the external environment, maintaining the hydration, and also regulating the temperature as the largest organ in the body. Because of the complex nature of the skin, it is particularly difficult for tissue engineers to develop a scaffold that can consistently improve healing in wound problems. One of the effective methods for wound repairing is to apply biomaterials because of their utility as scaffolds. Biomaterials that are used for this purpose can be classified into different categories. Synthetic biomaterials are also biocompatible and, flexible, and they can be synthesized in a way to produce physical and chemical properties. One of the synthetic copolymer biomaterials is polyurethane and its derivatives, which are used extensively to treat burns and wounds. One of the examples is Pellethane® 2363-80A, which can accelerate epithelialization (Wright et al. 1998). Teflon is also a non-carcinogenic polymer that fits in well with the injured area (Lee and Worthington 1999), and Silicone as a non-toxic, non-allergenic, and highly biocompatible polymer is resistant to biodegradation and can be used for as wound support material for soft tissue repairing and scar treatment (Whelan 2002). Natural polymer biomaterials are another category of biomaterial which is used for wound healing. Biomaterials with natural origin can be classified into several classes such as polysaccharide, protein, nanofiber-based biomaterials and also and marine biomaterials. Different Natural polymer biomaterials such as chitosan, collagen, elastin, and fibrinogen are biocompatible and also offer a therapeutic advantage in comparison to the synthetic biomaterials. However, its mechanical strength is low (Mogoşanu and Grumezescu 2014).

5 Artistic Design and Biomimetic Process

Biomimetics or the concept of bioinspiration relates to questions such as what can advance material science, or structural engineering learn from biological models, processes, and systems found in nature. The combination of fundamental natural methods with scientific methods and design will generate synergistic improvements due to multifaceted biomimetic processes. However, this section focuses on biomimetic art that is interested in exploring biomimetics in terms of natural phenomena abstraction creatively and not a direct mimicry of nature. The different approaches of representations and depiction of nature reveal various levels of abstraction that are dependent on the artist's technique and expression. In 1960, the term biomimetic with the concepts of bios (life) and mimesis (imitate) had just a basic discipline of science, but nowadays, it has become broadened as an interdisciplinary science because of the abstraction of useful ideas from nature. The main core of biomimetics is its integrative essence that brought knowledge from several disciplines to create a new body of knowledge by interdisciplinary quality. In art biomimetic processes, not only the natural phenomena are used as models, but also an artistic reflection that produces mental images is applied as models (Marom and Marom 2016).

To understand the relationship between art and biometrics, let's go-to term biomimetics. The concept of mimesis in the art world originated from the classical Greek aesthetic philosophy, and mimesis is an essential key for describing the main core of any artistic expression (painting, poetry, sculpture, etc.). The mimesis process is divided into two forms; reflection and expression. Both reflection and expression paths refer to an artist's ability, one is to receive images from reality or nature to form imaginative images in mind, and another is to materialize and transfer the mental images into expressive images in shapes, colors, and materials, respectively. To define the term art, we shall bring up a general definition, a definition that can refer to any intuitive, creative process. "Britannica Online" describes art as: "visual object or experience consciously created through an expression of skill or imagination." The depiction of nature by different visual forms and materials in works of art also would place in this definition, as well as drawing, painting, photography, sculpture and installation media. However, the different perceptions and insights of nature, along with the role of art, have been mainly dependent on various cultures and artistic evolution.

To show an artistic role in biomimetic processes, artistic design is presented below. This project exhibits an artistic demonstration of a natural mechanism incorporating engineering and art that presents the imitation by which reconstructed an artificial pet-BioMe from Venus flytrap mechanism (Marom and Marom 2016). This novel trapping mechanism of the carnivorous plants provides creative solutions for mimicry. According to the structure–function relationship as an important principle of the biomimetic approach, the nature images can be reduced to geometrical shapes based on the mechanical rules of biological systems.

A long-term study of scientists on the Venus flytrap shows that the leaves stick together in a fraction of a second to capture insects in reaction to the mechanical stimulus of trigger hairs (Burdon-Sanderson 1882). The too-quick speed of Venus flytrap leaves shut (about 40 ms) is not only explained by the potential-action in cells, but the leaf geometrical elastic deformations (convex to concave) could have a significant part in trap closing (Hodick and Sievers 1989). The mechanical and geometrical features of Venus plant closure provided the kinetic rule principles for mimicry and conversion into the biomimetic artificial trap-closing mechanism incorporated with artistic design (Fig. 3). This simple paper example provided a suitable model for understanding and testing the twisting geometry as a

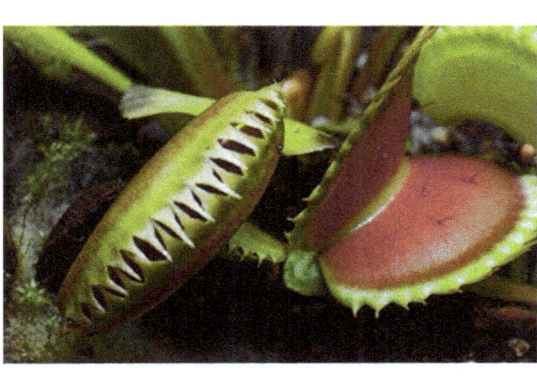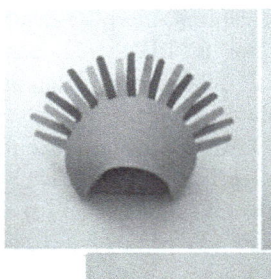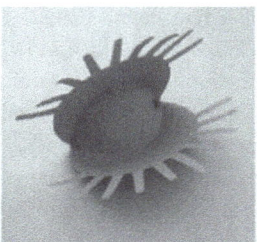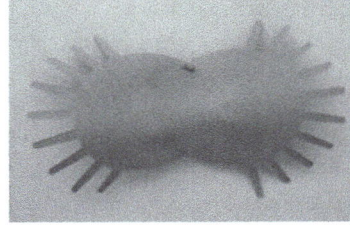

Fig. 3 Open-closed venus flytrap convex to concave states and the artistic model of bistable curvature mechanism

potential bistable procedure. However, the design of BioMe was a multidisciplinary process combined with biomimetic engineering areas, biology, and artistic mimesis.

Accordingly, the biomimetic procedure could be considered as a scientific process of transforming ideas from biology to feasible engineering solutions. In contrast, the biomimetic process in artistic design could be realized as converting ideas from biology into impractical and infeasible ideas. However, it contains the purpose of generating creative artistic experiences like conceptual, aesthetic feelings. See Fig. 3.

6 Interdisciplinary Education: Biological Inspiration

Biological inspiration presents a powerful and logical connection to multidisciplinary education. Scientists completely realize the function-design relationship general principles. However, both biologists and engineers approach the problem from their own point of view. Therefore, a biologically inspired design (BID) course was planned to promote relevant knowledge with all views. For this job, upper-level undergraduates majoring in biology, along with engineering was mixed in BID class to have practical training in techniques and methods that simplify the identification and conversion of biological principles into solutions for human problems. The final-output of the class is a design with a conceptual manner that comprises biology principles into a device or procedure along with a final project report with quantitative problem analysis to enable the quest for suitable biological principles. It is necessary that providing each student with field-specific technical training in the realization of such designs at the beginning of the BID course. The course should be designed in such a way that it develops an approach facilitates the implementation of BID, whilst the current practical topics in the fields of science, technology, engineering, and mathematical education (STEM) are new and applicable (Yen et al. 2016). So, the BID goals reflect the topic and problems to make challenges in interdisciplinary STEM education. BID course prepares a suitable environment in which to bring up interdisciplinary pedagogical operation and encourages the STEM education to overcome common problems (Baldwin 2009), like passive learning of students due to emphasis on memorizing or the absence of a basic concept to connect with real-world applications, etc.

There are several learning purposes for STEM-educating innovation by BID, which can be mentioned as (a) multidisciplinary correlation skills; (b) new procedure or techniques for innovative design; (c) new information about areas out of their main field; (d) using of available technology for a novel discipline; and (e) a particular interdisciplinary cooperative procedure. To achieve these learning goals, several BID course parts or components should be defined and developed.

One of the defined course parts is for invited bioinspired designers to have domain BID content lectures along with students' exercises that present the differences or resemblances of biological solutions against technological solutions of inspired designs. The expert practitioners talk about their work to illustrate the principles for using engineering procedures to realize the biological scheme and demonstrate the usage of mentioned principles to engineering design (French 1994; Vogel 1998). Profound biology-engineering content of lectures increase students' domain knowledge and prepare multidisciplinary relation examples (Handelsman et al. 2004; DeHaan 2005).

"Found object exercises" subject is another defined course component. First experience with nature solutions gained by investigating existing biological systems using a what–why–how (WWH) frame is similar to structure–behavior–function frame (Goel and Stroulia 2009; Goel et al. 2008). Students are introduced to a wide variety of nature-inspired systems by finding object exercises and the approach that each object represents certain functions. Here the WWH questions to analyze found objects are; (a) what the related components of the system are? (Due to the structure), (b) why does the system need the mechanism? (Due to the function), (c) how do the components interact to perform the mechanism? (Due to the behavior). The WWH analysis could be shared with the lecture-specialist if students ask about the lecture to recognize and analyze found objects that facilitate multidisciplinary interactions (Vincent and Mann 2002). Students should rethink on previous conclusions about the variety and utility of natural solutions. Therefore, this rethinking and reanalysis could be an origin of forthcoming designs.

Research Assignments are another component that improves students' understanding of biological systems relevant to their problem. They are introduced to search engines and strategies to find papers about their project. There is usually a problem that engineers and biologists have a different view and terminology of an identical process. This restricts the ability to find suitable biological models. Therefore, important strategies are needed to solve this problem. Primary literature sources can be helpful for this purpose. Therefore, students are led to use of general resources and then enter literature for wider searches, improving general processes. Current strategy aids in associating significant biological terms (biology) and specific function (engineering) relevant to a similar idea (Chiu and Shu 2007). To simplify the "search image" through the project, it is necessary that mentor teams meet with experts by appropriate specialty to receive design plans. This examines their designs from an interdisciplinary perspective and improves relationship abilities as well as deep learning comprehension and technical experiences understanding (Yen et al. 2016).

Social-cultural learning systems received the amount of attention in STEM education underline the collaborative structure of knowledge (Palincsar 1998). Therefore, the BID course with collaborative situations could remarkably increase mastering reality and learning quality of students and enhance their thinking process at finishing the course.

7 Biomimetic Approach in Architecture

Biomimetic is a tool for architectural innovation that could help decide contemporary problems in architecture and the environment. This new architecture field will facilitate a culture of active environmental design by transferring the biological attributes of life into architecture. The philosophy that utilizes biomimetics in architecture is to look for solutions for sustainability in nature via realizing the rules leading the natural forms. Here, sustainable design follows a set of bio-inspired principles from a multidisciplinary viewpoint. The intensive research indicates that "Sick Building Syndrome" could lead to "Sick Environment Syndrome"; therefore, more attention should be paid to this area on ecology in the future (Gruber 2011).

Architects have always been inspired by nature. Uncountable nature analogies could be found in architecture. There are two kinds of approaches for biomimetics applications in architecture. The first ones are approaches in a classical manner that study the overlaps among architecture and nature, and the second ones are the new kind of approaches on biology's life criterion in architecture (Gruber 2011).

From the classical perspective, it is mentioned that architecture is an integrated part of nature; nevertheless, it imitates nature in many ways. The subject of "natural constructions" is in the field of the classical approach; for example, the building of animals is one of those categories. There are various constructions of animals' buildings like caves, shells, massive huge buildings (termite mounds), beam assemblies (birds' nests), membrane constructions (spiderwebs), folded structures (bee-honeycomb structures), and vaults (ant-hills) (Gruber 2011). The technologies of animals' buildings that are widely genetically determined indicate the increasing complication and complexity of buildings with phylogenetic age. Older evolutionary species like insects have established more complicated or advanced constructions than younger species like vertebrates with primitive and simple constructions. The constructions could be compared via the procedure animals use materials from the environment to build domiciles, for instance, larval tubes of caddisfly; worm tubes, hermit crab shells; nests of fish, and mammals; beaver dams (Vogel 1998).

The use of biomimetic in architecture has a long history. Termite nest in Africa is a notable example of this kind of architecture. The unique feature of these six meter-tall constructions is that even if the outside temperature is hot and above 40 °C, the inside temperature remains cool and below 30 °C (Hwang et al. 2015). Eastgate Centre, located in Zimbabwe's capital, Harare, is modeled from a termite's nest with an all-natural cooling structure. Natural ventilation is accomplished by constructing holes on the roof and lower floors of the building, resembling a termite's nest. Exiting hot air from the roof and the entrance of cold air through the bottom will cool inside the building below 24 °C, while outside is above 38 °C. However, the rate of energy consumption is 10%.

Architecture with nature's feature is the other "natural construction" containing a long traditional use in buildings according to sustainability and ecology. Spatial notions, formal similarities, the geometry of nature, spirals in architecture are topics that fall into "aspects of nature in architecture". For instance, nature's geometry has been the purpose of the invention since the starting of scientific researches via the laws of symmetry and proportion. Harmony principles contain a significant role in architecture like that suitable aesthetic and proportioned places and arrangements could attain, especially by utilizing the module of nature. "Golden ratio" ($\varphi = 1.618$) that has been mentioned, "a divine proportion," has been applied in architecture in order to design specific harmonic proportions (Gruber 2011; Moosavi-Movahedi 2017).

The second approach, the presence of life criterion in architecture, will be making a huge architectural transformation. Here, architecture could be an urban structure, building, processes, or materials defined as the constructed environment, and it has been affected permanently by nature and living systems. Several significant biology's life features that could be utilized in architecture are mentioned as; order, energy processing, growth, sensing and reacting homeostasis and metabolism, and evolutionary development.

An Open system, a system that has a definite boundary while exchange occurs (Gruber 2011), can also be implemented in architecture as a living organism. "Openness" in ecological systems means exchanging energy and materials, while for life science includes the exchange of energy, resources, and information. "Openness" in architecture involves significant visibility, light, accessibility, and kinds of permeability. Transparent and visible urban buildings and structures could be an example of architectural openness. The kinds of issues; entering and absorbing materials and energy into the city and leaving urban waste and emissions, individual and public transportation, urban accessibility, design of openness buildings, the design of how buildings are adaptable to be open, etc. involved in architectural openness projects.

According to energy processing, the exchange of energy with the environment is open in architecture, similar to alive organisms. Depending on the forms of energy, the method of control is different. Light, kinetic energy, heat, electricity, and material bound energy are the primary energy forms that affect the building environment. The flow of energy management systems is developed and centralized based on energy utilization information about architecture. Living creatures are using information instead of extreme energy consumption in their technology (Vincent et al. 2006). By mimicking some of the technologies of nature (like photosynthesis), we should act to save and harvest the energy. Therefore, energy efficiency is a very significant issue in architecture in a way that could minimize building consumption from the central energy source.

Self-organization, as a characteristic of natural processes and living forms, can be exploited in architecture. According to architectural explanation, self-organization includes local independent activities in the absence of central control. Self-organized constructions can attain higher efficiency than traditional organizations (Bennett 2004). For example, unplanned settlements are self-organized patterns shaped via self-planned interaction that their structures are influenced by selecting factors based on environment, surface area, topography, accessibility, and transportation. Building minus unessential rules, but the strong regional planning structure could improve the constructed environment quality and help protect the spaces employed by other purposes instead of economy and industry necessities.

Self-organization for healing or self-healing as a valuable feature of living systems is especially significant in architectonic situations where limited damage causes an entire system collapse, as in airplanes or space-technology. Self-healing in current space technologies is dependent on the air-pressure factor to retain structural integrity.

Despite the living criteria brought in architecture, its technology is still far from making or creating artificial life. Not all of these living parameters have yet been found in one architecture project. The phenomena that have emerged today are that the architectural space for a gadget or car has become more important than activity or people. Creating artificial life is a tempting subject in interdisciplinary issues of architecture and life sciences. The major factor for "architectural aliveness" is how to architecture being used or high evaluated by residents. The subjects like "space usage for high-rate activity," "residents' satisfaction," "incorporating cultural and social people livings in architecture," etc. are indicated as high quality evaluating issues of life in architecture.

8 Conclusion

This work aims to provide a brief and helpful overview of the impact of biomimicry and bioinspiration in the human lifestyle. New technologies and great creations have been appeared looking toward nature for design inspiration. The use of biomimetic biomaterials is one of the most effective ways to treat many diseases via different methods, such as applying them as a suitable carrier system like various nano-platforms with controllable drug release and also their applications in physically replacements of soft, or hard tissues. Art, education and architecture are essential elements impressive in lifestyle. The biomimetic approach and mimesis of nature play key roles in deepening these concepts and improving the quality of individual and social life. This perspective is discussed in detail within this chapter considering art, education and architecture as important personal and social issues.

Acknowledgments This investigation is supported by Iran National Science Foundation (INSF) and the Institute of Biochemistry and Biophysics (IBB) University of Tehran. Chemistry & Chemical Engineering Research Center of Iran (CCERCI) and Kharazmi University are gratefully acknowledged.

References

Allen TM, Cullis PR (2013) Liposomal drug delivery systems: from concept to clinical applications. Adv Drug Deliv Rev 65(1):36–48

Alvarez-Lorenzo C, Concheiro A (2013) Bioinspired drug delivery systems. Curr Opin Biotechnol 24(6):1167–1173

Amini AR, Laurencin CT, Nukavarapu SP (2012) Bone tissue engineering: recent advances and challenges. Crit Rev™ Biomed Eng 40(5):363–408

Amoozgar Z, Yeo Y (2012) Recent advances in stealth coating of nanoparticle drug delivery systems. Wiley Interdisc Rev Nanomed Nanobiotechnol 4(2):219–233

Ang H, Xiao T, Duan W (2009) Flight mechanism and design of biomimetic micro air vehicles. Sci China Ser E Technol Sci 52(12):3722–3728

Baldwin RG (2009) The climate for undergraduate teaching and learning in stem fields. New Dir Teach LEarn 2009(117):9–17

Balmert SC, Little SR (2012) Biomimetic delivery with micro-and nanoparticles. Adv Mater 24(28):3757–3778

Bar-Cohen Y (2005) Biomimetics: mimicking and inspired-by biology. In: Smart structures and materials 2005: electroactive polymer actuators and devices (EAPAD). International Society for Optics and Photonics, pp 1–8

Bar-Cohen Y (2016) Biomimetics: nature-based innovation. CRC Press

Bar-Cohen Y (2006) Biomimetics—using nature to inspire human innovation. Bioinspiration Biomimetics 1(1):1–12

Batrakova EV, Gendelman HE, Kabanov AV (2011) Cell-mediated drug delivery. Expert Opin Drug Del 8(4):415–433

Bennett J (2004) Organisational strategy. In: Clements-Croome D (ed) Intelligent buildings: design, management and operation. Thomas Telford, London, p 237

Bensaude-Vincent B (2011) A cultural perspective on biomimetics. In: George A (ed) Advances in Biomimetics. InTech

Bianco A, Kostarelos K, Prato M (2005) Applications of carbon nanotubes in drug delivery. Curr Opin Chem Biol 9(6):674–679

Binyamin G, Shafi BM, Mery CM (2006) Biomaterials: a primer for surgeons. In: Seminars in pediatric surgery, vol 4. Elsevier, pp 276–283

Bogue R (2009) Inspired by nature: developments in biomimetic sensors. Sens Rev 29(2):107–111

Bohner M (2010) Design of ceramic-based cements and putties for bone graft substitution. Eur Cells Mater 20(1):3–10

Bombač D, Brojan M, Fajfar P, Kosel F, Turk R (2007) Review of materials in medical applications Pregled Materialov V Medicinskih Aplikacijah. RMZ Mater Geoenviron 54(4):471–499

Buhleier E, Wehner W, Vögtle F (1978) "Cascade"- and "Nonskid-Chain-Like" syntheses of molecular cavity topologies. Chemischer Informationsdienst 9(25):155–158

Burdon-Sanderson JS (1882) On the electromotive properties of the leaf of Dionæa in the excited and unexcited states. Philos Trans R Soc Lond 173:1–55

Carmona-Ribeiro AM (2010) Biomimetic nanoparticles: preparation, characterization and biomedical applications. Int J Nanomed 5:249

Chandrawati R, Caruso F (2012) Biomimetic liposome- and polymersome-based multicompartmentalized assemblies. Langmuir 28(39):13798–13807

Cheng Y, Wang J, Rao T, He X, Xu T (2008) Pharmaceutical applications of dendrimers: promising nanocarriers for drug delivery. Front Biosci 13(4):1447–1471

Chiu I, Shu LH (2007) Biomimetic design through natural language analysis to facilitate cross-domain information retrieval. Artif Intell Eng Des Anal Manuf 21(1):45–59

Choi SW, Kim WS, Kim JH (2003) Surface modification of functional nanoparticles for controlled drug delivery. J Dispersion Sci Technol 24(3–4):475–487

Cohen YH, Reich Y (2016) Biomimetic design method for innovation and sustainability, vol 10. Springer, Berlin

Cordon C, Piva M, Melo C, Pinhal M, Suarez E (2013) Nanoparticles as platforms of molecular delivery in diagnosis and therapy. OA Cancer 1:15–21

Davis J (2003) Overview of biomaterials and their use in medical devices. In: Handbook of materials for medical devices, pp 1–11

DeHaan RL (2005) The impending revolution in undergraduate science education. J Sci Educ Technol 14(2):253–269

De Witte T-M, Fratila-Apachitei LE, Zadpoor AA, Peppas NA (2018) Bone tissue engineering via growth factor delivery: from scaffolds to complex matrices. Regenerative Biomater 5(4):197–211

Dicks H (2016) The philosophy of biomimicry. Philos Technol 29(3):223–243

Dowson D (1992) Friction and wear of medical implants and prosthetic devices. Friction Lubr Wear Technol 18:656–664

Drotleff S, Lungwitz U, Breunig M, Dennis A, Blunk T, Teßmar J, Göpferich A (2004) Biomimetic polymers in pharmaceutical and biomedical sciences. Eur J Pharm Biopharm 58(2):385–407

Dubok VA (2000) Bioceramics-yesterday, today, tomorrow. Powder Metall Met Ceram 39(7–8):381–394

French M (1994) Invention and evolution. In: Design in nature and engineering, 2nd edn. Cambridge Press, Cambridge

Garg T, Singh O, Arora S, Murthy R (2011) Dendrimer—a novel scaffold for drug delivery. Int J Pharm Sci Rev Res 7(2):211–220

Goel AK, Stroulia E (2009) Functional device models and model-based diagnosis in adaptive design. Artif Intell Eng Des Anal Manuf 10(4):355–370

Goel AK, Rugaber S, Vattam S (2008) Structure, behavior, and function of complex systems: the structure, behavior, and function modeling language. Artif Intell Eng Des Anal Manuf 23(1):23–35

Gong Y-k, Winnik FM (2012) Strategies in biomimetic surface engineering of nanoparticles for biomedical applications. Nanoscale 4(2):360–368

Gruber P (2011) Biomimetics in architecture: architecture of life and buildings. Springer, Vienna, New York

Handelsman J, Ebert-May D, Beichner R, Bruns P, Chang A, DeHaan R, Gentile J, Lauffer S, Stewart J, Tilghman SM, Wood WB (2004) Education. Scientific teaching. Science 304(5670):521–522

Hanker JS, Giammara BL (1988) Biomaterials and biomedical devices. Science 242(4880):885–892

Hatakeyama H, Akita H, Harashima H (2013) The polyethyleneglycol dilemma: advantage and disadvantage of pegylation of liposomes for systemic genes and nucleic acids delivery to tumors. Biol Pharm Bull 36(6):892–899

Heini P, Berlemann U (2001) Bone substitutes in vertebroplasty. Eur Spine J 10(2):S205–S213

Hodick D, Sievers A (1989) On the mechanism of trap closure of venus flytrap (Dionaea Muscipula Ellis). Planta 179(1):32–42

Hwang J, Jeong Y, Park JM, Lee KH, Hong JW, Choi J (2015) Biomimetics: forecasting the future of science, engineering, and medicine. Int J Nanomed 10:5701–5713

Ingber DE, Mow VC, Butler D, Niklason L, Huard J, Mao J, Yannas I, Kaplan D, Vunjak-Novakovic G (2006) Tissue engineering and developmental biology: going biomimetic. Tissue Eng 12(12):3265–3283

Jang YL, Yun UJ, Lee MS, Kim MG, Son S, Lee K, Chae SY, Lim DW, Kim HT, Kim SH (2012) Cell-penetrating peptide mimicking polymer-based combined delivery of paclitaxel and sirna for enhanced tumor growth suppression. Int J Pharm 434(1–2):488–493

Jelinek R (2013) Biomimetics: a molecular perspective. Walter de Gruyter

Johnson E, Bonser R, Jeronimidis G (2009) Recent advances in biomimetic sensing technologies. Philos Trans Royal Soc Math Phys Eng Sci 367(1893):1559–1569

Kalyanasundaram K, Graetzel M (2010) Artificial photosynthesis: biomimetic approaches to solar energy conversion and storage. Curr Opin Biotechnol 21(3):298–310

Kato N, Kamimura S (2008) Bio-mechanisms of swimming and flying: fluid dynamics, biomimetic robots, and sports science. Springer Science & Business Media

Khan W, Muntimadugu E, Jaffe M, Domb AJ (2014) Implantable medical devices. In: Focal controlled drug delivery. Springer, Berlin, pp 33–59

Kimura S (2008) Molecular assemblies as biomimetic systems and their applications. Macromol Biosci 8(11):979–980

Kulinets I (2015) Biomaterials and their applications in medicine. In: Regulatory affairs for biomaterials and medical devices. Elsevier, pp 1–10

Kumar SS (2007) Biopolymers in medical applications. Tech Text, pp 1–15

Kuroda D, Kawasaki H, Hiromoto S, Hanawa T (2005) Annual Book of ASTM Standards, Section 13, Medical Devices and Services, 2000. Mater Trans 46(7):1532–1539

Langer K, Kohn J (1996) Bioresorbable and bioerodible materials. In: Biomaterials Science. Academic Press, New York, pp 64–72

Lee JJ, Worthington P (1999) Reconstruction of the temporomandibular joint using calvarial bone after a failed teflon-proplast implant. J Oral Maxillofac Surg 57(4):457–461

Lima AC, Custódio CA, Alvarez-Lorenzo C, Mano JF (2013) Biomimetic methodology to produce polymeric multilayered particles for biotechnological and biomedical applications. Small 9(15):2487–2492

Liu XY (2012) Bioinspiration: from nano to micro scales. Springer, Berlin

Lourenco M, Ferreira M, Branco S (2012) Molecules of natural origin, semi-synthesis and synthesis with anti-inflammatory and anticancer utilities. Curr Pharm Des 18(26):3979–4046

Mano JF (2013) Biomimetic approaches for biomaterials development. Wiley-VCH

Marom A, Marom G (2016) The biomimetic process in artistic creation. In: Bar-Cohen Y (ed) Biomimetics: nature-based innovation. CRC Press, Taylor & Francis Group, Boca Raton

Meyer RA, Sunshine JC, Green JJ (2015) Biomimetic particles as therapeutics. Trends Biotechnol 33(9):514–524

Mishra P, Nayak B, Dey R (2016) Pegylation in anti-cancer therapy: an overview. Asian J Pharm Sci 11(3):337–348

Mogoșanu GD, Grumezescu AM (2014) Natural and synthetic polymers for wounds and burns dressing. Int J Pharm 463(2):127–136

Moosavi-Movahedi F (2017) Perspective on golden ratio (Φ). Sci Cultivation 7:39–52

Newman DJ, Cragg GM (2007) Natural products as sources of new drugs over the last 25 years. J Nat Prod 70(3):461–477

Nosonovsky M, Rohatgi PK (2011) Biomimetics in materials science: self-healing, self-lubricating, and self-cleaning materials, vol 152. Springer Science & Business Media

Palincsar AS (1998) Social constructivist perspectives on teaching and learning. Annu Rev Psychol 49:345–375

Parida P, Behera A, Mishra S (2012) Classification of biomaterials used in medicine. Int J Adv Appl Sci 1:31-35

Peppas NA (2004) Intelligent therapeutics: biomimetic systems and nanotechnology in drug delivery. Adv Drug Deliv Rev 56(11):1529

Pina S, Oliveira JM, Reis RL (2015) Natural-based nanocomposites for bone tissue engineering and regenerative medicine: a review. Adv Mater 27(7):1143–1169

Ratner BD, Bryant SJ (2004) Biomaterials: where we have been and where we are going. Annu Rev Biomed Eng 6:41–75

Rodrigues L, Mota M (2016) Bioinspired materials for medical applications. Woodhead Publishing

Ruys AJ (2013) Biomimetic biomaterials: structure and applications. Elsevier

Sáenz A, Rivera E, Brostow W, Castaño VM (1999) Ceramic biomaterials: an introductory overview. J Mater Educ 21(5/6):267–276

Schmalz G, Arenholt-Bindslev D (2009) Biocompatibility of dental materials, vol 1. Springer

Sheikhpour M, Barani L, Kasaeian A (2017) Biomimetics in drug delivery systems: a critical review. J Control Release 253:97–109

Singh RA, Yoon E-S, Jackson RL (2009) Biomimetics: the science of imitating nature. Tribol Lubr Technol 65(2):40–47

Siraparapu YD, Bassa S, Sanasi PD (2013) A review on recent applications of biomaterials. Int J Sci Res 1:70–75

Stroble JK, Stone RB, Watkins SE (2009) An overview of biomimetic sensor technology. Sens Rev 29(2):112–119

Sumita M, Hanawa T, Teoh S (2004) Development of nitrogen-containing nickel-free austenitic stainless steels for metallic biomaterials. Mater Sci Eng, C 24(6–8):753–760

Toko K (2000) Biomimetic sensor technology. Cambridge University Press

Vaccaro AR, Madigan L (2002) Spinal applications of bioabsorbable implants. Orthopedics 25(10):S1115–S1120

Vauthier C, Labarre D (2008) Modular biomimetic drug delivery systems. J Drug Delivery Sci Technol 18(1):59–68

Venkatesh S, Byrne ME, Peppas NA, Hilt JZ (2005) Applications of biomimetic systems in drug delivery. Expert Opin Drug Delivery 2(6):1085–1096

Vert M, Doi Y, Hellwich K-H, Hess M, Hodge P, Kubisa P, Rinaudo M, Schué F (2012) Terminology for biorelated polymers and applications (Iupac Recommendations 2012). Pure Appl Chem 84(2):377–410

Vincent JF (2003) Biomimetic modelling. Philos Trans R Soc Lond B Biol Sci 358(1437):1597–1603

Vincent JF, Mann DL (2002) Systematic technology transfer from biology to engineering. Philos Trans Ser A Math Phys Eng Sci 360(1791):159–173

Vincent JF, Bogatyreva OA, Bogatyrev NR, Bowyer A, Pahl AK (2006) Biomimetics: its practice and theory. J R Soc Interface 3(9):471–482

Vogel S (1998) Cats' paws and catapults: mechanical worlds of nature and people. W. W. Norton & Company

Von Recum AF, Laberge M (1995) Educational goals for biomaterials science and engineering: prospective view. J Appl Biomater 6(2):137–144

Whelan J (2002) Smart bandages diagnose wound infection. Drug Discov Today 7(1):9–10

Whitesides GM (2015) Bioinspiration: something for everyone. Interface Focus 5(4):20150031–20150041

Wright KA, Nadire KB, Busto P, Tubo R, McPherson JM, Wentworth BM (1998) Alternative delivery of keratinocytes using a polyurethane membrane and the implications for its use in the treatment of full-thickness burn injury. Burns 24(1):7–17

Yen J, Weissburg MJ, Helms M, Goel AK (2016) Biologically inspired design: a tool for interdisciplinary education. In: Bar-Cohen Y (ed) Biomimetics: nature-based innovation. CRC Press, Taylor & Francis Group, Boca Raton

Nature's Generosity in Protecting Human Health

Nazanin Seighal Delshad, Bahareh Soleimanpour, and Peyman Salehi

Abstract

This chapter aims to demonstrate the high value of natural compounds in modern drug discovery. Although, in today's global market, the extraction of natural products does not count as a primary method to produce medicines, yet nature's selectivity toward producing specific stereoisomers makes this source an interesting target for further studies. The biological and chemical comparison between natural and synthetic chiral structures shows thoughtful selectivity of nature toward creating the isomer that possesses the highest therapeutic properties and least side effects. Thus, even the developments of modern techniques in synthetic chemistry and drug design could not replace or overshadow the importance of these natural treasures in the pharmaceutical industry. In this regard, we devoted this chapter to introduce the essential role of nature in all its forms (plants, bacteria, fungus, or even animals' organs) in the discovery of some critical therapeutic agents, including a few well-known drugs that saved the lives of many patients.

Keywords

Chirality · Bioselectivity · Natural product · Intelligent creation · Biosynthesis

1 Introduction

For millennia, humans' lives have mainly depended on nature as an essential source of food, shelter, clothing, and medicine. Nature also provides humans with natural products (i.e., products from plants, animals and minerals) that considered as the most decisive origins of drugs as well as the primary resources of therapeutic agents for the treatment of human disease for hundreds of years. The man has employed such products in various forms of traditional medicines, remedies, potions, and oils to cure his own as well as other living creatures' diseases (Morales et al. 2016; Newman et al. 2000; Kinghorn et al. 2011). However, throughout this long period, various systems evolved by different ancient cultures to use herbal medicines; amongst those primitive systems, some were developed in a more organized procedure, making them last for many years (e.g., Chinese herbal medicine, Ayurveda, Greek,

N. Seighal Delshad · B. Soleimanpour · P. Salehi (✉)
Department of Phytochemistry, Medicinal Plants and Drugs Research Institute, Shahid Beheshti University, Tehran, Iran
e-mail: p-salehi@sbu.ac.ir

N. Seighal Delshad
e-mail: n.seighaldelshad@mail.sbu.ac.ir

B. Soleimanpour
e-mail: b.soleymanpour@mail.sbu.ac.ir

etc.). The use of these herbal medicine systems is still so widespread that in 2013 the World Health Organization admitted that in many developing countries, traditional medicine is still considered as the primary type of health care for the population (Morales et al. 2016). This vast use of natural products makes them one of the most valuable non-wood forest products (Astutik et al. 2019). Apart from the large share of natural products in traditional medicine trades, medicinal plants also play a dominant role as the source of many well-known drugs, namely aspirin and quinine, digitoxin, morphine, and pilocarpine (Machairiotis et al. 2020).

Along with the dramatic development of medicinal plants and their high impact on the development of new drugs, they cannot be considered as the only source of natural medication. Discovery of "penicillin" by Fleming in 1928, and the re-isolation and clinical study of this compound by Chain Florey et al. is considered as the turning point for both drug companies and research groups to use microorganisms as a new source of drugs especially antibiotics. Although using microorganisms as a modern source was a big step for drug industries, it was not the only vital stage of drug discovery within this business (Butler 2004).

The discovery of chiral chemistry shared the story of the discovery of penicillin by Fleming; it was serendipitous. In 1848, Louis Pasteur accidentally noticed that crystals of tartaric acid were either left-handed or right-handed. As a matter of fact, this was not the only discovery made by Pasteur. In 1857 Pasteur discovered microorganisms distinguishing the two isomers of tartaric acid [(−) and (+) isomer] through metabolizing them at different ratios. This study was the debut for enantioselectivity in biological processes. Yet, it was not until 30 years after this discovery that the Italian chemist Arnaldo Piutti established his observations on the comparison between L and D isomers of asparagine. His study demonstrated that these two isolated enantiomers vary in taste, and his report was the commencement of a new field known as enantioselectivity in receptor-mediated biological activity (Gal 2012).

Pharmacologists and physicians may consider drugs as one single agent bearing a single action. However, this might be accurate for pure enantiomers. In most cases, racemic mixtures have different pharmacological outcomes depending on the pharmacological activity and deposition of each enantiomer in the body. Eventually, pharmacological and toxicological investigations in recent decades demonstrate that the biological activities of some isomeric pairs are dissimilar. Still, it aroused negligible concerns with synthesizing chiral pharmaceutical agents having two enantiomers until the tragedy of thalidomide, a sedative drug used by pregnant women in 1950. Unfortunately, this case resulted in 10,000 cases of phocomelia, caused by either of the two enantiomers of thalidomide. While one had the desired sedative effect, the other one showed a teratogenic outcome (Bentley 1995).

As mentioned earlier, most of the enantiomers vary in terms of pharmacological activities, and it is so rare to find a structure whose both enantiomers share the same pharmacodynamic activity as well as pharmacokinetic properties. Admittedly, this is not an unexpected matter since most natural compounds bear a specific enantiomeric form; all enzymes and receptors almost entirely composed of L-amino acids with stereoselective properties that react selectively toward different configurations. All proteins, enzymes, amino acids, carbohydrates, nucleosides, plus many alkaloids and hormones are all chiral compounds, and this makes chiral drugs the primary target for future medication. Drug chirality has become a significant aspect of the discovery of new drugs, drug design, and drug development, and stereochemistry has become an essential dimension of pharmacology. Now chiral drugs form about 60–70% of pharmaceuticals, and this would not be possible without the development of technologies that allowed us to prepare pure enantiomers. Asymmetric synthesis is one of the general methods to obtain a single enantiomer, and chiral catalysts play an essential role in this approach. Although, even in this method, natural compounds play a significant role as some these structures and their derivatives proved to be valuable chiral catalysts (Mohebbi et al. 2018a, b; Salehi et al. 2009; Dabiri et al. 2008; Song 2009; Marcelli and Hiemstra 2010). Although synthetic drugs play a central role in such matters, natural products are still considered as a source of new chiral chemical compounds. On the contrary to synthetic chiral structures, most of the natural compounds bear a specific enantiomeric form. For instance, natural amino acids are L-isomers, while natural sugars (carbohydrates) are D-isomers (Hyneck et al. 1990; Rentsch 2002; Nguyen et al. 2006; Sharma 2014; Eichelbaum et al. 2003).

As it has become clear that the human body is highly selective toward chiral compounds, the need for enantiomeric pure drugs has become an essential part of the research and development in pharmaceutical industries. Along the same line, since many bioactive structures produce in a single stereoisomer, nature considers a significant source of enantiomeric pure drugs. Following, we introduce you to a few well-known drugs that are provided in the single stereoisomeric form in nature, although they can be synthesized in more than one form.

The present chapter is designated so as to shed light on a number of natural compounds bearing universally recognized pharmaceutical properties. Moreover, it is to contrastively put on display their relative stereoisomers' function created synthetically in a laboratory environment showing either no or a lot less effective and, at times, indicating a catastrophic impression.

It is worthy of mentioning that the authors of the chapter primarily aimed at emphasizing on nature's generosity in catering essential pharmaceutical necessities for all living creatures which in fact is a flawless reflection of almighty God's gracious attention to all creatures' requirements regardless of how fundamental or trivial they might be.

2 Noradrenaline

Galen, one of the second century's greatest anatomists and physiologists, published the first report on the anatomical features of autonomic nerves and employed the term 'sympathetic nerve.' He explained that the chain of ganglia, alongside the spinal column, would transfer what was known as animal spirits throughout different organs, resulting in an event better known as sympathy (Goldstein 2001).

The sympathetic nervous system has a crucial responsibility in the human body by involuntary regulating cardiac activity, vascular tonicity, and also regulating the functional activity of the smooth muscles and glands. This regulation happens by releasing endogenic adrenergic substances, catecholines, from peripheral nerve endings into the synapses of the central nerve net (CNN). Three main endogenic catecholines are dopamine, noradrenaline, and adrenaline (Fig. 1). The mentioned compounds are mainly secreted by the adrenal glands and can be found all around the body (Nguyen et al. 2006).

In 1904, Stolz synthesized both adrenaline and its amino homologue, noradrenaline (Stolz 1904). In 1910 Barger and Dale explained that the injection of sympathomimetic primary amines like noradrenaline carefully stimulates the effects of sympathetic nerve system compared to the injection of adrenaline or other secondary amines (Roth 1962; Bennett 1999).

In 1946, Eluer, for the first time, discovered a sympathomimetic substance in extracts of splenic nerves of cattle, which showed the presence of (−)-noradrenaline by both colorimetrical (using iodine method) and biological analysis (Euler USv, 1946).

Noradrenaline, also known as noradrenaline, L-1-(3,4-dihydroxyphenyl)-2-aminoethanol, is a

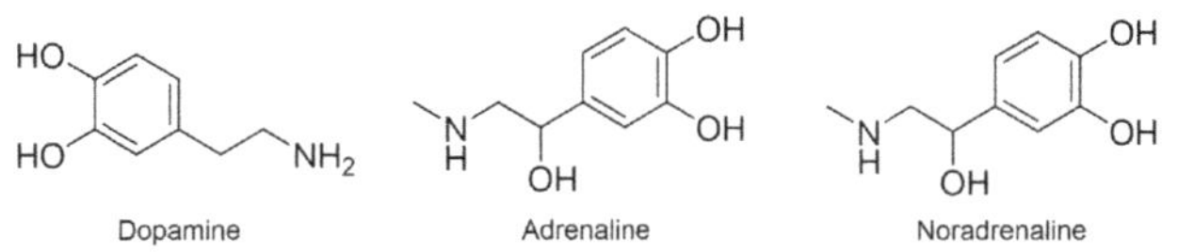

Fig. 1 Display of dopamine, adrenaline, and noradrenaline structure

monoamine neurotransmitter, found in ANS, being associated with the adaption of body conditions when facing stressful situations. As mentioned earlier, catecholines like noradrenaline are mainly secreted by adrenal glands from a general precursor, tyrosine, which further produces dopa, dopamine, and then noradrenaline, and act as a circulating hormone (Bryan and O'Donnell 1984; Musacchio et al. 1975).

Noradrenaline biosynthesis commences with the amino acid tyrosine, enzyme tyrosine hydroxylase (biopterin-dependent aromatic amino acid hydroxylase (AAAH)) converts tyrosine to dihydroxyphenylalanine (DOPA). This step is considered the rate-limiting step in the biosynthesis of L-noradrenaline and is tightly regulated at multiple levels. L-aromatic amino acid decarboxylase (AADC) would decarboxylate dopa to form dopamine. The first two steps in the biosynthesis of noradrenaline and epinephrine occur in the cytoplasm of the neuron. Then, dopamine is transported into storage vesicles in the nerve terminals via amine-specific transporters and then is hydroxylated to give noradrenaline by dopamine beta-hydroxylase (DBH) within the vesicles (shown in Scheme 1) (Bennett 1999; Euler USv, 1946; Bryan and O'Donnell 1984).

Noradrenaline affects the human body in numerous ways, the first and the foremost being responsible for the 'fight-or-flight' responses in stressful situations. Another significant effect of noradrenaline is its impact on increasing both systolic and diastolic blood pressure types, along with slowing the heartbeat rate, which makes this compound one of the vasopressor agents of choice in the treatment of shocks (LaPrairie et al. 2011; Wassall et al. 2009).

The comparison between noradrenaline and adrenaline showed that there are arrhythmic symptoms among the patients treated with dopamine. Furthermore, dopamine, compared to noradrenaline, was accompanied by higher death rates among patients suffering from cardiogenic shocks (LaPrairie et al. 2011; Wassall et al. 2009; Vardanyan et al. 2006; Backer et al. 2010; Bylund 2016).

Noradrenaline has two stereoisomers, (−)-noradrenaline (Fig. 2) that is produced naturally in the central nervous system (CNS) and (+)-noradrenaline, which is the synthetic type of this compound (Iversen et al. 1971).

Based on Iversen results on the accumulation of (−)-and (+)-noradrenaline or (−)- and (±)-adrenaline by extraneuronal uptake in the rats' hearts, it was believed that the extraneuronal uptake of catecholamines in tissues could not distinguish between the (−)- and (+)-isomers of these amines; on the other hand, they are not stereoselective (Iversen 1997). However, recent studies on the stereoselectivity of extraneuronal uptake of catecholamines in guinea-pig trachealis smooth muscle cells showed that the initial rates

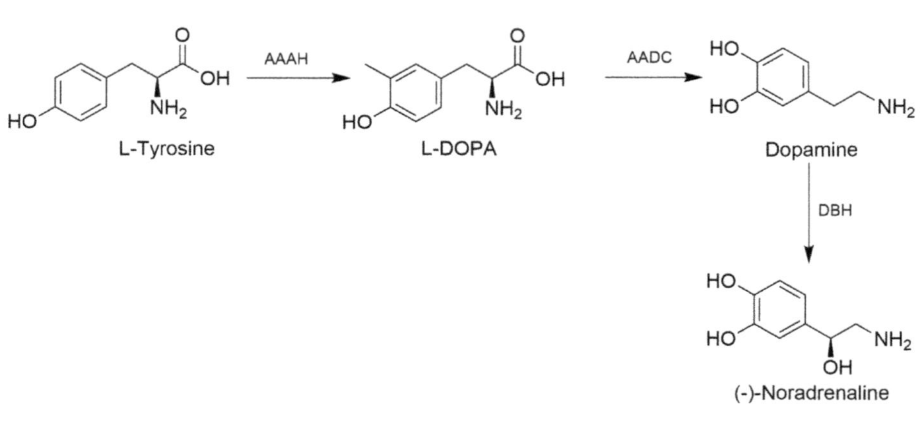

Scheme 1 Biosynthesis of (−)- Noradrenaline

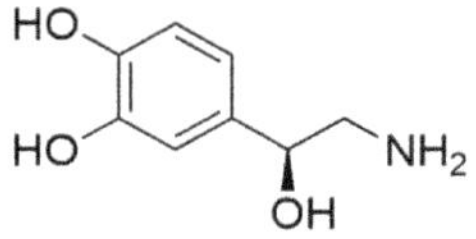

Fig. 2 (−)-Noradrenaline structure

Fig. 3 Calculated conformation of noradrenaline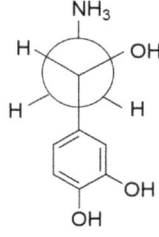

of absorption of the (−)-isomer of noradrenaline were almost 1.6 times higher than those of the (+)-isomer in tissues incubated in 25 μM noradrenaline (Bryan and O'Donnell 1984).

Another study of Iversen on differences in the uptake, storage, and metabolism of (+)- and (−)-noradrenaline bore significant outcomes. This study was performed on reserpine treated rats, mice and guinea-pigs' isolated perfused hearts. The rate of uptake of (+)- and (−)-noradrenaline measure by fluorimetric analysis of the removal of catecholamine from the perfusion medium. In rats and mice hearts, (−)-noradrenaline was taken up significantly more rapidly than (+)-noradrenaline, yet no stereochemical specificity find for noradrenaline uptake in guinea-pig hearts. It demonstrates that the absorption by noradrenaline terminals in the hypothalamus had a higher affinity for (−)-noradrenaline than for the (+)-isomer. Still, there is no difference in the affinity of these two isomers for uptake into dopamine terminals (Iversen et al. 1971).

Moreover, the in vivo studies on the metabolism pattern of (−)-noradrenaline and its (+)-isomer indicated that the pointed isomers have different metabolic fates. The study of the mouse samples suggested that the primary metabolites of (−)-noradrenaline were deaminated substances, with only a minor accumulation of (−)-normetanephrine. However, (+)-noradrenaline was metabolized almost entirely to (+)-normetanephrine shortly after injection, and (+)-normetanephrine remained the significant metabolite present for up to 1 h after injection. Likewise, investigation of the rat hearts and brains showed a higher amount of (+)-normetanephrine than (−)-normetanephrine at all times after injection of the isomers of noradrenaline (Iversen et al. 1971).

Moreover, a study was performed by Kier in 1969 on the preferred conformation of noradrenaline and a consideration of the α-adrenergic receptor, whose main focus was on the preferred conformation of noradrenaline based on calculated data using extended Hückel molecular orbital theory (shown in Fig. 3). Based on the study as mentioned above, the preferred conformation of noradrenaline is the same as what was previously calculated for (−)-ephedrine in respect to the relation of the quaternary and hydroxyl groups and the phenyl ring which is the same as (−)-noradrenaline (Kier 1969).

3 L-Dopa (Levodopa)

L-Dihydroxyphenylalanine, L-dopa, was first synthesized by Polish biochemist Casimir Funk in 1911 Funk (1911)). In 1913 Torquato Torquati, an Italian physician, found that broad bean, Vicia faba L, contains a catecholamine. Afterward, Marcus Guggenheim, who was a biochemist at The Hoffmann–La Roche isolated L-dopa from broad bean seeds (Vicia faba), characterized its chemical properties and introduced a practical method for synthesizing L-dopa. However, this compound thought to be inactive as Guggenheim could not detect any noticeable effect; he even self-ingests 2.5 g of this compound, which caused him to feel nauseous and vomit, yet showed no clinical use. This belief about L-dopa continued until the discovery of the role of dopamine as a neurohormone. Then L-dopa had been used as a medicine under the approved name of 'levodopa' (Fig. 4) (Guggenheim 1913; Ludin 2018).

L-dopa or 3,4-dihydroxyphenylalanine is an amino acid produced and used in humans, animals, and plants. During the tyrosinase function in melanogenesis, L-dopa is created from tyrosine (Scheme 2); this amino acid is also considered a

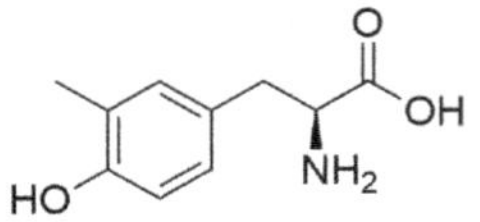

Fig. 4 L-dopa structure

precursor to dopamine, which further produces noradrenaline and adrenaline. The multistage biosynthetic pathway of this compound from L-tyrosine was suggested by both Peter Holtz and Hermann Blaschko (Hiroshima et al. 2014; Lopez et al. 2008; Broadley 2010; Holtz 1939; Blaschko 1939).

The pure solid L-dopa proved to be effective in reducing Parkinson's disease symptoms based on its ability to increase striatal dopamine content. This reaction occurred via decarboxylation of L-dopa by L-amino acid decarboxylase located primarily within DA axons. As a result, L-dopa can be considered a pro-drug for Parkinson's disease, since levodopa can correct the deficiency of dopamine by undergoing metabolic conversion to dopamine after entering the brain (Gjedde et al. 1993).

Although nature only produces L-dopa, the presence of D-dopa in the synthetic process is always one of the undesirable possibilities. Based on the stereospecificity of this enzyme, it was hard to believe that D-dopa could participate in the biosynthesis of dopamine. Although in the past, some other investigation on these two isomers revealed that in unilaterally striatal lesioned mice, D-dopa produces a similar turning behavior as L-dopa but at only one-tenth of the potency of L-dopa, with same efficacy of this amino acid in inducing circling. However, the later investigation of both in vivo and in vitro studies of these two revealed that in vivo studies, the inversion of D-dopa to L-dopa results in a better outcome. They suggested two pathways that lead to the conversion of D-dopa to L-dopa, the former involving oxidation of D-dopa to dihydroxyphenyl pyruvic acid by D-amino acid oxidase and the latter involving transamination of D-dopa to dihydroxyphenyl pyruvic acid. Further studies show that the use of sodium benzoate as an inhibitor of D-amino acid oxidase blocks D-dopa-induced circling while not affecting the circling induced by L-dopa, and the conversion of D-dopa to L-dopa dramatically relies on the oxidase activity. Now, it is clear that D-dopa not only has no effect on Parkinson's disease but also displays toxic side effects, like grave toxicity (agranulocytosis) (Coppi et al. 1972; Karoum et al. 1988; Wu et al. 2006a, b; Moses et al. 1996; Toussaint and Verniory 1969; Sumithira and Sujatha 2013).

4 Levothyroxine

Hypothyroidism is one of the most frequent chronic disorders in Western Communities and affects approximately 10% of the population worldwide. Today, using levothyroxine consuming is considered as a long-term thyroid replacement therapy (Hennessey 2015).

The discovery of a treatment for hypothyroidism fills with many physician discoveries and interventions. There are few documented reports of Chinese patients with hypothyroidism being treated using sheep thyroid (Slater 2011). There have been many studies on using sheep thyroid for hypothyroidism, namely transplanting sheep thyroid tissue into a myxedematous patient as well as the oral administration of fresh sheep thyroid glands, and last but not least injecting the myxedematous patient with thyroid extract that was obtained from sheep thyroids (Lindholm and Laurberg 2011; Murray 1891; Mackenzie 1892).

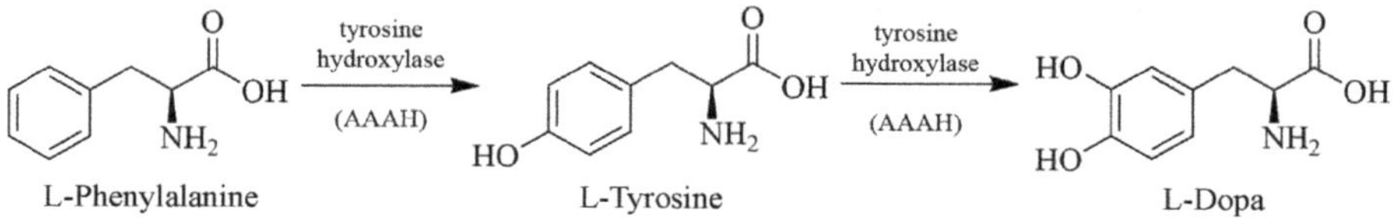

Scheme 2 Biosynthesis of L-dopa

As the oral use of these extracts was less time consuming and less costly, and oral preparation of extracts from ingested animal thyroid become more widespread, scientists were encouraged to identify those crucial ingredients that control the symptoms of hypothyroidism (Hennessey 2015); Kendall 1983).

It was in 1914 when Edward Calvin Kendall, for the first time, crystallized a substance containing 65.3% iodine. The substance was Levothyroxine (Fig. 5) or L-thyroxine or levothyroxine sodium, which was achieved by thyroxine (T4). However, it was not until 15 months later that he could obtain 33 g of this compound to investigate its physiologic properties (Kendall 1964). Moreover, the structural formula of this compound was discovered in 1926 by the same scientist. Barger and Harington were the first to synthesize thyroxine and published their employed procedure in 1927. They were also the ones who revealed the molecular structure of this compound, which then explained the link between dietary iodine and the thyroid gland as well as providing a mechanism for the regulation of growth, differentiation, and finally, the metabolism (Harington and Barger 1927).

The biosynthesis of thyroid hormone, as shown in Fig. 6, takes place on thyroglobulin (TG) in a series of eight major steps:

1. First, sodium-iodide symporter (NIS) transports Iodide to the cell. Construction of an electrochemical gradient generated by the Na^+, K^+-ATPase is a determinative factor for transporting Iodide in this step.
2. Afterward, pendrin (PDS/SLC26A4) transports Iodide into the follicular lumen.
3. Then TG is released in the follicular lumen, which is then used as the matrix for the synthesis of both thyroxine (T4) and triiodothyronine (T3).
4. Next, dual oxidase DUOX2 produces hydrogen peroxide (H2O2) that is crucial for the oxidation of Iodide. Dual oxidase DUOX2 is an enzyme requiring a specific maturation factor that is DUOXA2.
5. After that, the enzyme thyroperoxidase (TPO) oxidizes Iodide.
6. Consequently, TPO iodinates select tyrosyl residues on TG (organification or iodination), which further produces both mono- and diiodotyrosines (MIT, DIT). Afterward, TPO couples (coupling reaction) the iodotyrosines to form T4 or T3.
7. Then, iodinated TG is internalized by both micro- and macropinocytosis and is digested in lysosomes, and T4 and T3 are now secreted into the bloodstream through unidentified channels.
8. And finally, MIT and DIT are deiodinated in the cytosol by the iodotyrosine dehalogenase DEHAL1, and the released iodide is recycled for hormone synthesis (Kopp et al. 2009).

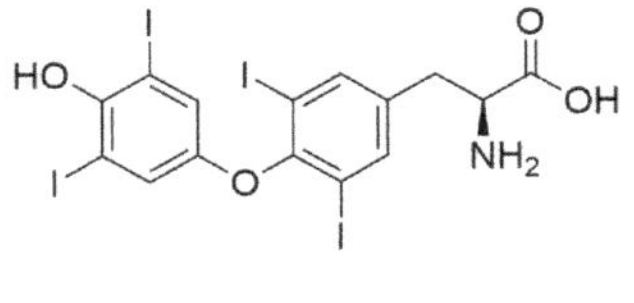

While L-thyroxine was used to supplement or replace thyroid hormone for the ones with hypothyroidism, it was also used to suppress TSH in persons with thyroid cancer or in those with nodular thyroid disease. Recently, synthetic L-thyroxine has been proved to be a well-established, convenient, safe, as well as inexpensive treatment modality and widely used for patients with hypothyroidism (Midgley et al. 2015).

While the natural form of thyroxine in mammals is the levo isomer, the process of alkaline hydrolysis of the gland in the first part of the extraction process, thyroxine, had undergone racemization into a mixture of optical isomers (Fig. 7). The dextro isomer of this compound is far less effective on hypothyroidism, unlike its levo isomer, but it lowers the levels of cholesterol, lipoprotein (a), beta-lipoproteins, and phospholipids in the serum. Although some studies say that it is effective without adverse thyromimetic effects or thyrocardiac side-effects, cholesterol levels) under the trade name of Choloxin. However, it was withdrawn from the market because of cardiac side effects (Steinberg

Fig. 5 Levothyroxine structure

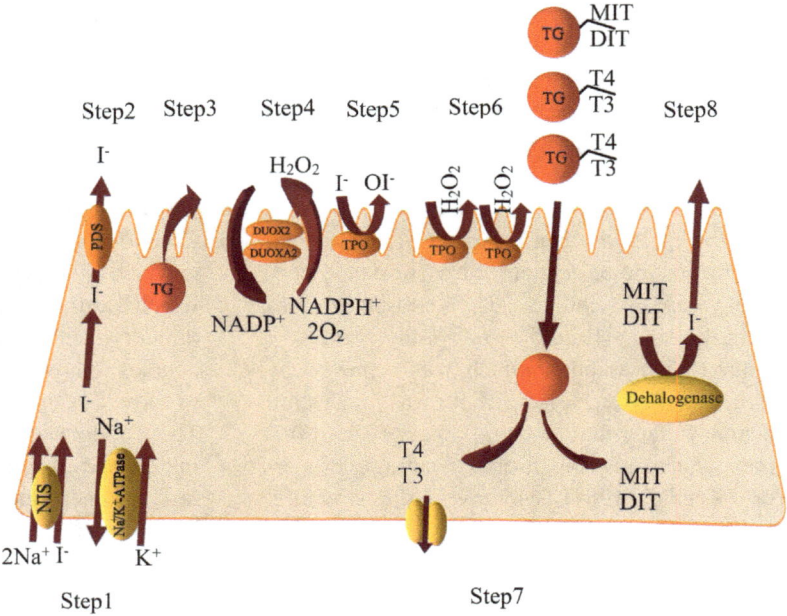

Fig. 6 Key steps in synthesis of thyroid hormone

and Steinberg 2007; Bantle et al. 1984; Wardle et al. 1974).

One of the interesting factors in these two isomers is their difference in their metabolism while investigating the two isomers of thyroxine in the dog; they figured D-thyroxine was inactivated more rapidly than L-thyroxine by the dog. Examination of their metabolism in rats also showed that D-thyroxine was metabolized more quickly by the rat than L-thyroxine (Midgley et al. 2015; Bantle et al. 1984; Wardle et al. 1974; Tekoa and King 2010; Sneader 2005; Kendall 1915; Vaidya and Pearce 2008; Krikler et al. 1971; Dufault et al. 1961; Shellabarger and Brown 1959; Flock et al. 1963).

In a study aiming at finding novel cholesterol-lowering drugs, D-thyroxine was used as one of the potential candidates by Canner et al. The initial investigations incorporating D-thyroxine indicated that, in contrary to its natural isomer, D-thyroxine did not display any noticeable impacts on the metabolism, blood pressure, and the heartbeat rate. However, this compound managed to maintain the cholesterol-lowering effect. Unfortunately, after 18 months from the initiation of this 5-year study, an increase in mortality rate was observed in patients diagnosed with pre-existing arrhythmias. In the following two years, the situation did not prove to get any better since the mortality rate in the group of patients prescribed with D-thyroxine as a whole kept increasing, which in turn resulted in discontinuation of this study. One of the main disadvantages of this study was that even the slightest increase in the amount of thyroid hormone activity was enough to provoke arrhythmias in

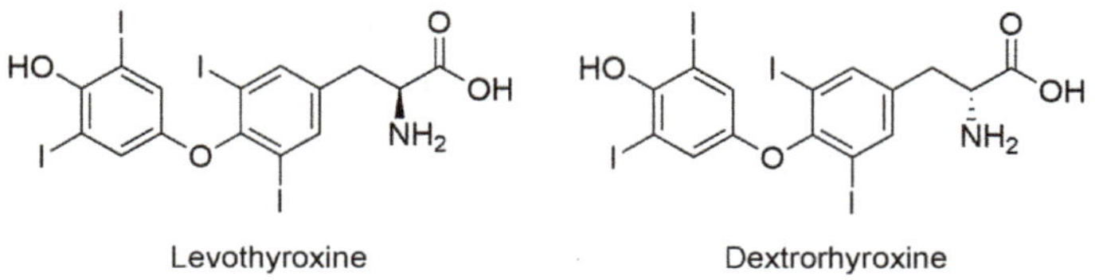

Fig. 7 Structures of two isomers of thyroxine

particular, and consequently endangering the cardiovascular system in general. On this account, it is safe to say that D-thyroxine barely influences hormonal activity—but it is not without noticeable impacts (Steinberg and Steinberg 2007; Canner et al. 1986).

Other studies suggested that after intravenous injection of the same amounts of the isomers in rats, the concentration of sodium dextrothyroxine became higher in the liver than sodium levothyroxine. However, in the heart, sodium levothyroxine was found in higher concentrations than its dextro enantiomer (Starr 1960). Despite the regional difference in the distribution of these two isomers, another study showed that the similarities in the effect of 4 mg dextrothyroxine and 0.15 mg levothyroxine persisted in such diverse functions as lowering serum TSH, cholesterol, triglyceride, and phospholipid levels and elevating basal metabolic rate (Gorman et al. 1979).

5 Physostigmine

The History of physostigmine (also known as serine, from the West African name of éséré, which refers to the Calabar bean) dates back to 1846 when William Daniell, who was a doctor in the British military at the time, published his first report on Calabar bean, *Physostigma venenosum Balf (Leguminosae)*. His report indicated that the locals would use the poisonous bean as an ordeal for criminals convicted of capital offenses in Old Calabar, Nigeria. Those criminals were forced to swallow the extract of beans. This strange method was used to recognize if someone is innocent. They believed that innocent prisoners with clear conscious would be able to swallow the beans, which only resulted in the sickness. However, the ones who are guilty would keep the beans in their mouths resulting in getting poisoned, and in some cases, it could take their lives. This ordeal-poison of the native tribes on the River Gambia, which comes from the bark of a leguminous tree, was first mentioned by M.M. Guillemin and Perottet, in their *Flore de Sénégambie* as *Fillcea suaveolens* (Christison 1855).

Daniell's report on Calabar beans motivated Robert Christison to investigate this bean; as a result, he cultivated the Calabar beans sent to him by the missionary, Probably William Daniell, and arranged animal experiments on the beans' extracts which stopped the heart of those animals and killed them. Afterward, he decided to explore the impacts of the beans on the human body by eating small pieces of the beans and recording the outcome. He experienced extreme weakness and atrial fibrillation and was lucky to survive (Sneader 2005); Christison 1855).

Afterward, Thomas Fraser, one of Christison's most prestigious students, isolated the active principle as an amorphous powder, which he called eserine. Then, Fraser investigated the extract and the pure alkaloid's effect on both voluntary and involuntary muscles of the body, including eye pupil, heart, CNS, glands, and intestines. The results of this experiment indicated that both alkaloid and extract result in mydriasis in eye pupil, and they both interfere with the effect of atropine on the heart rate. Later, Jobst and Hesse purified crystals of this compound in 1864 and named their product 'physostigmine' (Fig. 8) (Sneader 2005; Christison 1855; Jobst and Hesse 1864; Scheindlin 2010).

The first documented use of physostigmine as medicine dates back to 1875 when Ludwig Laqueur used this compound to cure blindness caused by glaucoma. Like Christison, he tested this drug on himself, although his experiment was quite more scientific and systematic. Physostigmine as an eye drop to caused loosening in the ciliary muscles and increased the outflow of aqueous humor, following decreased the elevated intraocular pressure. This drug is still used for the treatment of simple chronic glaucoma (Sneader 2005; Scheindlin 2010).

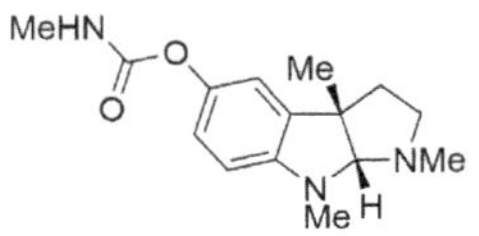

Fig. 8 Structure of (−)-physostigmine

Fraser was the first to describe physostigmine action in different organs and body systems. It enhances the salivary, bronchial secretions, and gastric increases intestinal tone and stimulates Gastrointestinal motility. Physostigmine also dilates the peripheral blood vessels, which decreases blood pressure, slows the heart rate, and finally constricts the pupil of the eye (Scheindlin 2010).

Otto Leowi investigated the biochemical mechanism of these effects on the body. He discovered acetylcholine and that physostigmine acted by preventing acetylcholine inhibition. Consequently, physostigmine is considered one of the pioneer drugs in blocking acetylcholinesterase. Further, In vitro studies indicate that besides being an acetylcholinesterase inhibitor (AChE), physostigmine can also inhibit butyrylcholinesterase (BChE) (Sneader 2005; Scheindlin 2010).

Biosynthesis of physostigmine in nature starts by C- alkylation at C-3 of tryptamine followed by ring formation involving the attack of the primary amine function onto the iminium ion (Scheme 3) (Dewick 2009).

Physostigmine contains two isomers from which (+)-physostigmine is a synthetic, unnatural isomer, and (−)-physostigmine is a natural isomer (Brossi and Pei 1998).

Julian, together with his colleague, Joseph Pikl, along with many other scientists around the world, were the competitors in the race to synthesize physostigmine. All scientists made an effort to simplify the synthetic process of this compound. Robert Robinson, as one of those scientists, published some reports on the partial synthesis of physostigmine, these reports paralleled with Julian's and Pikl's lab publications. These contemporary works on physostigmine led to revealing the last step of the synthesis pathway for physostigmine. Julian's full synthesis of physostigmine (Scheme 4) was considered one of the 25 most essential achievements in chemistry by the American Chemical Society (ACS) (Ault 2008; Julian and Pikl 1935a, b; Wilson and Willis 2010; Ravin and Higginbotham 2009).

Robinson's report on synthesizing unnatural (+)-physostigmine and (+)-physovenine is considered a big step to clarify the acetylcholine active centers' structures. Robinson's synthetic pathway for these artificial alkaloids closely resembled that of Julian and Pikl synthetic procedure. In this study, the enantiomeric resolution accomplished while treating eseroline with (+)-tartaric acid to acquire the (+)-eserethole. (+)-eseroline in this reaction was created by reacting (+)-eserethole with aluminum chloride, which further reacted with methylisocyanate to produce (+)-physostigmine. The alternative synthesis to create (+)-eseroline was also shown in this synthesis. Furthermore, the chemical resolution at this total synthesis was obtained by reacting carbinolamine with ditolyltartaric acid, which further provided them with optically active quaternary salts. Afterward, treating this salt with aqueous sodium hydroxide gave the desired optical active esermethole, which was O-demethylated to give eseroline (Scheme 5) Dewick 2009; Pallavicini et al. 1994; Pei et al. 1994; Dale and Robinson 1970).

The in vitro study performed by Robinson in 1970 on anti-acetylcholinesterase activities of

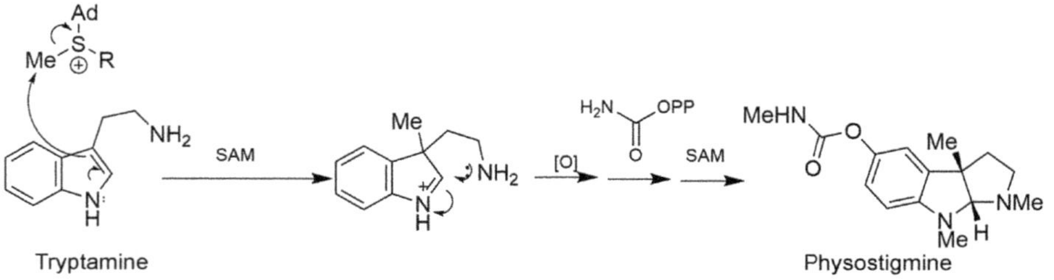

Scheme 3 Biosynthesis of physostigmine

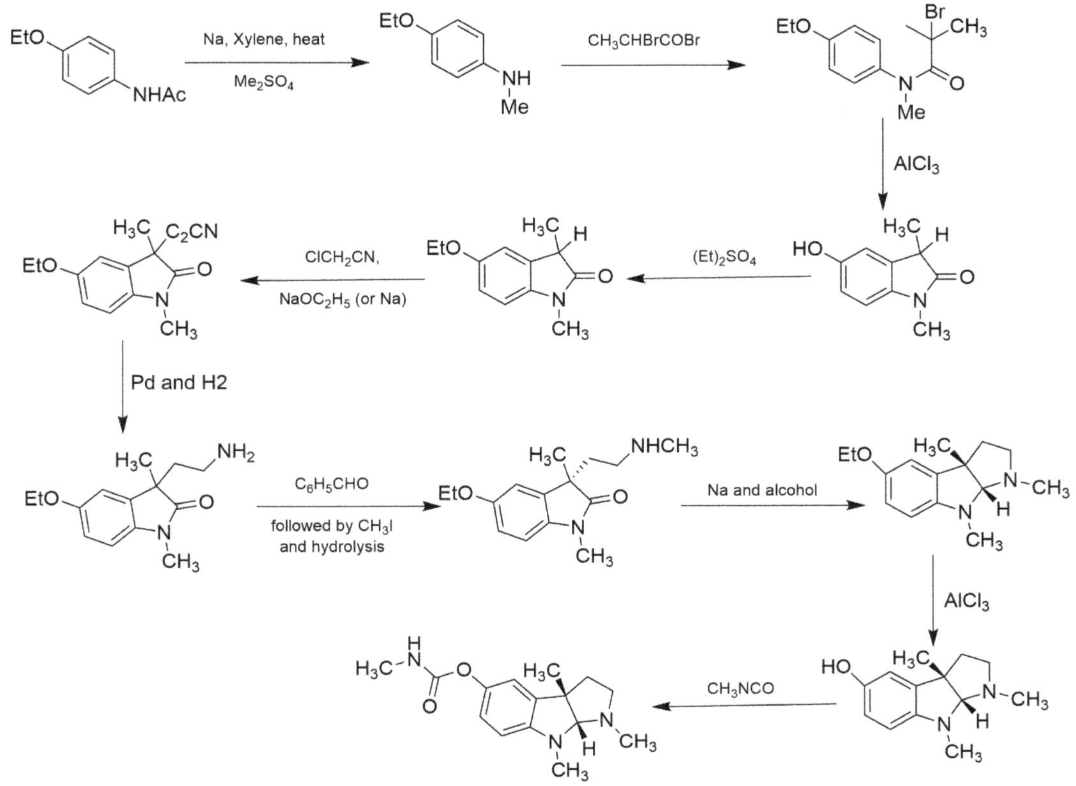

Scheme 4 First total synthesis of physostigmine suggested by Julian & Pikl

(+)-physostigmine and (+)-physovenine using erythrocyte acetylcholinesterase, showed that these two compounds have much lower anti-acetylcholinesterase activities than the alkaloids (−)-physostigmine and (−)-physovenine. The optical asymmetry of the enzyme surface or the receptor site can create a difference in inhibitory activities of the two enantiomers of these compounds (Dale and Robinson 1970).

Another study on inhibition of acetylcholinesterase from electric eel confirmed that inhibition of AChE in (+)-physostigmine is about 125 times less than its natural (−)-physostigmine. However, the (+)-physostigmine showed lower toxicity than its enantiomer (Brossi et al. 1986). Other studies on human tissue also confirm that the natural (−)-enantiomer of this compound is 1000 times more potent than the (+)-enantiomer (Triggle et al. 1998; Atack et al. 1989).

6 Morphine

Known as an alkaloid, Morphine is considered as one of the well-known plant-derived drugs obtained from the ancient medicinal herb, poppy (Brook et al. 2017).

Papaver somniferum L., poppy, is considered one of the first species cultivated by the man. Evidence of cultivating poppy was found in few historical sites, including closely related seeds of *P. somniferum subsp. Setigerum* was located in Danubian settlements, dated 4400–4000 BC. Also, some poppy seeds were found in northern France along with farming settlements on the shores of lakes in Switzerland that dated back to 3700–3625 BC (Brook et al. 2017).

P. somniferum and its subspecies setigerum are of few species capable of producing

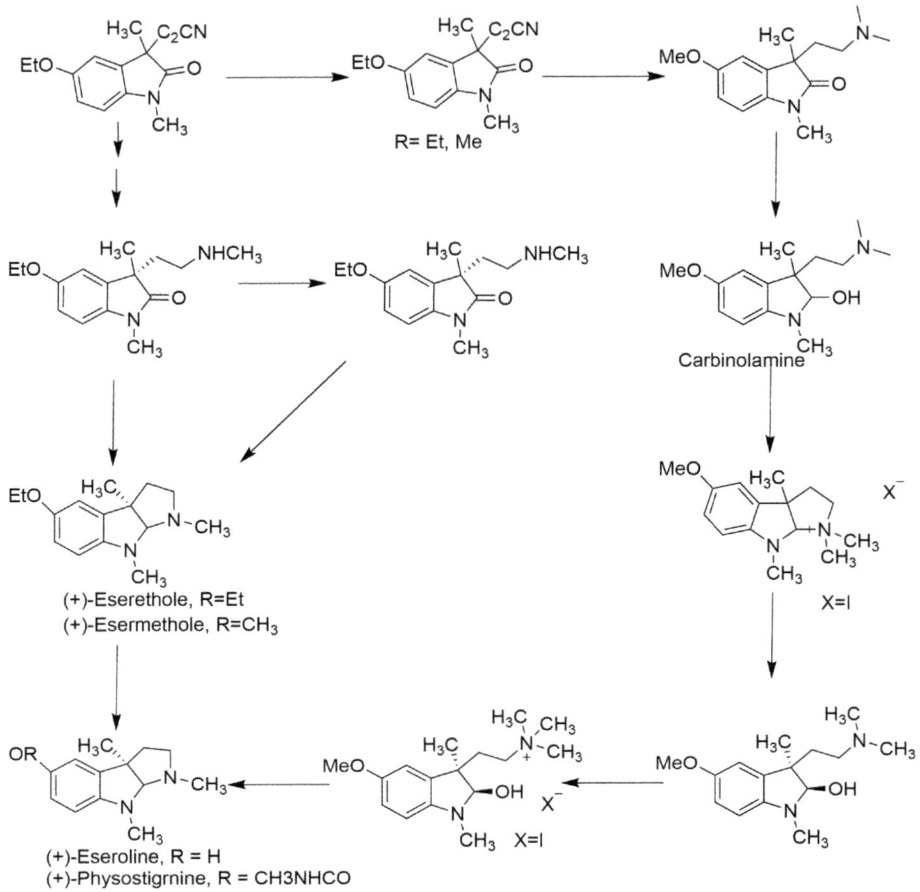

Scheme 5 Robinson Synthesis of (+)-physostigmine, and (+) eseroline

morphine and other narcotic compounds. However, the amount of those active compounds is meager, and they cannot provide any narcotic effects. The latex present in poppy's capsule includes the highest amount of these active alkaloids. These capsules should be dried for the use and preparation of the opium inside of them. However, it is still ambiguous how the man discovered the potential medicinal effects of this plant (Brook et al. 2017).

The early nineteenth century is considered the debut for one of the most revolutionary advancements in drug discovery, which was the development of new methods for the isolation of natural active compounds. Scientists, with the help of different solubility of compounds in various solvents, successfully separated active compounds like morphine. This method was first used by a French chemist, Nicolas Lémery, yet it is not precisely known when morphine was first extracted. However, it is possible that in mid-1600, Daniel Ludwig, the court physician of the Duke of Saxe-Gotha, was the one who extracted it for the first time. His method consists of dissolving opium in an acid and then saturated the solvent with an alkali And obtained a substance that was he called Magisterium Opii (Davenport-Hines 2003; Trease 1964).

Fig. 9 (−)-Morphine structure

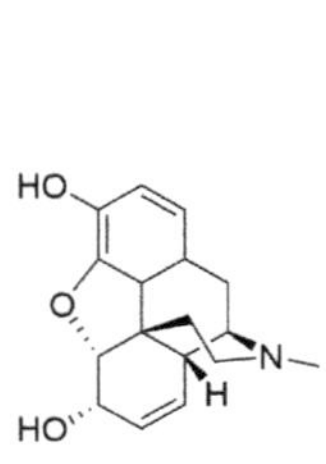

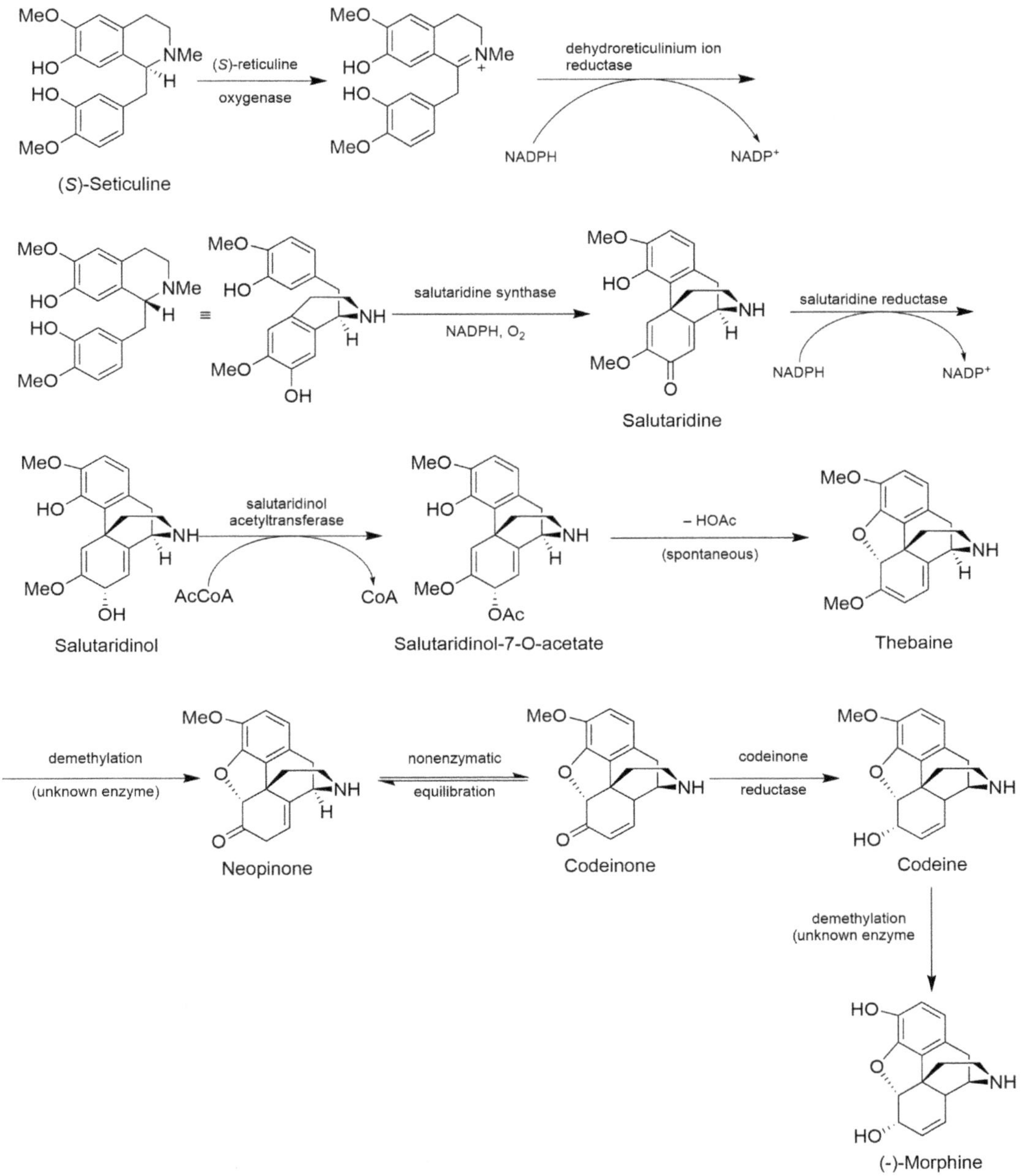

Scheme 6 Biosynthesis of (−)-morphine in opium poppy

A similar method was used by a few scientists to extract the active compound of opium. However, Friedrich Wilhelm Adam Sertürner was the one who published the first report on the isolation of opium's active compound in 1805. He also explained its properties, including solubility in acidic water, plus its precipitation by ammonia, and also identified this compound as a weak base. Afterward, he named this compound 'morphium' after Morpheus, the Greek God of dreams (Fig. 9) (Serturner 1805; Hodgson 2001).

After the Creation of the hypodermic needle by Charles-Gabriel Pravaz and Alexander Wood in 1850, morphine could be injected directly into blood vessels. This discovery gave morphine the ability to provide instant pain relief and put morphine in the front-line drugs used, especially for treating soldiers and warriors during wars (Brook et al. 2017; Hodgson 2001).

Two years after Sertürner's publication, Wilhelm Meissner identified morphine as an alkaloid (Meissner 1819). Following this event, Justus von Liebig in the 1820s and Henri Victor Regnault, in the 1830s, separately proposed the chemical formula for morphine, which was $C_{34}H_{36}N_2O_6$ and $C_{35}H_{40}N_2O_6$, respectively. Although these determinations were close, both proved to be inaccurate. It was in 1847; when August Lauren could deduce the correct chemical formula for morphine, $C_{34}H_{38}N_2O_6$, by creating morphine salt, excluding all moisture out of this salt, and using meticulous calculation (Blakemore and White 2002; Gates and Tschudi 1952; Laurent 1847).

The biosynthesis of this compound is almost entirely elucidated. Although, recent investigations confirmed that besides plants (*Papaver somniferum*) morphine and other alkaloids are also produced in mammalians with similar pathways. The biosynthesis of morphine (Scheme 6) starts with the conversion of (*S*)-reticuline into its (*R*)-enantiomer using (*S*)-reticuline-oxidase-mediated oxidation produced the 1,2- dehydroreticulinium ion followed by stereospecific reduction into to (*R*)-reticuline using 1,2- dehydroreticuline reductase. (*R*)-Reticuline then converted into salutaridine by an oxidative phenol coupling and created the morphinan structure with its specific stereochemistry. This reaction was catalyzed by salutaridine synthase, which is a microsomal NADPH-dependent cytochrome P-450 enzyme. Afterward, Salutaridine is reduced using NADPH dependent salutaridine reductase to produce salutaridinol. Then characteristic pentacyclic morphinan skeleton is built by creating the oxygen bridge between C4 and C5 to form the thebaine. This reaction is an S_N2-type reaction proceed by allylic alcohol moiety in the C ring. The hydroxyl group in Salutaridinol is activated by acetylation catalyzed by salutaridinol 7-*O*-acetyl transferase. Salutaridinol-7-*O*-acetate undergoes a spontaneous S_N2-type cyclization to produce thebaine. Afterward, thebaine is demethylated by thebaine 6-*O*-demethylase (T6ODM) to produce neopinone. Neopinone is in an equilibrium condition with its carbonyl-conjugated regioisomer, codeinone. Then codeinone is reduced by codeinone reductase (COR) to form codeine; this enzyme is so specific that it reduces only the C6 oxo group of codeinone. Then codeine is *O*-demethylated by codeine-*O*-demethylase (CODM) to produce morphine. There is a minor alternative pathway after the formation of thebaine (Scheme 7). In this rout, thebaine undergoes 3-*O*-demethylation by codeine-*O*-demethylase to produce oripavine, then it undergoes 6-*O*-demethylation by T6ODM to morphinone. In the end, morphinone is reduced to produce morphine by means of COR (Novak et al. (2000); Onoyovwe et al. 2013).

Twenty-seven years later, Robert Robinson suggested a structure for morphine, which was further confirmed by Marshall D. Gates, and his colleagues Gilg Tschudi. Then, Gates et al., proposed the first total synthesis procedure for morphine in 1952 (Scheme 8) after Otto Diels and Kurt Alder discovered the Diels–Alder reaction, since this reaction is a critical step of the synthesis of morphine (Blakemore and White 2002; Gates and Tschudi 1952).

There are many reports on the synthesis of unnatural (+)-morphine; However, one of the important ones was proposed by Rice et al. using commercially available (S)-tetrahydroisoquinolines as vital intermediates for this synthetic procedure. He also reported the unnatural alkaloids like (+)-codeine, and (+)-heroin (Scheme 9). Initial pharmacological studies in this report indicate that unnatural (+)-morphine did not show any analgesic activity in both the hot plate and tail-flick assays, on the contrary, (−)-morphine was highly potent in both assays (Hodgson 2001; Meissner 1819; Blakemore and White 2002).

Afterward, Rice established a report on stereospecific and nonstereospecific effects of

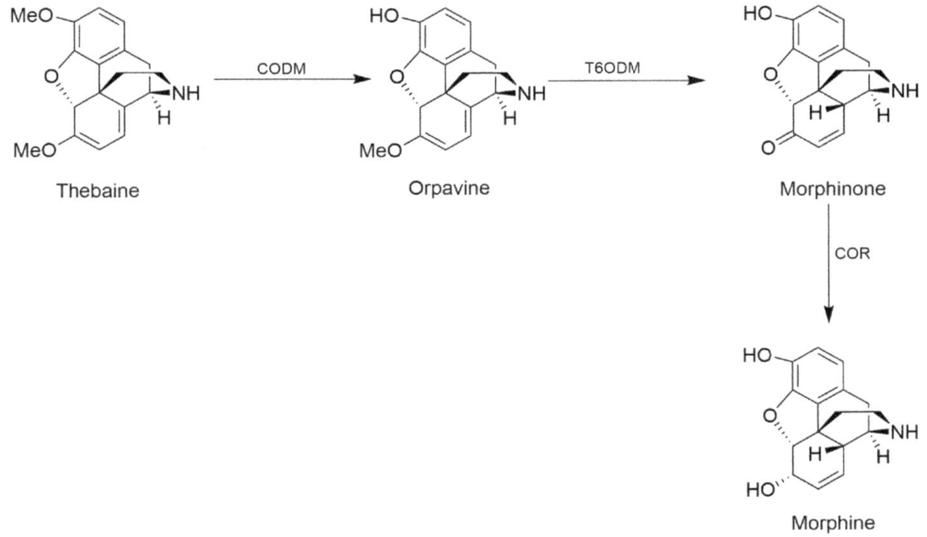

Scheme 7 An alternative route to producing (−)- morphine

both isomers of morphine. In his report, Rice compared two isomers of morphine by using three opiate assays. Both isomers were investigated in two levels of in vitro and in vivo. The results indicated that Morphine's effect on the body is based on its interaction with two distinct types of reaction. The first type possesses a high level of stereospecificity and mediates morphine analgesia, although the second type expresses a lower level of stereospecificity and mediates the hyperexcitability disorder. This type of receptor, after microinjecting morphine into CNS, causes explosive motor behavior. The results of in vitro studies showed the potency of unnatural (+)-morphine, in displacing [3H]-dihydromorphine from binding sites in rat brain homogenates is 10,000 folds lower than (−)-isomer. In the second assay, electrically stimulated guinea pig ileum, (+)-Morphine could not display effective inhibition for contractions even up to a hundred times more dosage than (−)-morphine, or (−)-normorphine. Also, (+)-isomer was unable to antagonize the action of (−)-isomer and (−)-normorphine. In the last assay, adenylate cyclase activity in neuroblastoma x glioma hybrid cell homogenates, (+)-morphine also presented 1000 times less potency of inhibitory than its (−)-isomer. Yet, it was unable to antagonize the action of natural morphine isomer (Brossi and Pei 1998; Goto et al. 1932; Goto and Shishido 1933; Jacquet et al. 1977). This report also shows that the injection of the unnatural morphine or (−)-morphine in the periaqueductal grey (PAG) resulted in explosive motor behavior (EMB) but not analgesia (Jacquet 1979).

7 Colchicine

Colchicine is an old drug that has been used for treating gout, rheumatism, and some other diseases. Colchicine was first isolated from *colchicum autumnale* in 1820 in the Colchis area located in the shore of the black sea; this plant grows in wet grasslands, open spaces in the forests, and shady rocky habitats that do not contain calcareous substrates (Akram et al. 2012).

This compound occurs in the corn, seeds, and flowers of saffron. Also, it can be isolated from meadow saffron, *colchicum autumnale*, and other related species (Shi et al. 1998).

This natural drug has been used to treat joint swelling since 1500 BC, although, nowadays, it has been useful for the treatment of Gout disease (Echteld et al. 2014). Gout disease is considered

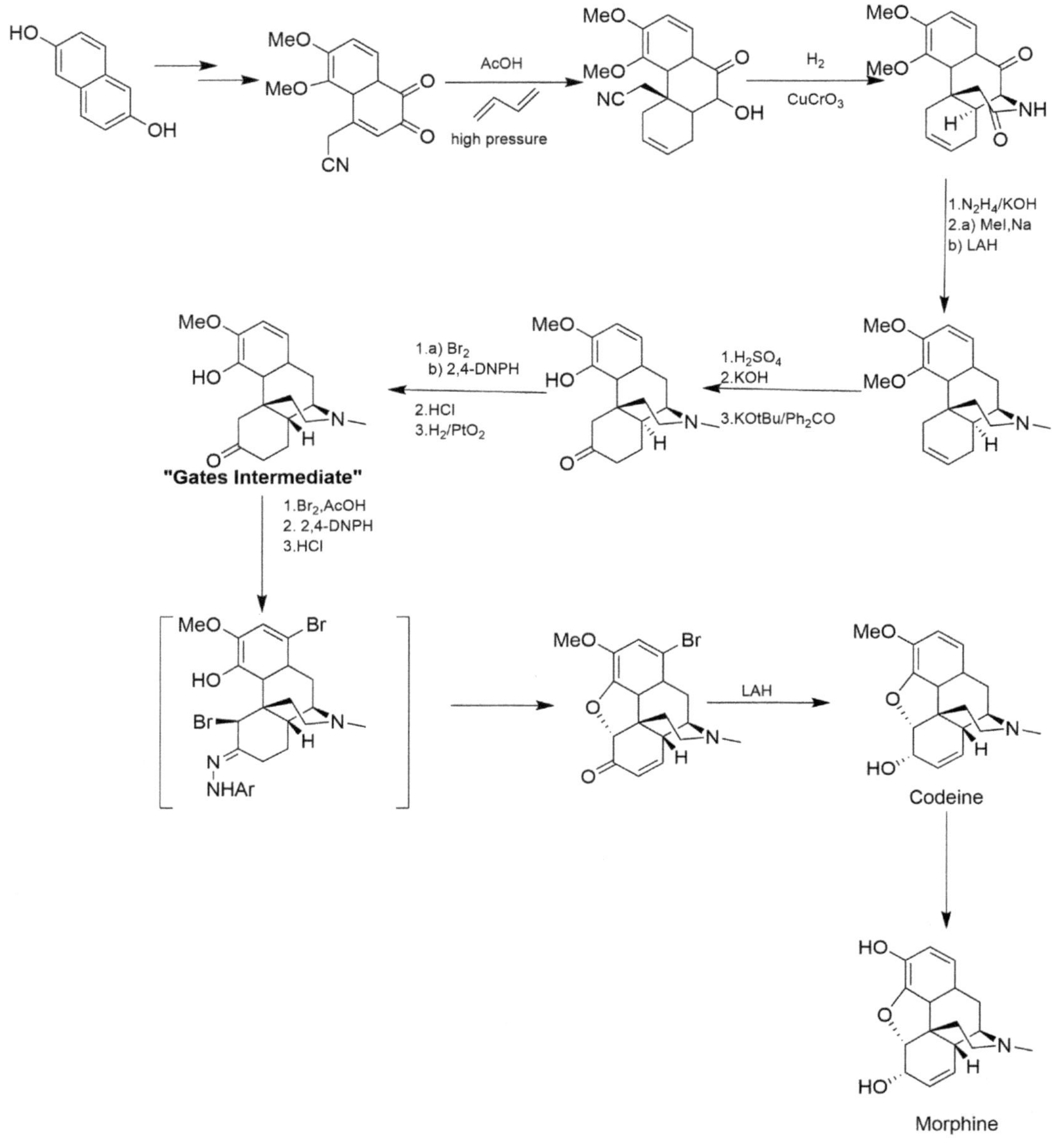

Scheme 8 Gates total synthesis of (−)-morphine

the type of inflammatory arthritis with a high level of pain. The low dose of colchicine proved to be beneficial for reducing the pain and other symptoms of Gout disease (Dalbeth et al. 2016).

Colchicine is a tricyclic alkaloid, having a unique structure with a trimethoxyphenyl ring (ring A), a seven-member ring (ring B) that contains acetamide at the seventh position of this ring, and finally a tropolonic ring (ring C) (Fig. 10) (Cerquaglia et al. 2005).

Different studies show that colchicine biosynthesis can occur in two different ways. Phenylalanine and tyrosine are two precursors involved in the biosynthesis of colchicine (Leete

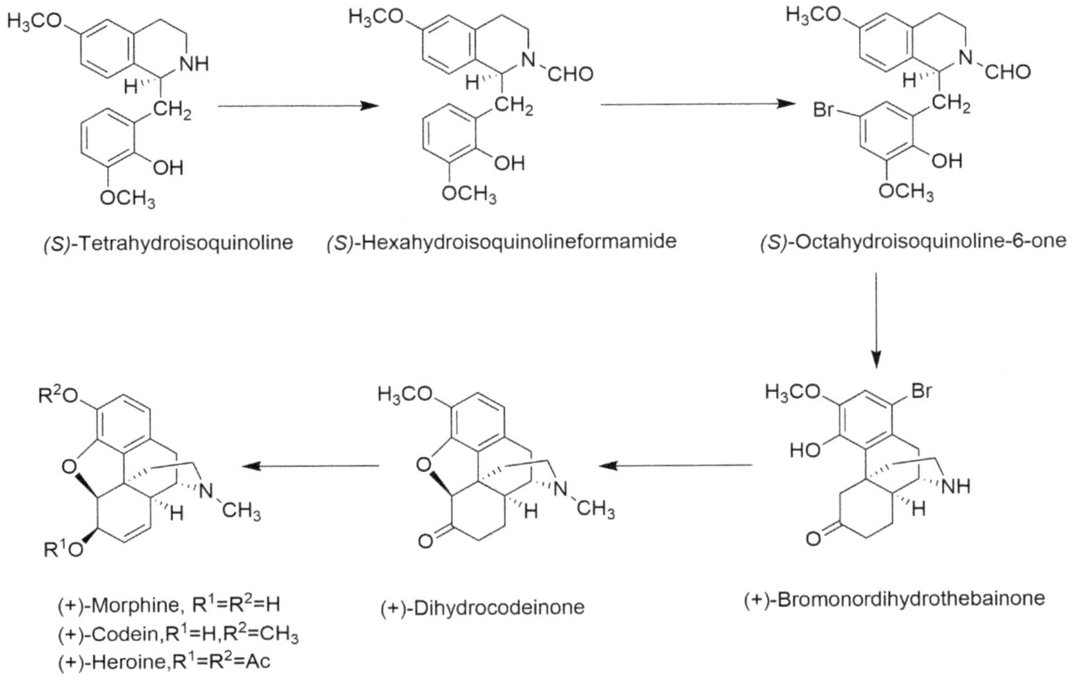

Scheme 9 Main compounds in the Rice total synthesis of (+)-morphine, (+)-codeine, and (+)-Heroine

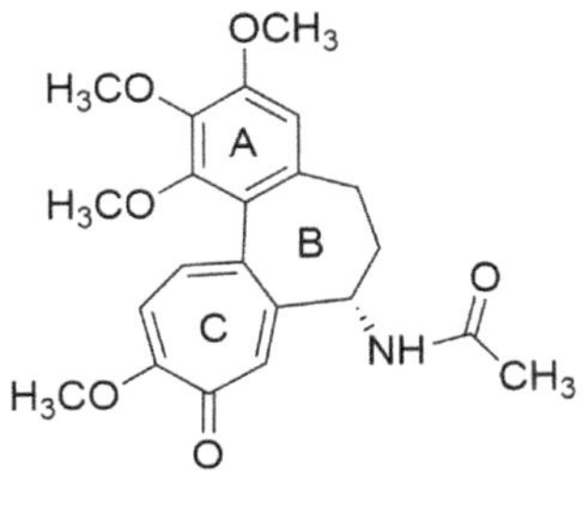

Fig. 10 Colchicine structure

1963). Moreover, there is another way showing that colchicine can be produced biosynthetically from an alkaloid compound, i.e., (S)-autumnaline. This biosynthesis starts with the coupling reaction that involves an intermediate named isoandrocymbine. Later, S-adenosylmethionine preforms O-methylation on the obtained molecule. Afterward, two oxidation steps took place and followed by the cleavage of the cyclopropane ring, which results in the formation of the tropolone ring contained by N-formyldemecolcine. Then, N-formyldemecolcine hydrolyzes and produces the molecule demecolcine, which further goes through oxidative demethylation results in deacetylcolchicine. The molecule of colchicine appears finally after the addition of acetyl-coenzyme A to deacetylcolchicine (Maier and Zenk 1997)).

Scheme 10 illustrates the biosynthetic formation of colchicine from (S)-autumnaline, alternatively via *para-para* coupling involving isoandrocymbine or via *ortho-para* with the isomer as an intermediate (Maier and Zenk 1997).

According to studies, colchicine has antimitotic properties to stop cell growth by inhibiting mitosis; as a result, it is useful for cancer treatment and antitumor activities. Colchicine binds to tubulin, which is a protein involves in the cytoskeleton structure and plenty of cellular functions such as cell division through mitosis. There are a lot of natural and synthetic compounds that inhibit or promote microtubules in mitosis. Colchicine is one of those compounds that bind at the interphase of α and β subunits of the tubulin and then blocks the cell division. The best stage for adding high concentrations of colchicine is metaphase, since, in this step of

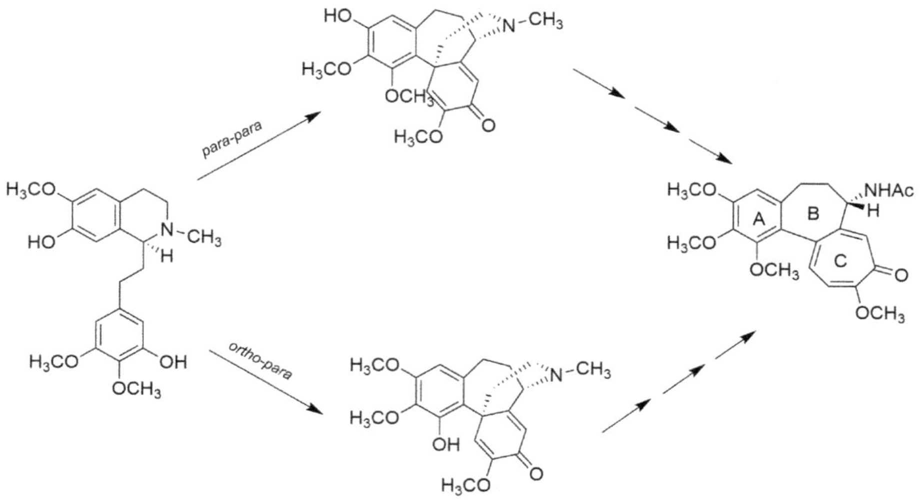

Scheme 10 Biosynthetic formation of (−)-colchicine from (S)-autumnaline

division, the action will be stopped immediately. In conclusion, this function causes the anticancer property of colchicine (Bhattacharyya et al. 2008).

Colchicine has two stereoisomers, (−)-colchicine, the natural enantiomer that has been isolated from *colchicum autumnale*, and its unnatural enantiomer is (+)-colchicine (Brossi 1985). This unnatural enantiomer was first synthesized from natural colchicine in 1957 by Corrodi and Hardegger (Shi et al. 1998). When they studied its antimitotic function in vitro, they found out that this unnatural enantiomer has 1% of the natural alkaloid potency.

Besides, when the researchers injected (+)-colchicine intramuscularly to mice, it was much less potent in comparison with the natural (−)-colchicine. Also, they comprise each other for their affinity in coupling deacetylcolchisine to bovine serum albumin, and finally, the results showed that lower potency of the natural enantiomer is the same here (Julian and Pikl 1935b).

8 Nicotine

Nicotine is a potent alkaloid that has been studied during history by physiologists and pharmacologists since it was isolated from tobacco in 1828 by Posselt and Reimann (Drobnik and Drobnik 2016). Nicotine is regarded as both a sedative and a stimulant with plenty of neurological effects (Clarke and Kumar 1983; Foulds et al. 1997). Nicotine has a wide range of pharmacological and psychodynamic impacts on the body. Nicotine stimulates releasing adrenaline and dopamine in the body (Artalejo et al. 1985). Moreover, it makes the pancreas produce less amount of insulin. Also, it has an increasing effect on heart-rate and heart-stroke volume (Gilbert et al. 1989).

(−)-Nicotine or 3-(1-methylpyrrolidin.2-yl) pyridine naturally isolated from tobacco; however, the (+)-nicotine, which consider a synthetic enantiomer, has been prepared during a four-step method (Fig. 11) (Chiribau et al. 2004).

The most critical step in this process is a hydroboration cycloalkylation reaction. The mentioned step starts with the hydroboration of the double bond, then creates a boron-nitrogen

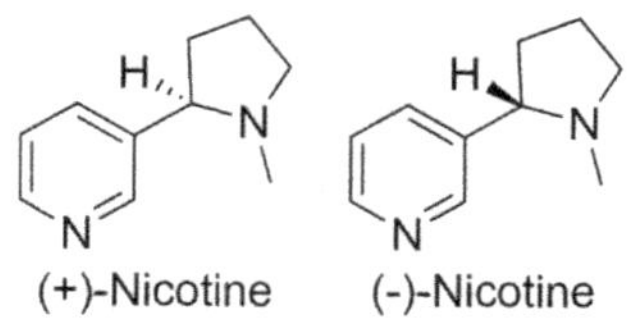

Fig. 11 Two isomers of nicotine

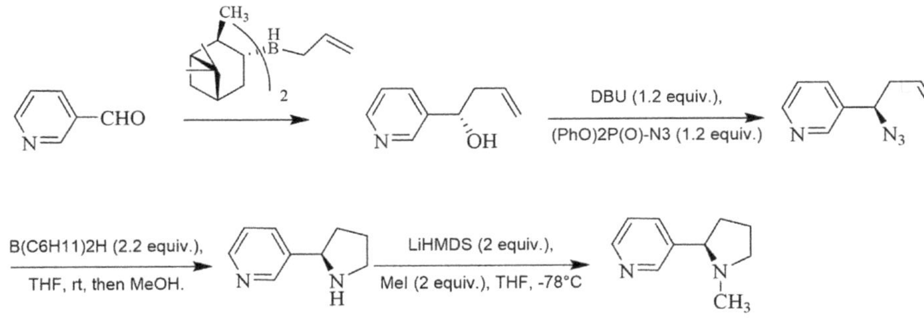

Scheme 11 Synthesis of (+)-nicotine

bond between the azide and the trialkylborane. Finally, ring closure takes place by hydroboration with concomitant loss of nitrogen (Scheme 11) (Chiribau et al. 2004; Girard et al. 2000).

The different pharmacological outcomes of (−)-nicotine and (+)-nicotine in the human body have been the subject of study between different groups. As a result, researchers found out that (−)-nicotine is 28 times more potent than (+)-nicotine in discriminative stimulus effects on squirrel monkeys (Takada et al. 1989). Furthermore, the results of other investigations also demonstrate that the effect of (−)-nicotine on schedule behavior in rats is 10–20 times more potent than (+)-nicotine (Zhang et al. 1994).

(−)-Nicotine biosynthesis in the plant starts with the stereospecific reduction of nicotinic acid by NADPH to produce 3,6-dihydronicotinic acid. In scheme 12, tritium is placed at C-6 of the nicotinic acid structure to highlight the stereochemistry of these reactions. The hydride anion from NADPH enters the pro-R position at C-6. The illustrated stereochemistry at C-3 is optional, but the reason behind this decision was the biological and chemical features of dienes.; mainly, the reduction of dienes results in the cis addition of the two hydrogens. Later, transferring of a proton from the carboxyl group to the nitrogen produces the zwitterion, which is a β iminium carboxylate. This compound easily decarboxylates, resulting in 1,2-dihydropyridine. The obtained compound functions as a nucleophile and attacks the 1- methyl-Δ1- L-pyrrolinium salt on its Re face to produce (2′S)-3,6-dihydronicotine. The reaction of 1,2-dihydropyridine takes place at its C-5 position instead of its C-3, and is consistent with the reaction of dienamines with electrophilic reagents. The final step of this biosynthesis is oxidation (with NADP$^{+)}$ that includes stereospecific elimination of the hydrogen at C-6 in the pro-S position (Scheme 12) (Leete 1992).

According to some studies, researchers comprised these isomers' effects on rat blood pressure and showed that the maximal results of the (+)-nicotine were considerably weak and only about 40% of the (−)-isomer. Along the same line, another study presented that the potency of (+)-nicotine effects on cat autonomic ganglions were about 0.2 of the (−)-nicotine (Laurent 1847).

One other study of the same nature demonstrated that (+)-nicotine has no impact on the secretion of noradrenaline from the adrenergic nerve terminals of the isolated rabbit pulmonary artery. On the other hand, (−)-nicotine produces sympathomimetic effects by releasing noradrenaline from those terminals (Laurent 1847).

9 Dextrorphan

Racemorphan is a racemic mixture of two stereoisomers, including levorphanol, which was first approved to be used in the United States in 1953 and dextrorphan that is a morphinane alkaloid; levorphanol is the synthetic isomer that was first described in Germany in 1946 (Fig. 12) (Fischer et al. 2010).

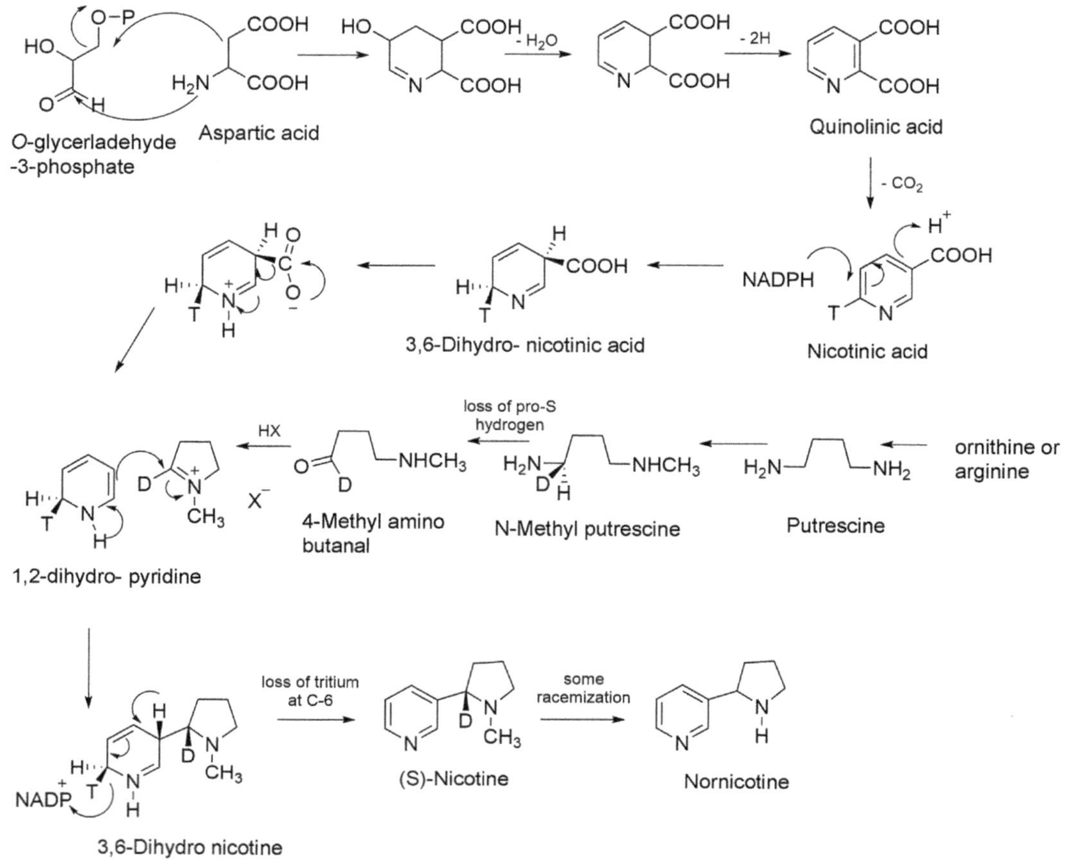

Scheme 12 Summary of enzymic reaction involved in biosynthesis of (+)-nicotine

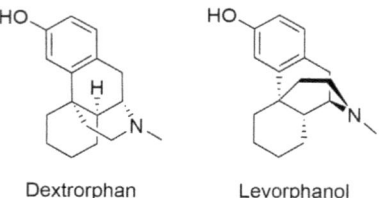

Fig. 12 Two isomers of racemorphan

Levorphanol or (−)-3-hydroxy-N-methyl morphinane's synthesis (Scheme 13) starts from the condensation of cyclohexanone with cyanoacetic acid (Knoevenagel reaction), along with this step simultaneous decarboxylation takes place, which results in 1-cyclohexenylacetonitrile. The nitrile group is reduced by hydrogen in the presence of Raney cobalt leading in 2-(1-cyclohexenyl) ethylamine. Later, 4-methoxyphenylacetyl chloride acylates the obtained amine to form 2-(1-cyclohexenyl) ethyl-4-methoxyphenylacetamide. Cyclization of the produced amide using phosphorous oxychloride creates 1-(4-methoxybenzyl)-3,4,5,6,7,8- hexahydroquinoline. The imine bond in the resulted compound is further hydrogenated in the presence of Raney nickel, producing 1-(4-methoxybenzyl)-1,2,3,4,5,6,7,8- octahydroquinoline, which is then methylated by formaldehyde in the presence of Raney nickel and results in 1- (4-methoxybenzyl)-2-methyl-1,2,3,4,5,6,7,8-octahydroquinolin. In

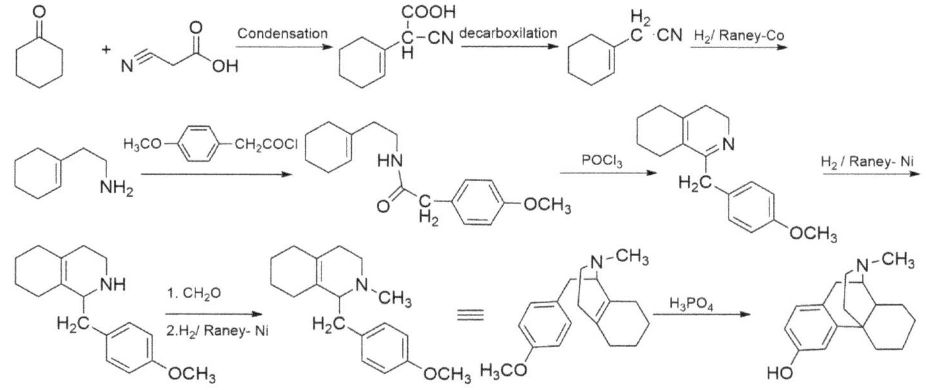

Scheme 13 Synthesis of levorphanol

the last step, the obtained compound undergoes cyclization and demethylation at the same time to produce 3-hydroxy-N-methylmorpinane or levorphanol (Casy and Parfitt 2013).

Levorphanol is using for treating pain, and also it is the agonist of different receptors as well as antagonists for the NMDA receptor (Gudin et al. 2016).

The natural isomer of racemorphan, dextrorphan, is produced by the O-demethylation of dextromethorphan by the CYP2D6 enzyme in the body (Scheme 14) (Fischer et al. 2010).

Both of these stereoisomers are NMDA antagonists, and according to the studies, this likelihood has been raised that NMDA antagonists can be effective based on their therapeutic functions in different clinical situations (Choi et al. 1987).

Church et al. in 1985 reported that both racemorphan enantiomers are NMDA antagonists, and the investigators showed that the natural dextrorphan is more potent and selective than levorphanol, which is the synthetic enantiomer in antagonizing NMDA (Choi et al. 1987).

Choi et al. in 1987 studied this function of dextrorphan and levorphanol on cortical cells that prepared from fetal mice, and the results showed that dextrorphan is the potent enantiomer (Choi et al. 1987).

NMDA receptor is a glutamate receptor that exists in the Central nervous system of mammalians and is an ion channel receptor, and when glycine and glutamate bind to this receptor, it will be activated. This receptor is too essential for memory and plasticity, and also it involves in different neurodegenerative diseases such as Parkinson, Huntington, and schizophrenia (Furukawa et al. 2005).

According to other investigations, the effect of dextrorphan and levorphanol compared with each other for their effects on HPA axis

Scheme 14 Biosynthesis of Dextrorphan

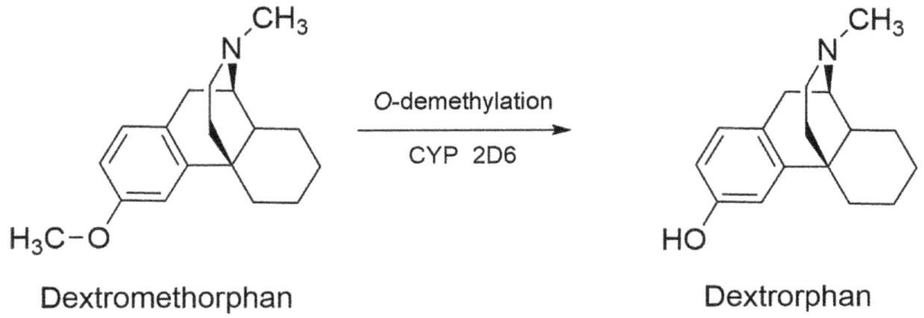

(Hypothalamus-pituitary -adrenal) and the result showed that dextrorphan stimulates this axis more than levorphanol (Pechnick and Poland 2004).

10 Glyceollin

Glyceollin is a novel group of pterocarpan isoflavonoids of phytoalexins, which isolated from soybean (*Glycine max*) (Tilghman et al. 2010).

Soybean is a type of legumes natively found in Eastern Asia, and during history, it has been used by the Chinese and other nations to treat varieties of cancer like breast and prostate cancers, and by the eighteenth century, it was introduced to Europe and America (Hymowitz and Newell 1981).

The name of the genus, glycine, comes from the Greek word glykós, which means sweet (Hymowitz and Newell 1981). This plant contains different nutrients, and it has been clinically proved that eating foods containing soybean may lower the risk of cancer in humans (Tse and Eslick 2016).

Burden and Bailey discovered that when soybean tissues face a microbial or physical stimulus like fungal infections, UV exposure, or sudden changes in temperature, they start producing a class of compounds called glyceollins (Bamji and Corbitt 2017).

Glyceollin biosynthesis in soy plants starts with phenylalanine, then followed by a cascade of enzymatic processes, which results in producing all three types of glyceollins (types I, II, and III) all of these types of glyceollin have

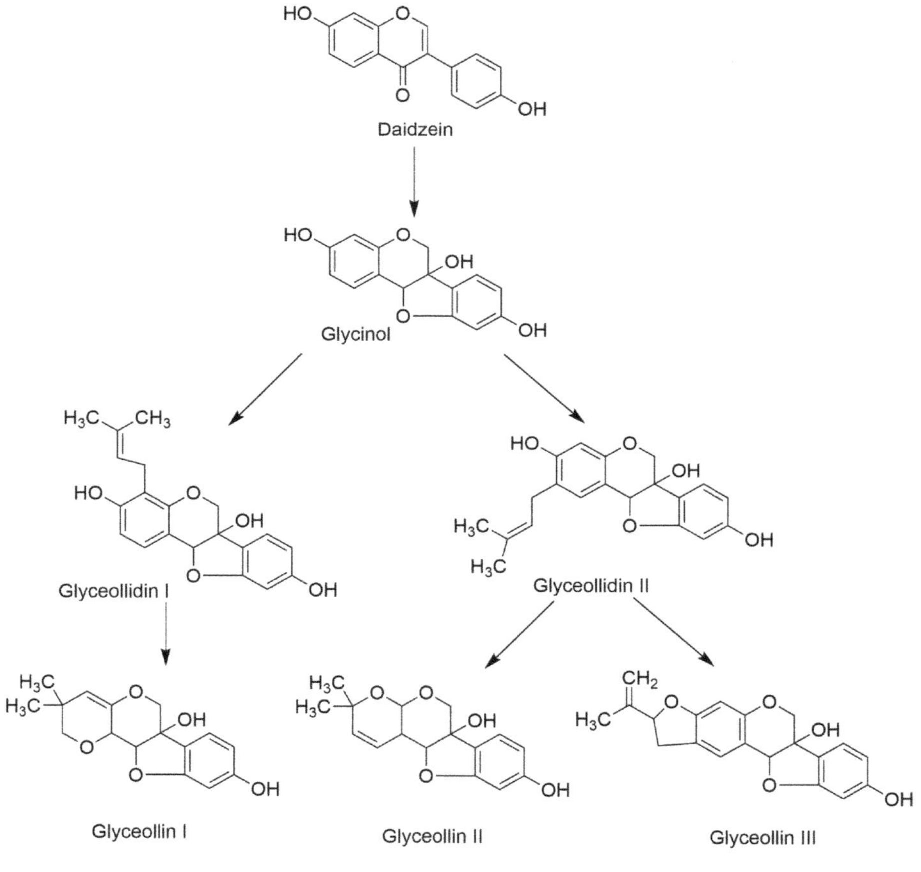

Scheme 15 Glyceollin biosynthesis in soy plants

similar core structure, and all of them are isolated from daidzein through different steps (Scheme 15) (Bamji and Corbitt 2017).

These compounds have several different effects like antimicrobial, antitumor, and antiestrogenic activities. Few studies investigated the antiestrogenic effects of the first type of glyceollin, which is considered as the most common type of this natural compound. In addition to Its Antiestrogenic effect, this compound is regarded as the selective estrogen receptor modulators, or SERMs (Bamji and Corbitt 2017; Riggs and Hartmann 2003). These Estrogen receptors (ER) can be found in both men's and women's tissues in two different types of α and β (Lecomte et al. 2017).

The comparison between three types of glyceollin indicates which type is the most potent and most prevalent type of glyceollin. Glyceollin I showed high antiestrogenic activity, and also it is useful for breast cancer treatment (Payton-Stewart et al. 2010).

Glyceollin I has two isomers, from which the (+)-glyceollin I was first synthesized by Khuspe and Erhardt (Fig. 13). Recent studies within which both isomers of glyceollin I (natural (−)-glyceollin I and unnatural (+)-glyceollin I) were compared for their antiestrogenic activity causing different biological activities, showed that (+)-glyceollin I increased estrogen response element (ERE) transcriptional activities of both estrogen receptors (ERs) without antiestrogenic activity. On the other hand, (−)-glyceollin I, decreased the activity of both receptors with potent antiestrogenic activity. The researchers used human cancer cells from the breast to study this property (Payton-Stewart et al. 2010).

11 Epibatidine

Epibatidine (exo-2-(6-chloro-3-pyridil)-7-azabicyclo- [2.2.1] heptane) is a natural potent alkaloid which was first discovered by John W. Daly in 1974. Daly found this compound in the skin of the Ecuadoran frog: scientifically known as *Epipedobates Anthonyi*. Searching for the best resource for this alkaloid, the highest amounts were detected in the population *of Epipedobates tricolor, E. tricolor*, that existed in grasslands, and cacao fields, in roadsides of mountains, plus drainage area in the pacific versant of the Andes in Ecuador. The lowest level of Epibatidine was discovered in highland populations of E.tricolor near the small rivers, while the grassland population that was found in banana fields did not contain any amount of Epibatidine (Salehi et al. 2018; Daly et al. 2005).

Daly and Charles collected the samples of about 300 frogs that their skins were the source of epibatidine, and according to their studies, injection of this new compound caused analgesic properties in mice (Daly et al. 2000).

The frog as mentioned earlier, was used by the Ecuador natives as a means of applying poison to their gadgets during their hunts. However, there is no evidence that confirms people used this specie for medical purposes up until 1993 that epibatidine was first synthesized. Afterward, this compound attracted considerable attention in scientific communities to investigate its properties as an active compound (Daly et al. 2000).

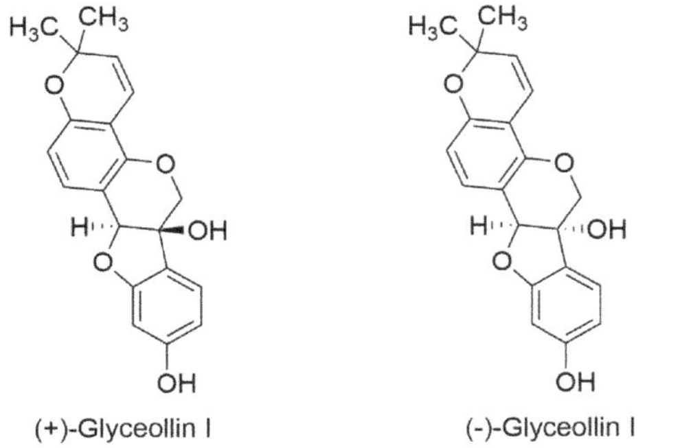

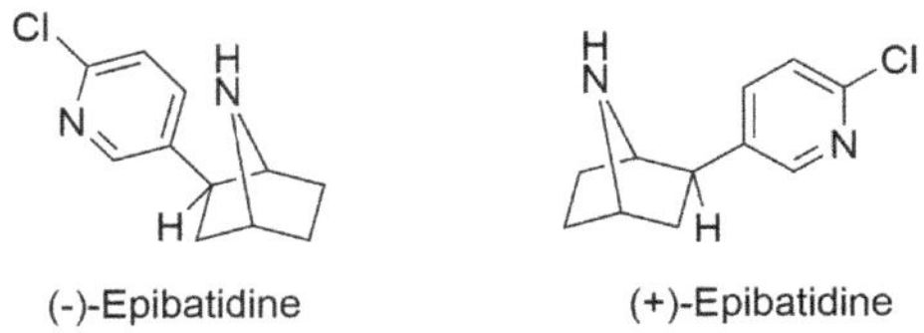

Fig. 13 Two isomers of glyceollin I

Fig. 14 Two isomers of epibatidine

Epibatidine is a pyridinederivatives that is structurally akin to nicotine (Fig. 14). Moreover, it has non-similar mechanisms of action, such as binding to nicotinic acetylcholine receptors and muscarinic acetylcholine receptors. Furthermore, because of the low affinity of epibatidine to the proteins of plasma, it is highly potent of metabolism (Qian et al. 1993).

Epibatidine also binds to the nicotinic receptors and causes analgesic properties (Salehi et al. 2018). Studies show that analgesic potency of epibatidine is 200 times greater than morphine and 120 times more potent than nicotine, making it a highly potent alkaloid. In contrary to morphine and nicotine, epibatidine is non-opioid and is considered as a lead compound in developing pain management medicines. It is also used as medical care for disorders whose pathogenesis involves nicotinic receptors (Carroll 2004).

This compound attracted much attention and has been synthesized in different ways. The enantioselective synthesis of (+) and (−)-epibatidine by Elias James Corey is presented in Scheme 16 (Corey et al. 2010).

(−)-Epibatidine is the unnatural enantiomer of (+)-epibatidine, and according to several studies, the natural enantiomer is two times more potent

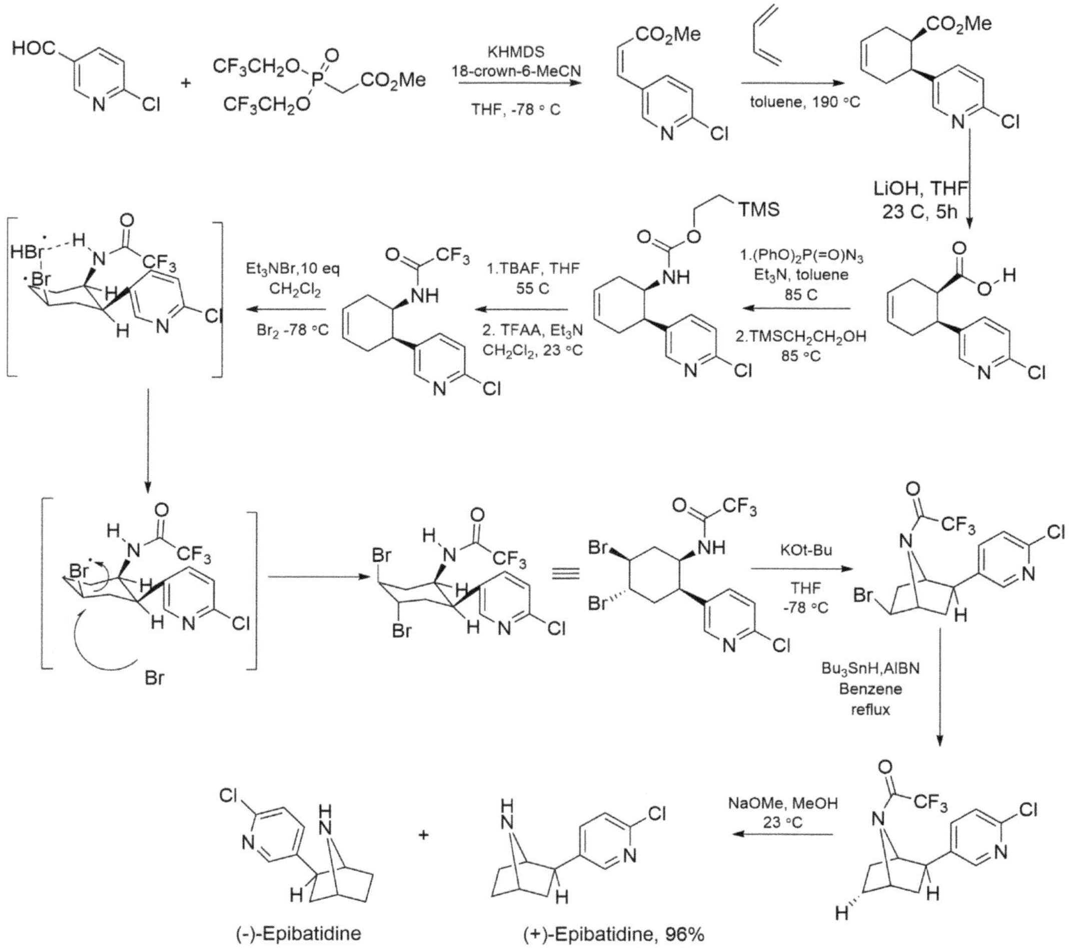

Scheme 16 Enantioselective synthesis of (+ and -)-epibatidine

than unnatural one for their analgesic potency. Also, both of the isomers are ganglionic-type nicotinic receptors and muscle-type central nicotinic receptors agonist, at the same time, another study shows that (−)-epibatidine is five times less potent than the natural one regarding this property (Damaj et al. 1994).

12 Conclusion

This chapter has been dedicated to depicting a number of natural compounds examples possessing pharmaceutical properties that are beneficial to humans' health whilst proving that their stereoisomers not only lack the pharmaceutical effects of these molecules but also are harmful to the man in some cases. Even though the biosynthesis pathways of such compounds are known to the experts today, nobody knows why the mother nature has synthesized and provided creatures with what they exactly yearn for. Nobody's ever found out how individual plants can take advantage of very primitive substances found in soil and air in the presence of water and sun to produce complicated compounds with chiral centers and precise stereochemistry to fend for themselves against their foes. No one knows how a monosexual flower is aware of scattering what sort of molecule or pigment in an effort to attract specific insects to perform the pollination duties.

The answers must be sought not in the realm of sciences but within the intelligence that lies behind the creation. Mighty God, with his inimitable graciousness, has assigned the nature the mission of providing the man with the pharmaceutical compounds he requires and inspiring him to make what he needs. However, the man disrespects nature by polluting the environment.

References

Akram M, Alam O, Usmanghani K, Naveed A, Asif M (2012) Colchicum autumnale: a review. J Med Plants Res 6:1489–1491

Artalejo A, Garcia A, Montiel C, Sanchez-Garcia P (1985) A dopaminergic receptor modulates catecholamine release from the cat adrenal gland. J Physiol 362(1):359–368

Astutik S, Pretzsch J, Ndzifon Kimengsi J (2019) Asian medicinal plants' production and utilization potentials: a review. Sustainability 11(19):5483

Atack JR, Yu QS, Soncrant TT, Brossi A, Rapoport SI (1989) Comparative inhibitory effects of various physostigmine analogs against acetyl- and butyryl-cholinesterases. J Pharmacol Exp Ther 249(1):194–202

Ault A (2008) Percy Julian, Robert Robinson, and the identity of eserethole. J Chem Educ 85(11):1524

Bamji SF, Corbitt C (2017) Glyceollins: soybean phytoalexins that exhibit a wide range of health-promoting effects. J Funct Foods 34:98–105

Bantle JP, Hunninghake DB, Frantz ID, Kuba K, Mariash CN, Oppenheimer JH (1984) Comparison of effectiveness of thyrotropin-suppressive doses of D- and L-Thyroxine in treatment of hypercholesterolemia. Am J Med 77(3):475–481

Bennett MR (1999) One hundred years of adrenaline: the discovery of autoreceptors. Clin Auton Res 9(3):145–159

Bentley RJ (1995) From optical activity in quartz to chiral drugs: molecular handedness in biology and medicine, vol 38. Johns Hopkins University Press, Baltimore

Bhattacharyya B, Panda D, Gupta S, Banerjee M (2008) Anti-mitotic activity of colchicine and the structural basis for its interaction with tubulin. Med Res Rev 28(1):155–183

Blakemore PR, White JD (2002) Morphine, the proteus of organic molecules. Chem Commun 11:1159–1168

Blaschko H (1939) The specific action of L-Dopa decarboxylase. J Physiol 96(50):50–51

Broadley KJ (2010) The vascular effects of trace amines and amphetamines. Pharmacol Ther 125(3):363–375

Brook K, Bennett J, Desai SP (2017) The chemical history of morphine: an 8000-year journey, from resin to de-novo synthesis. J Anesth Hist 3(2):50–55

Brossi A (1985) Further explorations of unnatural alkaloids. J Nat Prod 48(6):878–893

Brossi A, Pei X-F (1998) Biological activity of unnatural alkaloid enantiomers. In: The alkaloids: chemistry and biology, vol 50. Elsevier, pp 109–139

Brossi A, Schönenberger B, Clark OE, Ray R (1986) Inhibition of acetylcholinesterase from electric eel by (−)- and (+)-physostigmine and related compounds. FEBS Lett 201(2):190–192

Bryan LJ, O'Donnell SR (1984) Stereoselectivity of extraneuronal uptake of catecholamines in guinea-pig trachealis smooth muscle cells. Br J Pharmacol 82(3):757–762

Butler MS (2004) The role of natural product chemistry in drug discovery. J Nat Prod 67(12):2141–2153

Bylund DB (2016) Norepinephrine. In: Reference module in biomedical sciences. Elsevier

Canner PL, Berge KG, Wenger NK, Stamler J, Friedman L, Prineas RJ, Friedewald W (1986) Fifteen year mortality in coronary drug project patients: long-term benefit with niacin. J Am Coll Cardiol 8(6):1245–1255

Carroll FI (2004) Epibatidine structure-activity relationships. Bioorg Med Chem Lett 14(8):1889–1896

Casy AF, Parfitt RT (2013) Opioid analgesics: chemistry and receptors. Springer Science & Business Media

Cerquaglia C, Diaco M, Nucera G, La Regina M, Montalto M, Manna R (2005) Pharmacological and clinical basis of treatment of familial mediterranean fever (Fmf) with colchicine or analogues: an update. Curr Drug Targets Inflamm Allergy 4:117–124

Chiribau CB, Sandu C, Fraaije M, Schiltz E, Brandsch R (2004) A Novel Γ-N-methylaminobutyrate demethylating oxidase involved in catabolism of the tobacco alkaloid nicotine by arthrobacter nicotinovorans Pao1. Eur J Biochem 271(23–24):4677–4684

Choi DW, Peters S, Viseskul V (1987) Dextrorphan and levorphanol selectively block N-methyl-D-aspartate receptor-mediated neurotoxicity on cortical neurons. J Pharmacol Exp Ther 242(2):713–720

Christison R (1855) On the properties of the Ordeal-Bean of Old Calabar Western Africa. Monthly J Med (edinb) 20(3):193–204

Clarke P, Kumar R (1983) Characterization of the locomotor stimulant action of nicotine in tolerant rats. Br J Pharmacol 80(3):587–594

Coppi G, Vidi A, Bonardi G (1972) Quantitative determination of D-Dopa present in levodopa samples. J Pharm Sci 61(9):1460–1461

Corey EJ, Kürti L (2010) Examples of enantioselective synthesis. In: Corey EJ, Kürti L (eds) Enantioselective chemical synthesis. Academic Press, Boston, pp 179–326

Dabiri M, Salehi P, Kozehgary G, Heydari S, Heydari A, Esfandyari M (2008) Enantioselective addition of diethylzinc to aromatic aldehydes catalyzed by 14-hydroxylsubstituted morphinans. Tetrahedron Asymmetry 19(16):1970–1972

Dalbeth N, Merriman TR, Stamp LK (2016) Gout. The Lancet 388(10055):2039–2052

Dale FJ, Robinson B (1970) The synthesis and anti-acetylcholinesterase activities of (+)-physostigmine and (+)-physovenine. J Pharm Pharmacol 22(12):889–896

Daly JW, Garraffo MH, Spande TF, Decker MW, Sullivan JP, Williams M (2000) Alkaloids from frog skin: the discovery of epibatidine and the potential for developing novel non-opioid analgesics. Natural Product Reports 17(2):131–135

Daly J, Spande T, Garraffo H (2005) Alkaloids from amphibian skin: a tabulation of over eight-hundred compounds. J Nat Prod 68:1556–1575

Damaj M, Creasy K, Grove A, Rosecrans J, Martin B (1994) Pharmacological effects of epibatidine optical enantiomers. Brain Res 664(1–2):34–40

Davenport-Hines R (2003) The pursuit of oblivion: a global history of narcotics. WW Norton & Company

De Backer D, Biston P, Devriendt J, Madl C, Chochrad D, Aldecoa C, Brasseur A, Defrance P, Gottignies P, Vincent J-L (2010) Comparison of dopamine and norepinephrine in the treatment of shock. N Engl J Med 362(9):779–789

Dewick PM (2009) Alkaloids. In: Medicinal natural products: a biosynthetic approach. 3rd edn. Wiley & Sons, pp 311–420

Drobnik J, Drobnik E (2016) Timeline and bibliography of early isolations of plant metabolites (1770–1820) and their impact to pharmacy: a critical study. Fitoterapia 115:155–164

Dufault C, Tremblay G, Nowaczynski W, Genest J (1961) Influence of dextro-thyroxine and androsterone on blood clotting factors and serum cholesterol in patients with atherosclerosis. Can Med Assoc J 85(19):1025–1031

Eichelbaum MF, Testa B, Somogyi A (2003) Stereochemical aspects of drug action and disposition. In: Handbook of experimental pharmacology, vol 153, 1st edn. Springer, Berlin Heidelberg

Euler USv, (1946) A specific sympathomimetic ergone in adrenergic nerve fibres (sympathin) and its relations to adrenaline and nor-adrenaline. Acta Physiol Scand 12(1):73–97

Fischer J, Ganellin CR, Ganesan A, Proudfoot J (2010) Analogue-based drug discovery, 1st edn. Wiley-VCH

Flock EV, David C, Hallenbeck GA, Owen CA, JR. (1963) Metabolism of D-thyroxine. Endocrinology 73(6):764–774

Foulds J, Stapleton JA, Bell N, Swettenham J, Jarvis MJ, Russell MA (1997) Mood and physiological effects of subcutaneous nicotine in smokers and never-smokers. Drug Alcohol Depend 44(2–3):105–115

Funk C (1911) Lxv.—synthesis of Dl-3: 4-dihydroxyphenylalanine. J Chem Soc Trans 99:554–557

Furukawa H, Singh SK, Mancusso R, Gouaux E (2005) Subunit arrangement and function in Nmda receptors. Nature 438(7065):185–192

Gal J (2012) The discovery of stereoselectivity at biological receptors: Arnaldo Piutti and the taste of the Asparagine Enantiomers—history and analysis on the 125th anniversary. Chirality 24(12):959–976

Gates M, Tschudi G (1952) The syntheis of morphine. J Am Chem Soc 74(4):1109–1110

Gilbert DG, Robinson JH, Chamberlin CL, Spielberger CD (1989) Effects of smoking/nicotine on anxiety, heart rate, and lateralization of eeg during a stressful Movie. Psychophysiology 26(3):311–320

Girard S, Robins RJ, Villiéras J, Lebreton J (2000) A short and efficient synthesis of unnatural (R)-nicotine. Tetrahedron Lett 41(48):9245–9249

Gjedde A, Léger GC, Cumming P, Yasuhara Y, Evans AC, Guttman M, Kuwabara H (1993) Striatal L-Dopa decarboxylase activity in Parkinson's Disease in Vivo: implications for the regulation of dopamine synthesis. J Neurochem 61(4):1538–1541

Goldstein DS (2001) Adrenaline and noradrenaline. In: Encyclopedia of life science. Wiley

Gorman CA, Jiang NS, Ellefson RD, Elveback LR (1979) Comparative effectiveness of dextrothyroxine and levothyroxine in correcting hypothyroidism and lowering blood lipid levels in hypothyroid patients. J Clin Endocrinol Metab 49(1):1–7

Goto K, Shishido H (1933) Über Dihydro-Sinomenilan Und Seinen Abbau. Justus Liebigs Annalen Der Chemie 507(1):296–300

Goto K, Shishido H, Takubo K (1932) Über 1-Brom-Sinomenilsäure Und 1-Brom-Sinomenilon. Justus Liebigs Annalen Der Chemie 495(1):122–132

Gudin J, Fudin J, Nalamachu S (2016) Levorphanol use: past, present and future. Postgrad Med 128(1):46–53

Guggenheim M (1913) Dioxyphenylalanin, Eine Neue Aminosäure Aus Vicia Faba. Hoppe-Seyler' s Zeitschrift für Physiologische Chemie 88(4):276–284

Harington CR, Barger G (1927) Chemistry of thyroxine: constitution and synthesis of thyroxine. Biochem J 21(1):169

Hennessey JV (2015) Historical and current perspective in the use of thyroid extracts for the treatment of hypothyroidism. Endocrine Pract 21(10):1161–1170

Hiroshima Y, Miyamoto H, Nakamura F, Masukawa D, Yamamoto T, Muraoka H, Kamiya M, Yamashita N, Suzuki T, Matsuzaki S, Endo I, Goshima Y (2014) The protein ocular albinism 1 is the orphan Gpcr Gpr143 and mediates depressor and bradycardic responses to dopa in the nucleus tractus solitarii. Br J Pharmacol 171(2):403–414

Hodgson B (2001) In the Arms of Morpheus: The Tragic History of Laudanum, Morphine, and Patent Medicines. Firefly Books

Holtz P (1939) Dopadecarboxylase. Die Naturwissenschaften 27(43):724–725

Hymowitz T, Newell C (1981) Taxonomy of the genus glycine, domestication and uses of soybeans. Econ Bot 35(3):272–288

Hyneck M, Dent J, Hook JB (1990) Chirality: pharmacological action and drug development. In: Brown C (ed) Chirality in drug design and synthesis. Academic Press, pp 1–28

Iversen L (1997) The uptake of catechol amines at high perfusion concentrations in the rat isolated heart: a novel catechol amine uptake process. Br J Pharmacol 120(S1):267–282

Iversen LL, Jarrott B, Simmonds MA (1971) Differences in the uptake, storage and metabolism of (+)- and (−)-noradrenaline. Br J Pharmacol 43(4):845–855

Jacquet YF (1979) Morphine: exogenous endorphin? In: Endorphins in mental health research. Springer, pp 325–334

Jacquet Y, Klee W, Rice K, Iijima I, Minamikawa J (1977) Stereospecific and nonstereospecific effects of (+)- and (−)-morphine: evidence for a new class of receptors? Science 198(4319):842–845

Jobst J, Hesse O (1864) Ueber Die Bohne Von Calabar. Justus Liebigs Annalen Der Chemie 129(1):115–121

Julian PL, Pikl J (1935) Studies in the indole series. V. The complete synthesis of physostigmine (eserine). J Am Chem Soc 57 (4):755–757

Julian PL, Pikl J (1935) Studies in the Indole Series. Iii. On the Synthesis of Physostigmine. Journal of the American Chemical Society 57 (3):539–544.

Karoum F, Freed WJ, Chuang L-W, Cannon-Spoor E, Wyatt RJ, Costa E (1988) D-Dopa and L-Dopa similarly elevate brain dopamine and produce turning behavior in rats. Brain Res 440(1):190–194

Kendall EC (1915) The isolation in crystalline form of the compound containing iodin, which occurs in the thyroid: its chemical nature and physiologic activity. J Am Med Assoc LXIV 25:2042–2043

Kendall E (1964) Reminiscences on the isolation of thyroxine. In: Mayo clinic proceedings, p 548

Kendall EC (1983) The isolation in crystalline form of the compound containing iodin, which occurs in the thyroid: its chemical nature and physiologic activity. J Am Med Assoc 250(15):2045–2046

Kier LB (1969) The preferred conformation of noradrenaline and a consideration of the A-adrenergic receptor. J Pharm Pharmacol 21(2):93–96

King TL, Brucker MC (2010) Pharmacology for women's health. Jones & Bartlett Publishers

Kinghorn AD, Pan L, Fletcher JN, Chai H (2011) The relevance of higher plants in lead compound discovery programs. J Nat Prod 74(6):1539–1555

Kopp P, Solis-S JC (2009) Thyroid hormone synthesis. In: Wondisford FE, Radovick S (eds) Clinical management of thyroid disease. saunders, Philadelphia, W. B, pp 19–41

Krikler D, Lefevre D, Lewis B (1971) Dextrothyroxine with propranolol in treatment of hypercholesterolaemia. The Lancet 297(7706):934–936

LaPrairie JL, Schechter JC, Robinson BA, Brennan PA (2011) Perinatal risk factors in the development of aggression and violence. In: Huber R, Bannasch DL, Brennan P (eds) Advances in genetics, vol 75. Academic Press, pp 215–253.

Laurent A (1847) Sur La Composition Des Alcalis Organiques Et De Quelques Combinaisons Azotées. Annales De Chimie Et De Physique 19:359–377

Lecomte S, Chalmel F, Ferriere F, Percevault F, Plu N, Saligaut C, Surel C, Lelong M, Efstathiou T, Pakdel F (2017) Glyceollins trigger anti-proliferative effects through estradiol-dependent and independent pathways in breast cancer cells. Cell Commun Signal 15(1):26

Leete E (1963) The biosynthesis of the alkaloids of colchicum. Iii. The incorporation of phenylalanine-2-C14 into colchicine and demecolcine. J Am Chem Soc 85(22):3666–3669

Leete E (1992) The biosynthesis of nicotine and related alkaloids in intact plants, isolated plant parts, tissue cultures, and cell-free systems. In: Secondary-metabolite biosynthesis and metabolism. Springer, pp 121–139

Lindholm J, Laurberg P (2011) Hypothyroidism and thyroid substitution: historical aspects. J Thyroid Res 2011:809341

Lopez VM, Decatur CL, Stamer WD, Lynch RM, McKay BS (2008) L-Dopa Is an endogenous ligand for Oa1. PLoS Biol 6(9):236

Ludin H (2018) The L-Dopa story: translational neuroscience ante verbum. Clin Transl Neurosci 2:1876540–2514183

Machairiotis N, Vasilakaki S, Kouroutou P (2020) Natural products: potential lead compounds for the treatment of endometriosis. Eur J Obstet Gynecol Reprod Biol 245:7–12

Mackenzie HW (1892) A case of myxoedema treated with great benefit by feeding with fresh thyroid glands. BMJ 2(1661):940

Maier UH, Zenk MH (1997) Colchicine is formed by para-para phenol coupling from autumnaline. Tetrahedron Lett 38(42):7357–7360

Marcelli T, Hiemstra H (2010) Cinchona alkaloids in asymmetric organocatalysis. Synthesis 2010(08):1229–1279

Meissner W (1819) Ueber Ein Neues Pflanzenalkali (Alkaloid). Journal Für Chemie Und Physik 25:379–381

Midgley JEM, Larisch R, Dietrich JW, Hoermann R (2015) Variation in the biochemical response to L-Thyroxine therapy and relationship with peripheral thyroid hormone conversion efficiency. Endocrine Connect 4(4):196–205

Mohebbi M, Bararjanian M, Ebrahimi SN, Smieško M, Salehi P (2018a) Noscapine derivatives as new chiral catalysts in asymmetric synthesis: highly enantioselective addition of diethylzinc to aldehydes. Synthesis 50(09):1841–1848

Mohebbi M, Salehi P, Bararjanian M, Ebrahimi SN (2018b) Noscapine-derived B-amino alcohols as new organocatalysts for enantioselective addition of diethylzinc to aldehydes. J Iran Chem Soc 15(1):47–53

Morales F, Padilla S, Falconí F (2016) Medicinal plants used in traditional herbal medicine in the Province of Chimborazo, Ecuador. Afr J Tradit Complement Altern Med 14(1):10–15

Moses J, Siddiqui A, Silverman PB (1996) Sodium Benzoate differentially blocks circling induced by D- and L-Dopa in the Hemi-Parkinsonian Rat. Neurosci Lett 218(3):145–148

Murray GR (1891) Note on the treatment of myxoedema by hypodermic injections of an extract of the thyroid gland of a sheep. BMJ 2(1606):796

Musacchio JM (1975) Enzymes Involved in the Biosynthesis and Degradation of Catecholamines. In: Iversen LL, Iversen SD, Snyder SH (eds) Biochemistry of biogenic amines. Springer, US, Boston, MA, pp 1–35

Newman DJ, Cragg GM, Snader KM (2000) The influence of natural products upon drug discovery. Natural Product Rep 17(3):215–234

Nguyen L, He H, Pham-Huy C (2006) Chiral drugs: an overview. Int J Biomed Sci IJBS 2:85–100

Novak BH, Hudlicky T, Reed JW, Mulzer J, Trauner D (2000) Morphine synthesis and biosynthesis-an update. Curr Org Chem 4(3):343–362

Onoyovwe A, Hagel JM, Chen X, Khan MF, Schriemer DC, Facchini PJ (2013) Morphine biosynthesis in opium poppy involves two cell types: sieve elements and laticifers. Plant Cell 25(10):4110

Pallavicini M, Valoti E, Villa L, Lianza P (1994) Synthesis of (−)- and (+)-esermethole via chemical resolution of 1,3-dimethyl-3-(2-aminoethyl)-5-methoxyoxindole. Tetrahedron: Asymmetry 5(1):111–116

Payton-Stewart F, Khupse RS, Boué SM, Elliott S, Zimmermann MC, Skripnikova EV, Ashe H, Tilghman SL, Beckman BS, Cleveland TE, McLachlan JA, Bhatnagar D, Wiese TE, Erhardt P, Burow ME (2010) Glyceollin I enantiomers distinctly regulate er-mediated gene expression. Steroids 75(12):870–878

Pechnick RN, Poland RE (2004) Comparison of the effects of dextromethorphan, dextrorphan, and levorphanol on the hypothalamo-pituitary-adrenal axis. J Pharmacol Exp Ther 309(2):515–522

Pei X-F, Greig NH, Flippen-Anderson JL, Bi S, Brossi A (1994) Total synthesis of racemic and optically active compounds related to physostigmine and ring-C Heteroanalogues from 3-[2′-(dimethylamino)ethyl] 2,3-dihydro-5-methoxy-1,3-dimethyl-1h-indo L-2-Ol. Helv Chim Acta 77(5):1412–1422

Qian C, Li T, Shen T, Libertine-Garahan L, Eckman J, Biftu T, Ip S (1993) Epibatidine is a nicotinic analgesic. Eur J Pharmacol 250(3):R13–R14

Ravin JG, Higginbotham EJ (2009) The story of Percy Lavon Julian: against all odds. Arch Ophthalmol 127(5):690–692

Rentsch KM (2002) The importance of stereoselective determination of drugs in the clinical laboratory. J Biochem Biophys Methods 54(1):1–9

Riggs BL, Hartmann LC (2003) Selective estrogen-receptor modulators—mechanisms of action and application to clinical practice. N Engl J Med 348(7):618–629

Roth GM (1962) The role of the catecholamines in hypertension: a review. Am J Cardiol 9(5):724–730

Salehi P, Dabiri M, Kozehgary G, Baghbanzadeh M (2009) An efficient method for catalytic enantioselective addition of diethylzinc to aryl aldehydes by a C2-symmetric chiral imino alcohol. Tetrahedron Asymmetry 20(22):2609–2611

Salehi B, Sestito S, Rapposelli S, Peron G, Calina D, Sharifi-Rad M, Sharopov F, Martins N, Sharifi-Rad J (2018) Epibatidine: a promising natural alkaloid in health. Biomolecules 9(1)

Scheindlin S (2010) Episodes in the story of physostigmine. Mol Interventions 10(1):4

Serturner F (1805) Darstellung Der Reinen Mohnsaure (Opiumsaure) Nebst Einer Chemischen Untersuchung Des Opiums Mit Vorzuglicher Hinsicht Auf Einen Darin Neu Entdeckten Stoff Und Die Darin Gehorigen Bemerkungen. Trommsdorffs Journal Der Pharmazie 14(1):47–98

Sharma B (2014) Nature of chiral drugs and their occurrence in environment. J Xenobiotics 4(1):14–19

Shellabarger CJ, Brown JR (1959) The biosynthesis of thyroxine and 3:5:3′-triiodothyronine in larval and adult toads. J Endocrinol 18(1):98

Shi Q, Chen K, Morris-Natschke SL, Lee K-H (1998) Recent progress in the development of tubulin inhibitors as antimitotic antitumor agents. Curr Pharm Des 4(3):219–248

Slater S (2011) The discovery of thyroid replacement therapy. Part 3: a complete transformation. J R Society of Med 104 (3):100–106.

Sneader W (2005) Drug discovery: a history. Wiley & Sons

Song CE (2009) Cinchona alkaloids in synthesis and catalysis : ligands, immobilization and organocatalysis, pp 107–128.

Starr P (1960) Sodium dextrothyroxine and sodium levothyroxine: results of their use in an athyreotic patient with angina pectoris and hypercholesteremia. JAMA 173(17):1934–1935

Steinberg D (2007) The search for cholesterol-lowering drugs. In: Steinberg D (ed) The cholesterol wars. Academic Press, Oxford, pp 125–142

Stolz F (1904) Über Adrenalin Und Alkylaminoacetobrenzcatechin. Ber Dtsch Chem Ges 37(4149):416

Sumithira G, Sujatha M (2013) Drug chirality & its clinical significance evident, future for the development/separation of single enantiomer drug from racemates-the chiral switch. Int J Pharm Geniun Res 1(1):1–19

Takada K, Swedberg M, Goldberg S, Katz J (1989) Discriminative stimulus effects of intravenous L-nicotine and nicotine analogs or metabolites in squirrel monkeys. Psychopharmacology 99(2):208–212

Tilghman S, Boue S, Burow M (2010) Glyceollins, a novel class of antiestrogenic phytoalexins. Mol Cell Pharmacol 2:155–160

Toussaint C, Verniory A (1969) Serum renin levels and postnephrectomy blood pressure. N Engl J Med 281 (5):272–273

Trease GE (1964) Pharmacy in history, vol 784. Baillière, Tindall and Cox

Triggle DJ, Mitchell JM, Filler R (1998) The pharmacology of physostigmine. CNS Drug Rev 4(2):87–136

Tse G, Eslick GD (2016) Soy and isoflavone consumption and risk of gastrointestinal cancer: a systematic review and meta-analysis. Eur J Nutr 55(1):63–73

Vaidya B, Pearce SHS (2008) Management of hypothyroidism in adults. BMJ 337:a801

Van Echteld I, Wechalekar MD, Schlesinger N, Buchbinder R, Aletaha D (2014) Colchicine for Acute Gout. Cochrane Database of Systematic Reviews (8).

Vardanyan RS, Hruby VJ (2006) Adrenergic (sympathomimetic) drugs. In: Vardanyan RS, Hruby VJ (eds) Synthesis of essential drugs. Elsevier, Amsterdam, pp 143–159

Wardle EN, Schardt W, Uldall PR, Brown A, Jonfiah D, Moore A, Park R, Wood E (1974) Study of the lipid-lowering action of choloxin and nilevar in patients with chronic renal failure. Postgrad Med J 50 (590):737–740

Wassall RD, Teramoto N, Cunnane TC (2009) Noradrenaline. In: Squire LR (ed) Encyclopedia of neuroscience. Academic Press, Oxford, pp 1221–1230

Wilson BA, Willis MS (2010) Percy Lavon Julian: pioneer of medicinal chemistry synthesis. Lab Med 41(11):688–692

Wu M, Zhou X-J, Konno R, Wang Y (2006a) D-Dopa is unidirectionally converted to L-Dopa by D-amino acid oxidase, followed by dopa transaminase. Clin Exp Pharmacol Physiol 33:1042–1046

Wu M, Zhou X-J, Konno R, Wang Y-X (2006b) D-Dopa is unidirectionally converted to L-Dopa by D-Amino acid oxidase, followed by dopa transminase. Clin Exp Pharmacol Physiol 33(11):1042–1046

Zhang X, Gong Z-H, Nordberg A (1994) Effects of chronic treatment with (+)-and (−)-nicotine on nicotinic acetylcholine receptors and N-methyl-D-aspartate receptors in rat brain. Brain Res 644(1):32–39

Biodiversity and Drug Discovery Approach to Natural Medicine

Mansooreh Mazaheri and Ali Akbar Moosavi-Movahedi

Abstract

Biodiversity is the same as a variety of life on earth. It has direct and indirect benefits for supporting the needs of humans and is critical to ecosystem functions and human's health. Human health depends on ecosystem products. Biodiversity has a crucial role in life because if there are a higher number of plant species, animals' species, and other kinds of living organisms, it ensures natural sustainability for all life forms and healthy ecosystems. The sources of many drug products are living organisms include plants, animals and marine. Also, some of the metabolites of microbial organisms are used in drug products. So, they provide natural drugs against various diseases and have a high importance function in health care. By increasing the protection of biodiversity, global health will increase by discovering new biomedical relevant compounds. Proceeded with access to living organisms are the prerequisites of drug discovery from natural sources. These days, maintaining natural products is a difficult task versus a modernized pharmaceutical industry and modified biodiversity. So, the establishment of best practices for the sustainable production of natural products is essential. This chapter presents an overview of drug discovery and the significance of some natural products for biodiversity protection.

Keywords

Biodiversity · Drug discovery · Health · Natural sources

1 Introduction

According to WHO reports, primary health care of 80% of the world's residents depends on traditional medicines (Cragg et al. 1995). Plants, minerals, and other natural matter are biological sources of natural products (Grover et al. 2002). It reports that practically the origin of half of the new drugs presented from 1981 until 2006 were natural products. Natural products are the primary sources of many anti-cancer and anti-infective materials (McChesney et al. 2007). Many researchers highlighted the importance of ecosystems and natural substances to the drug discovery process (Kingston and Newman 2002, 2005; Butler 2008; Baker et al. 2007; Butler and

M. Mazaheri (✉)
Standard Research Institute, Research Center of Food Technology and Agricultural Products, Karaj, Iran
e-mail: m_mazaheri@standard.ac.ir

A. A. Moosavi-Movahedi
Institute of Biochemistry & Biophysics, University of Tehran, Tehran, Iran
e-mail: moosavi@ut.ac.ir

Newman 2008; Cragg et al. 2009). The interest in using natural products referred to more than thousands of years ago (Scartezzini and Speroni 2000).

Plants and animals have essential value in human health. In traditional medicines, plants and animals widely use. Also, in modern medicines, they are used as raw materials. In many countries, using herbal medicines is popular, and plant products have significant attention in the system of health care (Cragg and Newman 2005). In chemical studies, it reports that from more than 100 drugs derived from almost 90 plants that used in traditional medicine, near 75% of them were had been found by the isolation of the active materials from plants (Cragg et al. 1999). A large number of drugs have originated from active materials of plants or have been developed from microbial species, have clinically usage, especially for their anti-infective properties. Some famous drugs such as aspirin as a popular treatment for fever and pain, penicillin as an antibiotic, quinine for malaria, vincristine and paclitaxel as chemotherapeutic agents, artemisinin for malaria, morphine for pain control, etoposide for anti-tumor activity, and the digoxin for heart failure are some examples of natural products derived plants. Some examples of sources of these drugs shown in Table 1.

Other examples of high-value bioactive compounds as sources for natural drugs are microorganisms founded in soil, water and air. Stauros-porine, vancomycin, rapamycin, dinoflagellates (saxitoxin), myxobacteria (epothiloneandtubulysins), cyanobacteria (apratoxin A and jamaicamide), sponges (discodermolide), hemiasterlin. And dinoflagellates (saxitoxin) are some examples of them (Basso et al. 2005).

Over thousands years, we used natural products as medicine. They have a particular chemical diversity. It led to their biological activities, diversity, and differences in therapeutic properties. They will have a significant effect on drug discovery to create new medicines for treating human diseases (Galm and Shen 2007). Their incomparable novel mechanisms of action and chemical diversity of natural products assume a critical task in many medication advancements and research projects. These days, they have experienced an interesting expansion in their capability to communicate with various and distinctive biological targets, and some of them are popular as the most effective drugs for human health (Winter and Tang 2012; Li and Vederas 2009).

2 Medicinal Plants with Bioactive Compounds

Despite scientific progress in the medicine industry, plants have considered an essential part of traditional medicine in many countries and different cultures. Bioactive compounds regard as secondary metabolites in plants. They are critical organic compounds at healthy growth and development stages of plants. The products of biochemical in the plant cells are named side tracks and include lipids, carbohydrates, proteins and amino acids. The plant does not need them for daily functioning. These products are classified into different groups. These groups are flavonoids, glycosides, tannins, alkaloids, steroids and other compounds. Many kinds of research show their effects against many serious diseases. Some of these bioactive compounds have been mentioned in Table 2.

The essential specifications of herbal medicines are their multi-component systems that target multi-targets. In addition to Table 2, there are many plants such as turmeric, saffron, cinnamon, turmeric, ginger, and liqurice that have traditional medical applications. In many diseases, inflammation plays an important role (Paul et al. 2006). Several species of Curcuma grow in different areas ranging from sea level to very high elevations (Dymock and Hooper 1980). Many species of the genus Curcuma are there with enormous diversity and enormous medicinal usage. Biological activities, including anti-inflammatory and antioxidant properties of Curcuma, causes for using it as a remedy for cancer, diabetes and amyloidosis diseases. Also,

Table 1 Some natural products and their sources (Kingston 2011; Haynes 2001; Butler 2004; Okello et al. 2004; Sharma and Gupta 2015; Mofidi-Najjar 2019; Mazaheri et al. 2015a,b; Chin 2016; Rahban et al. 2020; Oh and Kwon TKJIi, 2009; Hashimoto et al. 1996; Min et al. 1999; Li et al. 2009)

Natural products	Sources	Usage
Morphine	Opium (*Papaversomniferum* L., Papaveraceae)	Treat severe pain
Quinine	*Cinchona officinalis* L. (Rubiaceae)	Anti-malarial drugs
Artemisinin	*Artemisia annua* L. (Asteraceae),	Anti-malarial drugs
Cardenolide digitoxin	Leaves of foxglove, *Digitalis purpurea* L. (Scrophulariaceae)	Anti-cancer activity
Antihypertensive indole alkaloid Drug reserpine	Indian snakeroot, *Rauuvolfiaserpentina* (L.) Benth. ex Kurz (Apocynaceae)	High blood pressure
Physostigmine	African plant Physostigmavenenosum Balf. f. (Fabaceae)	Memory enhancement
Paclitaxel	Yew *Taxusbrevifolia* Nutt. (Taxaceae)	Chemotherapeutic drug in breast and lung cancer treatment
Paclitaxel	Yew *Taxuscanadensis*	Chemotherapeutic drug in breast and lung cancer treatment
Curcumin	Tumeric and curry spice	Antioxidant, anti-inflammation, inhibition of protein fibrillation In many diseases such as Alzheimer's disease
Artemisinin	Qinghao (*Artemisia annua*)	Fevers
Galantamine (Reminyl)	*Galanthus* spp. and *Narcissus* spp.	Alzheimer's disease
Vinblastine	*Catharanthusroseus*	Anti-cancer agents
Plasmepsin II	*Albiziaadinocephala*	Antimalarial
Camellia sinensis L. extract	Tea	Anti-cholinesterase and β-secretase activities for Alzheimer's disease
Metformin	*Galegaofficinalis*	Diabetes treatment
Vincristine	*Vincarosea*	Cancer treatment
Taxol	*Taxusbrevifolia*	Cancer treatment
Acetyldigoxin	*Digitalis lanata*	Cardiovascular disease treatment
Digitoxin	*Digitalis purpurea*	Cardiovascular disease treatment
Berberine	*Berberis vulgaris*	Bacillary dysentery treatment
Atropine	*Atropa belladonna*	Neurological disorders treatment
Withanolides	*Withania somnifera*	Inhibitor of angiogenesis, inflammation and oxidative stress
3-o-gallate	*Tea polyphenolics*	Lipase inhibitor activity
Theasinensin	*Tea (thea sinensis)*	Antiviral activity
Gallic acid	*Terminalia Chebula*	HIV integrase inhibitory activity
Colchicine	*Saffron*	Anti-inflammation

Table 2 Examples of bioactive compounds isolated from natural sources (Sharma et al. 2006; Gupta et al. 2009; Harinantenaina et al. 2006; Sugihara et al. 2000; Hemalatha et al. 2010; Langcake and Pryce 1976; Dixon and Ferreira 2002; Rao 1993; Noble 1990; Prabhakar 2013; Aggarwal et al. 2011; Bucolo et al. 2012; Zang et al. 2015; Häkkinen et al. 1999; Skates et al. 2018; Egert et al. 2009; Johnson et al. 2012; Stan et al. 2008; Park et al. 2012; Singh et al. 2019; Basnet and Skalko-Basnet 2011)

Name of plant	Active compound
For diabetes	
Morus (Berries)	Resveratrol
Aloe vera, kiwi fruits, lettuce and banana	Emodin
Lemon	Eriodictyol
Grapefruit, tea cruciferous vegetables and some edible berries	Kaempferol
Eugenia jambolana	α-Hydroxysuccinamic acid
Glycine max	Guanidium derivative
Cassia auriculata	Coumarin derivative
Momorandica charantia	Charantin
Gymnemasylvestris	Gymnemic acid
For cardiovascular diseases	
Morus (Colored berries)	Anthocyanins
Broccoli, rocket, cauliflower, Brussels sprouts, cabbage	Isothiocyanates
Eugenia jambolana	α-Hydroxysuccinamic acid
Glycine max	Genistein
Terminaliaarjuna	Arjunolic acid
Vitisvinifera Resveratrol	
Tea	Quercetin
Green and black tea	Catechins
For cancer	
Tumeric and curry spice	Curcumin
Ginseng or winter cherry	Withaferin A
Glycine max	Genistein
Taxusbrevifolia	Taxol
Vincarosea	Vincristine
Magnolia officianalis	Magnolol
Grapes (Vitis vinifera), blueberries, mulberries, soy, pomegranate and peanuts	Resveratrol

antibiotic and antiviral activities of Curcuma report in many studies (Mazaheri et al. 2015b; Zhang et al. 2018; Barzegar and Moosavi-Movahedi 2011).

Curcumin is a product obtained from turmeric. Using it in food as a spice, in medical and in the textile industry and other various areas, has a long history in Asia (Maheshwari et al. 2006). Curcuma longa is cultivated considerably in the countries with a tropical climate. India and China are producers of turmeric. In traditional Indian medicine, turmeric has been recommended for use as a medicine. In Iran, turmeric use in many Persian dishes as a starter ingredient. Some studies suggest that curcumin acts as a neuroprotective factor in neurodegenerative disorders because of antioxidant and inhibitory effects of it against fibrillation of proteins. Also, the cytotoxicity of fibrils inhibits by curcumin (Mazaheri et al. 2015b).

Most species of Curcuma are very much sensitive to low temperatures, grown as an unirrigated crop in dense rainfall area, and as an irrigated crop in a moderate rainfall area. The crop requires well-drained, loose and friable loamy or alluvial soil. Heavy black or clayey soils are unsuitable as rhizome development is not proper. It cannot stand in waterlogged or alkaline soil (Pemba and Bhutia 2017).

Saffron is another sustainable crop that contains many novel bioactive molecules. Saffron is cultivated extensively in Iran, Spain, India, Greece, Azerbaijan, Morocco, and Italy. It is used as a spice to flavor foods and as a medical herb. Cancer preventive of saffron and anti-tumor effects of it has been reported in many related types of research. The practical material of saffron is carotenoids include crocin, crocetin and dimethylcrocetin. Their anticarcinogenic action of these compounds has been recognized because of the effect on H1 structure and H1-DNA interaction (Ashrafi et al. 2005).

Because of its particular biological action, physiological and agronomic specifications, saffron can be used to overcome adverse conditions and can offer good production in sustainable agriculture. The loss of the land surface of saffron cultivation in some areas of the world is led to a corresponding genetic erosion of this crop.

Ginger is another plant used as a food additive. Also, ginger has many uses to cure different human diseases, such as diabetes, cancer, fever, frequent colds, motion sickness, gastrointestinal complications, and rheumatic disorders (Kundu et al. 2009). It has been distributed across the tropics of Asia, Africa, America and Australia.

The root of *Glycyrrhiza glabra* is named liquorice which a sweet flavor can be extracted from it. It is a legume native to Western Asia and southern Europe and used in traditional medicine. Liquorice extract is rich in bioactivities compounds. Expectorant activities include antioxidant properties, antiviral, antibacterial, antidiabetic, anti-cancer, anti-inflammatory, antithrombic, antifungal, antimalarial, antiulcer, estrogenic, immunostimulant, and antiallergenic activities report in the literature. The biological compounds have classified into flavonoids, coumarins, triterpenoids, stilbenoids, and others (Hao et al. 2015).

The extract from the liquorice root has shown antimicrobial activity. In many third world populations, countries don't have suitable health care systems. In these countries, the essential sources of disease are viruses and bacteria. Due to the biological activity of liqurice root extract, liqorice-related medicines are useful for curing the many common diseases of people in undeveloped countries (Wang et al. 2015).

Aloe Vera is another plant that is found in tropical climates and has medicinal benefits. It is used in the cosmetic industry too. It is known safe and named as the wonder plant because of the numerous properties it possesses. It can help treat inflammatory conditions because of potent anti-inflammatory properties. In Homoeopathic and Allopathic, Aloe Vera uses widely too.

The plant leaves contain numerous bioactive compounds. The potential of this plant for the treatment of burns such as sunburns and minor cuts and are reported for skin cancer (Sahu et al. 2013). Aloe Vera provides 20 of the 22 required amino acids and 7 of the 8 essential ones as basic building blocks of proteins in the body and muscle tissues. It has anthraquinones that provide Aloe-emodin, Aloetic acid, alovin, anthracine with Analgesic, antibacterial properties. The enzymes of anthranol, barbaloin, chrysophanic acid, smodin, ethereal oil, ester of cinnamonic acid, isobarbaloin and resistannol of Aloe Vera have antifungal and antiviral activity but toxic at high concentrations. Auxins and gibberellins are hormones in them with wound healing and anti-inflammatory activities. Minerals, salicyclic acid, saponins, steroids and vitamins are other Chemical compositions of it (Rodriguez et al. (2005)).

In addition to plants mentioned above, other plants such as grape, pomegranate, tea, garlic, parsley, mint, jujube, hollyhock, milk thistle, rosemary, calendula, basil, nuts, pineapple, and many other plants and their products such as olive oil have wonderful medical properties. For example, anti-cancer and antioxidant activities of walnut peptides prove their possible therapeutic advantage in inhibition of cancer (Jahanbani et al. (2016)).

Remarkable percent of the medicines endorsed in the world originate from plants, so they are considered as crucial and vital by the WHO (Rates 2001).

Most of the medicinal plants have been in existence since ancient times, and the use of them for the treatment of diseases is not a new issue. In China, Egypt and India, and in the new world' tropics, there are many evidences about using medical plants (Cragg et al. 1995).

These drugs are just valuable if they are made accessible to the individuals who need them and are utilized appropriately. Unfortunately, changes in ecosystem services affect tropical forests, and they have been reduced (Cao and Kingston 2009).

The decreasing rate of tropical rainforests led to a catastrophic loss of biodiversity. Suppling of medicinal plants is possible through obtaining and gathering from wild populations and cultivation. Numerous communities living in the world depend on plant products collected from ecosystems. They use plants for food and curing diseases and also for cultural purposes, so preserving the biodiversity of plants is fundamental for the insurance of life.

3 Microbial Sources as Natural Drugs

These days, developing in microbial molecular biology and microbial genetic studies have been led to the improvement of the metagenomics pathway. It has happened by the expression of biosynthetic pathways in a direct manner gained from environmental DNA and cloned in a suitable host. Industrial and academic groups have been focused on filamentous organisms such as bacteria and fungi from the actinomycetales. Each day scientists discover new species and even major taxa of fungi and actinomycetes. The number of medicines derived from secondary metabolites of these organisms is too much, and

its effects proved for numerous therapeutic areas, including infectious diseases and also for oncology, immunosuppression, atherosclerosis (Bérdy 2005).

Some examples of microbial natural products in pharmaceutical industry are *Penicillium* spp., *Aspergillus* spp., *Acremonium* spp., *Emericellopsis* spp., *Amycolatopsis lactamdurans, Streptomyces Clavuligerus, Streptomyces Cattleya, Saccharopolyspora erythraea, Streptomyces Orientalis, Streptomyces Griseus, Micromonospora Purpurea, Streptomyces* spp., *Dactosporangium* spp., *Actinomadura Brunnea* with antibiotic activities, *Streptomyces Nodosus* and *Glarealozoyensis* with antifungal activities, *Streptomyces Tsukubaensis, Streptomyces Hygroscopicus, Penicillium* spp., *Verticicladiella Abientina, Septoria Nodorum* with Immunosuppressant activities and *Streptomyces Verticillus, Streptomyces Peucetius,* and other *Streptomyces* spp. with antitumor properties. Also *Aspergillus Terreus, Monascusruber* and *Penicillium* spp. can help to Cholesterol lowering (Bérdy 2005).

Microorganism, also show biogeographic models of diversity. Many species of microorganisms are specialized ecologically and restricted geographically too. For example, in the tropics area, many of the fungi can be found, but they never observe in temperate regions (Polishook et al. 2001). So, changing the attention to the isolation efforts for different kinds of natural substrata geographic sources and ecological niches make it conceivable to discover substantially other fungal species.

4 Marine Sources as Natural Medicine

Ocean occupies almost 70% of planet earth's surface. More than 8500 marine natural products found, and It has been proven that the vast numbers of these compounds have excellent pharmacological activity (Bhakuni and Rawat 2006). Many types of research about the marine environment, especially in invertebrates, have been shown that sponges, bryozoans, tunicates, and mollusks are good sources of bioactive compounds. Marine natural products have important roles in biomedical research and the medical industry. As indicated by the US National Cancer Institute about natural compounds as medicine, the most applicable bioactive compounds, particularly antitumor compounds such as discodermolide, bryostatin, aplidine, kahalalide F and ecteinascidin 743 and several others obtained from the marine environment have passed clinical trials (Simmons et al. 2005).

Ziconotide (Prialt®, Elan Corporation) is another example of natural products with unique bioactive specifications. It is a peptide that previously obtained from a tropical cone snail and is useful in pain treatment. Another example is Plitidepsin (Aplidin®, Pharma Ma), adepsi peptide was isolated from the Mediterranean *Tunicat Aplidium Albicans* (Rinehart and Lithgow-Berelloni 1991; Urdiales et al. 1996). This drug is used for curing some of the cancers, such as small cell and non-small cell lung, melanoma, acute lymphoblastic leukemia, and non-Hodgkin lymphoma (Mayer et al. 2010). Another anticancer drug is ecteinascidin 743 (ET743; Yondelis™). Its source is ascidian *Ecteinascidia Turbinate* (Cuevas and Francesch 2009).

Spisulosine is another example that displayed particular significant property against tumor cells contrasted with ordinary cells. This compound has been separated from the marine clam *Spisula Polynyma* (Alvarez-Miranda et al. 2003).

Also, *Cryptophycin* is another marine source drug for recognizing cancerous tumor cells. This drug can be used for tumors in the colon, pancreas, ovarian, brain, prostate, breast and lung cancers. Also, it is destroying agents for the multi-drug resistant (MDR) tumor cells (Folmer et al. 2010).

Antitumor activities and anti-microbial properties of the brown algae, antibacterial and antifungal activities of green, brown and red algae are other examples of medicine activities of marine sources (Trimurtulu et al. 1994).

Spongouridine and spongothymidine from the Caribbean sponge *Cryptothecacrypta* are biologically active compounds from marine sponge sources with antiviral activity. Cytosine arabinoside (Ara-C) and (Ara-A) are prepared by the synthesis of structural analogues of them and used as an anti-cancer and antiviral drug, respectively (Faulkner 1988).

Another example is the bryologs class of synthetic derivative from bryostatin one that is used in biomedicine as anti-cancer agents, anti-AIDS/HIV and anti-Alzheimer's. Their origin comes back to marine bryozoan *Bugula neritina*, and the bacterial symbiont of *B. neritina* (Mayer et al. 2010; Faulkner 1988; McConnell et al. 1994). Halichondrin B has been separated from a kind of marine sponge, is another biomedicine for the treatment of breast carcinoma (Chin et al. 2006).

Posidonia oceanica (L.) Delile is a compound originated from grass-like marine plants of the Mediterranean Sea. It is used in traditional medicine for diabetes and hypertension. In recent researches, it has shown that *Posidonia oceanica* leaves extract has wonderful bioactivities, including the ability to weaken human cancer cell migration (Vasarri et al. 2020).

Marine bacteria are also invaluable resources as bioactive compounds. The isolated strain of Micrococcus genus from the Persian Gulf is another example of marine sources that revealed a valuable source to access worth medicinal ingredients when cultured under optimized conditions (Karbalaei-Heidari et al. 2020).

5 Animal Sources as Natural Medicine

Other sources of some drugs are animals. For example, the skin of an Ecuadorian poison frog has some compounds, such as Epibatidine. It is recorded that this compound is more potent than morphine (Aicher et al. 1992). Another example is Teprotide, a bioactive product extracted from Brazilian viper. Researchers used it for the development of anti-hypertensive medicines such as cilazapril and captopril (Spande et al. 1992).

Many animal products and ingredients derived from animal products are used as food and medicine too. Milk, honey, egg, and insulin made from animal's tissue, are some examples of animal products for medical use. Camel is a particular animal with magical natural products. Its products have unique medicinal properties as well as a source of nutrients. Therapeutic actions have been described in many studies. Its bioactive agents have novel immunological activities against pathogenic agents and pathological conditions (Ali et al. 2019).

Inhibitor action of camel urine for cancer, lactoferrin's properties in the treatment of hepatitis C virus, and antidiabetics agent function of camel milk were reported (Ali et al. 2019). In the future, researches may also prove camel product's role in the treatment of other diseases.

In many regions of Asia and Africa, camel milk as a traditional drug is used for the treatment of various diseases such as diabetes, asthma and edema. Bioactive compounds of camel's milk can cure diabetes. Also, it is reported that camel milk doesn't have β-LG, so it doesn't have allergic effects (Khalesi et al. 2017). After consuming and digestion of the camel milk, the produced peptides start to act as natural antioxidants and angiotensin-converting enzyme inhibitors (Salami et al. 2011).

Honey has been known as a traditional medicine for centuries (Chowdhury 1999). Scientists also introduce honey as a new effective medicine for many kinds of diseases. For the treatment of heal wounds, gastric ulcers, hepatic and gastrointestinal disorders, the effects of honey have been proved.

The most remarkable of its property is the antibacterial activity that mentions in numerous studies (Emsen 2007; Medhi and Kaman 2008).

In some in vitro studies, it shows that honey has the ability to exhibiting useful cardiovascular protection because of its power to inhibit reactive oxygen species-induced low-density lipoprotein (LDL) oxidation. Also, honey has the capability of inhibiting the development of tumors in bladder cancer (Ahmad et al. 2009; Hegazi and Abd El-Hady 2009; Swellam et al. 2003).

According to FAO experts report, insect pollination is an essential effective factor in the production of many plants such as fruits, nuts, seeds, and berries, and bees have an important role among the pollinating insects. Flowering plants life depends on bees and many bioactive plants originate from the flowering plants (Bradbear 2009).

6 Natural Products and Biodiversity Conservation

Governments, agricultural authorities, and farmers will require to pay attention to the relationship between biodiversity and natural resources such as gardening and marine products, because of their continuing and growing demand. Overhunting, overfishing, and the results of destructive events in the environment and other factors can have an adverse effect on biodiversity.

For developing drug discovery, it needs to promote molecular diversity, and it relates to biodiversity preservation. Different species include wild species, have been the source of drug discovery from old-time, and using them is critical for the treatment of many diseases, and they are essential in human health (Cragg et al. 1995). So, plants and marine organisms are considered as the base of development of clinical drugs and drug discovery, and there is a need to build the concept of sustainability into research models of resources and knowledge about synthetic and natural drug discovery programs.

Also, chemical reagents are non-renewable, and using them depletes future resources. According to some estimates, our planet is losing at least one valuable drug every two years (Scannell and Bosley 2016). Biodiversity loss is irreversible and leads to a loss of knowledge about the traditional medicines and medicinal use of natural products and their derivatives and then the loss of molecular diversity by destroying ecosystems.

So, biodiversity conservation is very critical to future drug discovery, and the sustainable development of all types of natural products will relate to considering biodiversity conservation.

7 Effects of Biodiversity Loss on Human Health

Human health depends on the well-functioning ecosystems and also the health of native species. Each disturbance of natural habitat alters the biodiversity of both structurally and functionally. It leads to a reduction of abundances of some organisms while causing an increase in the population of others. Biodiversity losses can threaten the survival of humans by the effect on biomedical research.

Any change in flora and faunal given region leads to modification of interaction among the biota which in turn lead to altered relationship between the organisms and their physical environments and it leads to diseases transmission in the given region (Scannell and Bosley 2016; Pimm et al. 1995; Walter et al. 2005; Anantha Kumar Duraiappah 2005; Stearns 2009). Biodiversity loss has been reported by different estimates; It is estimated is that only about 7 million square kilometers of humid tropical forests (50%) remain in all of the world, and we lose 1 million square kilometers of rainforest every 5–10 years (Stearns 2009). It is predicted that a reduction and demolition rate of species extinctions and existing large blocks of tropical forest are considerable (Pimm and Raven 2000). Some regions in the world have been known as "Biodiversity Hotspots" because of the highest risk for biodiversity loss Jenkins 2003). Biodiversity loss can have adverse effects on human life. Loss of biodiversity changes ecosystem functions and has an impact on producing goods and services for human health.

Disrupting ecosystem function causes biodiversity loss, and it results in less ability of an ecosystem to respond to a disturbance, more susceptible to demolition and perturbation, and it is a danger to human demand. Many natural disasters in continents, especially in North America and Asia, are some examples of them (Myers et al. 2000). Biodiversity loss decreases the supplies of raw materials, and it affects the expansion of drug discovery. Reducing the medical models because of the reduction of raw materials is another result of losing biodiversity that has limitation effect on the discovery of potential medicines and can spread human diseases (Pushpangadan 2005).

Taxol and the Pacific yew are examples of the effects of biodiversity loss. It was found that Pacific yew contains the compound Taxol, that can kill cancer tumors. Its function differs from the mechanisms of chemotherapeutic agents. Taxol can inhibit the disassembly of the mitotic spindle and prevents cell division. Synthesis of several Taxol-like compounds that are even more effective than the natural compound designed after the discovery of the complex molecule Taxol and its mechanism of action (E C (2002). It is proven that Taxol is one of the most important drugs that can be used for the treatment of breast cancer and ovarian cancer (Nicolaou et al. 1996).

There are some peptide compounds in the venom of cone snails in tropical coral reefs with vast diversity that is used as natural medicine. Some of these peptide compounds can act as a barrier in neuromuscular systems for a wide variety of ion channels and receptors (Abraham and Lewis 2018). So, these peptide compounds have an essential role in neurophysiological research.

In developing countries, plants are used for the treatment of disorders and have remarkable particular medicinal value. In these countries, exploring biodiversity for drug discovery is considerable for indigenous people. By gathering medicinal plants or purchasing lands by large pharmaceutical companies in order to make new drugs, these drugs and the plants themselves can become unavailable or unaffordable to the local people who cannot afford the products from these sources, and it can effect on their health because biodiversity can provide benefits to protect against many diseases and also plays a crucial role in human nutrition.

8 Conclusion

Plants and animals are rich sources of medicinal compounds, and using them to cure illness has history ancient. So, their existence is significant for health care. The utility of these products and their biological function in discovering compounds is considerable and supported by a history of successes.

The interconnections between natural medicine and environment conservation are related to the health interest derived from the existence of a full complement of species and genetic diversity. The need for biodiversity conservation is urgent because it provides our fundamental needs for goods and services such as food, health and has a remarkable role in research and development of medicines for developing countries with large populations. Natural products may be efficient therapeutics in comparison with synthetic drugs, so special attention to preserve them is required.

It seems that the establishment of best practices for sustainable production of natural products and also collection, storage, and preparation with special attention are essential. The construction of regulatory measures is another task for the involvement of stakeholders; that maybe there is a need for specific training them about conservation of the natural resource. Other suggestions are raising awareness of the long-term economic benefits of protecting biodiversity over the short-term benefits of habitat destruction and unsustainable resource extraction. Promotion of the best practices in sustainable commercialization of natural products and considering the balance of ecosystems and population are necessary to help biodiversity conservation.

Also, authorities, organizations, other partners must help each other to identify regional biodiversity conservation priorities and preserve the remaining hotspots of biodiversity through a collaborative approach as well as the activities include the collation and generation of knowledge about the regions and also the species in the areas. Potentials preserving biodiversity shall be in self-interest of all people. Also promoted awareness and information exchange about agricultural biodiversity and rural sustainability are essential for maintaining biodiversity. By sufficient funding, acceptable and in time support from decision-makers, governments worldwide, NGOs and industries, the formation of international partnerships and assistance programs, we can preserve our planet's worthy and incredible biodiversity.

References

Abraham N, Lewis RJ (2018) Neuronal nicotinic acetylcholine receptor modulators from cone snails. Marine Drugs 16(6):208

Aggarwal BB, Prasad S, Reuter S, Kannappan R, Yadav V, Park B, Hye Kim J, Gupta S, Phromnoi K, Sundaram C, Prasad S, Chaturvedi M, Sung B (2011) Identification of novel anti-inflammatory agents from ayurvedic medicine for prevention of chronic diseases: "reverse pharmacology" and "bedside to bench" approach. Current. Drug Targets 12(11):1595–1653

Ahmad A, Khan RA, Mesaik MA (2009) Anti inflammatory effect of natural honey on bovine thrombin-induced oxidative burst in phagocytes. Phytotherapy Res PTR 23(6):801–808

Aicher TD, Buszek KR, Fang FG, Forsyth CJ, Jung SH, Kishi Y, Matelich MC, Scola PM, Spero DM, Yoon SK (1992) Total synthesis of Halichondrin B and Norhalichondrin B. J Am Chem Soc 114(8):3162–3164

Ali A, Baby B, Vijayan R (2019) From desert to medicine: a review of camel genomics and therapeutic products. Front Genet 10(17)

Alvarez-Miranda MR-GA, Ptero G, Lacal JC (2003) Characterization of the mechanism of action of Es-285, a novel antitumor drug from mactomeris polynyma. Clin Cancer Res 9:17

Anantha Kumar Duraiappah SN (2005) Ecosystems and human well-being: biodiversity synthesis, Millennium ecosystem assessment

Ashrafi M, Bathaie SZ, Taghikhani M, Moosavi-Movahedi AA (2005) The effect of carotenoids obtained from Saffron on histone H1 structure and H1-DNA interaction. Int J Biol Macromol 36(4):246–252

Baker DD, Chu M, Oza U, Rajgarhia V (2007) The value of natural products to future pharmaceutical discovery. Natural Prod Rep 24(6):1225–1244

Barzegar A, Moosavi-Movahedi AA (2011) Intracellular Ros protection efficiency and free radical-scavenging activity of curcumin. PLoS ONE 6(10):e26012

Basnet P, Skalko-Basnet NJM (2011) Curcumin: an anti-inflammatory molecule from a curry spice on the path to cancer treatment. Molecules 16(6):4567–4598

Basso LA, Silva LHPd, Fett-Neto AG, Azevedo Junior WFd, Moreira ÍdS, Palma MS, Calixto JB, Astolfi Filho S, Santos RRd, Soares MBP, Santos DS (2005) The use of biodiversity as source of new chemical entities against defined molecular targets for treatment of malaria, tuberculosis, and T-cell mediated diseases: a review. Memórias Do Instituto Oswaldo Cruz 100:475–506

Bérdy J (2005) Bioactive microbial metabolites. J Antibiotics 58(1):1–26

Bhakuni DS, Rawat DS (2006) Bioactive marine natural products. Springer Science & Business Media

Bradbear N (2009) Bees and their role in forest livelihoods: a guide to the services provided by bees and the sustainable harvesting, processing and marketing of their products, vol 19. Food and Agriculture Organization of the United Nations (FAO)

Bucolo C, Leggio GM, Drago F, Salomone S (2012) Eriodictyol prevents early retinal and plasma abnormalities in streptozotocin-induced diabetic rats. Biochem Pharmacol 84(1):88–92

Butler MS (2004) The role of natural product Chemistry in drug discovery. J Nat Prod 67(12):2141–2153

Butler MS (2008) Natural products to drugs: natural product-derived compounds in clinical trials. Natural Prod Rep 25(3):475–516

Butler MS, Newman DJ (2008) Mother nature's gifts to diseases of man: the impact of natural products on anti-infective, anticholestemics and anticancer drug discovery. Progress in Drug Research Fortschritte Der Arzneimittelforschung Progres Des Recherches Pharmaceutiques 65(1):3–44

Cao S, Kingston DGI (2009) Biodiversity conservation and drug discovery: can they be combined? The Suriname and Madagascar experiences. Pharma Biol 47(8):809–823

Chin KY (2016) The spice for joint inflammation: anti-inflammatory role of curcumin in treating osteoarthritis. Drug Design Devel Therapy 10:3029–3042

Chin YW, Balunas MJ, Chai HB, Kinghorn AD (2006) Drug discovery from natural sources. AAPS J 8(2):E239-253

Chowdhury MM (1999) Honey: is it worth rubbing it in? J R Soc Med 92(12):663

Cragg GM, Newman DJ (2005) Biodiversity: a continuing source of novel drug leads. Pure Appl Chem 77(1):7–24

Cragg GM, Boyd MR, Grever MR, Schepartz SA (1995) Pharmaceutical prospecting and the potential for pharmaceutical crops. Natural product drug discovery and development at the United States National Cancer Institute. Annals Missouri Botanical Garden 82(1):47–53

Cragg GM, Boyd MR, Khanna R, Kneller R, Mays TD, Mazan KD, Newman DJ, Sausville EA (1999) International collaboration in drug discovery and development: the NCI experience. Pure Appl Chem 71(9):1619–1633

Cragg GM, Grothaus PG, Newman DJ (2009) Impact of natural products on developing new anti-cancer agents. Chem Rev 109(7):3012–3043

Cuevas C, Francesch A (2009) Development of Yondelis (Trabectedin, Et-743). A semisynthetic process solves the supply problem. Natural Prod Rep 26(3):322–337

de Rodriguez DJ, Hernandez-Castillo D, Rodriguez-Garcia R, Angulo-Sanchez JL (2005) Antifungal activity in vitro of aloe vera pulp and liquid fraction against plant pathogenic fungi. Ind Crops Prod 21(1):81–87

Dixon RA, Ferreira D (2002) Genistein. Phytochemistry 60(3):205–211

Dymock W, Hooper D (1980) Pharmacographia Indica, Reprinted by Singh B, Singh MP. Dehradun, India

EC (2002) Biodiversity, its importance to human health center for health and the global environment. Center for Health and the Global Environment, Harvard Medical School

Egert S, Bosy-Westphal A, Seiberl J, Kürbitz C, Settler U, Plachta-Danielzik S, Wagner AE, Frank J, Schrezenmeir J, Rimbach G, Wolffram S, Müller MJ (2009) Quercetin reduces systolic blood pressure and plasma oxidised low-density lipoprotein concentrations in overweight subjects with a high-cardiovascular disease risk phenotype: a double-blinded, placebo-controlled cross-over study. Br J Nutr 102(7):1065–1074

Emsen IM (2007) A different and safe method of split thickness skin graft fixation: medical honey application. Burns J Int Soc Burn Injuries 33(6):782–787

Faulkner DJ (1988) Marine natural products. Natural Prod Rep 5(6):613–663

Folmer F, Jaspars M, Dicato M, Diederich M (2010) Photosynthetic marine organisms as a source of anticancer compounds. Phytochem Rev 9(4):557–579

Galm U, Shen B (2007) Natural product drug discovery: the times have never been better. Chem Biol 14(10):1098–1104

Grover JK, Yadav S, Vats V (2002) Medicinal plants of India with anti-diabetic potential. J Ethnopharmacol 81(1):81–100

Gupta S, Sharma SB, Prabhu KM (2009) Ameliorative effect of Cassia Auriculata L. leaf extract on glycemic control and atherogenic lipid status in alloxan-induced diabetic rabbits. Indian J Exp Biol 47(12):974–980

Häkkinen SH, Kärenlampi SO, Heinonen IM, Mykkänen HM, Törrönen AR (1999) Content of the flavonols quercetin, myricetin, and kaempferol in 25 edible berries. J Agric Food Chem 47(6):2274–2279

Hao D-C, Gu XJ, Xiao P-G (2015) Medicinal plants: Chemistry, Biology and Omics, pp 1–681

Harinantenaina L, Tanaka M, Takaoka S, Oda M, Mogami O, Uchida M, Asakawa Y (2006) Momordica Charantia constituents and antidiabetic screening of the isolated major compounds. Chem Pharm Bull 54(7):1017–1021

Hashimoto F, Kashiwada Y, Nonaka G-i, Nishioka I, Nohara T, Cosentino LM, Lee KH (1996) Evaluation of tea polyphenols as anti-HIV agents. Bioorg Med Chem Lett 6(6):695–700

Haynes RK (2001) Artemisinin and Derivatives: the future for malaria treatment? Curr Opin Infect Diseases 14(6):719–726

Hegazi AG, Abd El-Hady FK (2009) Influence of honey on the suppression of human low density lipoprotein (Ldl) peroxidation (in Vitro). Evidence Complement Alternative Med 6(1):113–121

Hemalatha T, Pulavendran S, Balachandran C, Manohar BM, Puvanakrishnan R (2010) Arjunolic acid: a novel phytomedicine with multifunctional therapeutic applications. Indian J Exp Biol 48(3):238–247

Jahanbani R, Ghaffari SM, Salami M, Vahdati K, Sepehri H, Sarvestani NN, Sheibani N, Moosavi-Movahedi AA (2016) Antioxidant and anticancer activities of walnut (Juglans Regia L.) protein hydrolysates using different proteases. Plant Foods Human Nutrition 71(4):402–409

Jenkins M (2003) Prospects for biodiversity. Science (new York, NY) 302:1175–1177

Johnson R, Bryant S, Huntley AL (2012) Green tea and green tea catechin extracts: an overview of the clinical evidence. Maturitas 73(4):280–287

Karbalaei-Heidari HR, Partovifar M, Memarpoor-Yazdi M (2020) Evaluation of the bioactive potential of secondary metabolites produced by a new marine micrococcus species isolated from the Persian Gulf. Avicenna J Med Biotechnol 12(1):61–65

Khalesi M, Salami M, Moslehishad M, Winterburn J, Moosavi-Movahedi AA (2017) Biomolecular content of camel milk: a traditional superfood towards future healthcare industry. Trends Food Sci Technol 62:49–58

Kingston DGI (2011) Modern natural products drug discovery and its relevance to biodiversity conservation. J Nat Prod 74(3):496–511

Kingston DGI, Newman DJ (2002) Mother nature's combinatorial libraries; their influence on the synthesis of drugs. Curr Opin Drug Discov Devel 5(2):304–316

Kingston DGI, Newman DJ (2005) The search for novel drug leads for predominately antitumor therapies by utilizing mother nature's pharmacophoric libraries. Curr Opin Drug Discov Devel 8(2):207–227

Kundu JK, Na HK, Surh YJ (2009) Ginger-derived phenolic substances with cancer preventive and therapeutic potential. Forum Nutrition 61:182–192

Langcake P, Pryce RJ (1976) The production of resveratrol by Vitis Vinifera and other members of the Vitaceae as a response to infection or injury. Physiol Plant Pathol 9(1):77–86

Li JW, Vederas JC (2009) Drug discovery and natural products: end of an era or an endless frontier? Science (new York, NY) 325(5937):161–165

Li JJ, Lee SH, Kim DK, Jin R, Jung D-S, Kwak S-J, Kim SH, Han SH, Lee JE, Moon SJ, Ryu DR, Yoo TH, Han DS, Kang SW (2009) Colchicine attenuates inflammatory cell infiltration and extracellular matrix accumulation in diabetic nephropathy. Am J Physiol Ren Physiol 297(1):F200–F209

Maheshwari RK, Singh AK, Gaddipati J, Srimal RC (2006) Multiple biological activities of curcumin: a short review. Life Sci 78(18):2081–2087

Mayer AM, Glaser KB, Cuevas C, Jacobs RS, Kem W, Little RD, McIntosh JM, Newman DJ, Potts BC, Shuster DE (2010) The Odyssey of marine pharmaceuticals: a current pipeline perspective. Trends Pharmacol Sci 31(6):255–265

Mazaheri M, Moosavi-Movahedi AA, Saboury AA, Rezaei MH, Shourian M, Farhadi M, Sheibani N (2015a) Curcumin mitigates the fibrillation of human serum albumin and diminishes the formation of reactive oxygen species. Protein Pept Lett 22(4):348–353

Mazaheri M, Moosavi-Movahedi AA, Saboury AA, Khodagholi F, Shaerzadeh F, Sheibani N (2015b) Curcumin protects B-lactoglobulin fibril formation and fibril-induced neurotoxicity in Pc12 cells. PLoS ONE 10(7):e0133206

McChesney JD, Venkataraman SK, Henri JT (2007) Plant natural products: back to the future or into extinction? Phytochemistry 68(14):2015–2022

McConnell OJ, Longley RE, Koehn FE (1994) The discovery of marine natural products with therapeutic potential. Biotechnology (reading, Mass) 26:109–174

Medhi B, Puri A, Upadhyay S, Kaman L (2008) Topical application of honey in the treatment of wound healing: a metaanalysis. JK Sci 10(4):166–169

Min BS, Jung HJ, Lee JS, Kim YH, Bok SH, Ma CM, Nakamura N, Hattori M, Bae K (1999) Inhibitory effect of triterpenes from crataegus pinatifida on HIV-I protease. Planta Med 65(04):374–375

Mofidi-Najjar F (2019) Remediation effect of curcumin as a natural antioxidant on damaged glycated catalase. In: Paper presented at the 12th EBSA, 10th ICBP-IUPAP biophysics congress, Madrid, Spain, 24–26 July 2019

Myers N, Mittermeier RA, Mittermeier CG, da Fonseca GA, Kent J (2000) Biodiversity hotspots for conservation priorities. Nature 403(6772):853–858

Nicolaou KC, Guy RK, Potier P (1996) Taxoids: new weapons against cancer. Sci Am 274(6):94–98

Noble RL (1990) the discovery of the vinca alkaloids—chemotherapeutic agents against cancer. Biochem Cell Biol 68(12):1344–1351

Oh JH, Kwon TK (2009) Withaferin A inhibits tumor necrosis factor-alpha-induced expression of cell adhesion molecules by inactivation of Akt and NF-kappaB in human pulmonary epithelial cells. Int Immunopharmacol. 9(5):614–619

Okello EJ, Savelev SU, Perry EK (2004) In vitro anti-beta-secretase and dual anti-cholinesterase activities of Camellia Sinensis L. (Tea) relevant to treatment of dementia. Phytotherapy Res PTR 18 (8):624–627

Park JB, Lee MS, Cha EY, Lee JS, Sul JY, Song IS, Kim JY (2012) Magnolol-induced apoptosis in Hct-

116 colon cancer cells is associated with the amp-activated protein kinase signaling pathway. Biol Pharm Bulletin 35(9):1614–1620

Paul AT, Gohil VM, Bhutani KK (2006) Modulating Tnf-alpha signaling with natural products. Drug Discov Today 11(15–16):725–732

Pemba H, Bhutia AS (2017) Promising curcuma species suitable for hill regions towards maintaining biodiversity. J Pharmacogn Phytochem 6(6):726–731

Pimm S, Raven P (2000) Biodiversity-extinction by numbers. Nature 403:843–845

Pimm SL, Russell GJ, Gittleman JL, Brooks TM (1995) The future of biodiversity. Science (new York, NY) 269(5222):347–350

Polishook JD, Ondeyka JG, Dombrowski AW, Peláez F, Platas G, Teran AM (2001) Biogeography and relatedness of nodulisporium strains producing nodulisporic acid. Mycologia 93(6):1125–1137

Prabhakar O (2013) Cerebroprotective effect of resveratrol through antioxidant and anti-inflammatory effects in diabetic rats. Naunyn Schmiedebergs Arch. Pharmacol. 386(8):705–710

Pushpangadan P, Behl HM (2005) Environment & biodiversity: agenda for future. In: Paper presented at the third international conference on plants & environmental pollution (ICPEP-3)

Rahban M, Habibi-Rezaei M, Mazaheri M, Saso L, Moosavi-Movahedi AA (2020) Anti-viral potential and modulation of Nrf2 by curcumin: pharmacological implications. Antioxidants 9(12):1228:1–24

Rao KV (1993) Taxol and Related Taxanes. I. Taxanes of Taxus Brevifolia Bark. Pharm Res 10(4):521–524

Rates SM (2001) Plants as source of drugs. Toxicon 39 (5):603–613

Reid WV, Mooney HA, Cropper A, Capistrano D, Carpenter SR, Chopra K, Dasgupta P, Dietz T, Duraiappah AK, Hassan R, Kasperson R, Leemans R, May RM, McMichael AJ, Pingali P, Samper C, Scholes R, Watson RT, Zakri AH, Shidong Z, Ash NJ, Bennett E, Kumar P, Lee MJ, Raudsepp-Hearne C, Simons H, Thonell J, Zurek MB (2005) Ecosystems and human well-being: synthesis, millennium ecosystem assessment. Island Pres, Washington, DC

Rinehart KL, Lithgow-Berelloni AM (1991) Novel antiviral and cytotoxic agent. Chem Abstract 115:2480–2486

Sahu P, Giri D, Singh R, Pandey P, Gupta S, Shrivastava A, Kumar A, Pandey K (2013) Therapeutic and medicinal uses of aloe vera: a review. Pharmacol Pharm 4:599–610

Salami M, Moosavi-Movahedi AA, Moosavi-Movahedi F, Ehsani MR, Yousefi R, Farhadi M, Niasari-Naslaji A, Saboury AA, Chobert JM, Haertlé T (2011) Biological activity of camel milk casein following enzymatic digestion. J Dairy Res 78(4):471–478

Scannell JW, Bosley J (2016) When quality beats quantity: decision theory, drug discovery, and the reproducibility crisis. PLoS ONE 11(2):e0147215

Scartezzini P, Speroni E (2000) Review on some plants of Indian traditional medicine with antioxidant activity. J Ethnopharmacol 71(1–2):23–43

Sharma SB, Gupta R (2015) Drug development from natural resource: a systematic approach. Mini Rev Med Chem 15(1):52–57

Sharma SB, Nasir A, Prabhu KM, Murthy PS (2006) Antihyperglycemic effect of the fruit-pulp of Eugenia Jambolana in experimental diabetes mellitus. J Ethnopharmacol 104(3):367–373

Simmons TL, Andrianasolo E, McPhail K, Flatt P, Gerwick WH (2005) Marine natural products as anticancer drugs. Mol Cancer Ther 4(2):333–342

Singh AP, Singh R, Verma SS, Rai V, Kaschula CH, Maiti P, Gupta SC (2019) Health benefits of resveratrol: evidence from clinical studies. Med Res Rev 39 (5):1851–1891

Skates E, Overall J, DeZego K, Wilson M, Esposito D, Lila MA, Komarnytsky S (2018) Berries containing anthocyanins with enhanced methylation profiles are more effective at ameliorating high fat diet-induced metabolic damage. Food Chem Toxicol 111:445–453

Spande TF, Garraffo HM, Edwards MW, Yeh HJC, Pannell L, Daly JW (1992) Epibatidine: a novel (chloropyridyl)azabicycloheptane with potent analgesic activity from an ecuadoran poison frog. J Am Chem Soc 114(9):3475–3478

Stan SD, Hahm E-R, Warin R, Singh SV (2008) Withaferin a causes foxo3a-and bim-dependent apoptosis and inhibits growth of human breast cancer cells in vivo. Can Res 68(18):7661–7669

Stearns SC (2009) Sustaining life: how human health depends on biodiversity. Environ Health Perspect 117 (6):A266–A266

Sugihara Y, Nojima H, Matsuda H, Murakami T, Yoshikawa M, Kimura I (2000) Antihyperglycemic effects of gymnemic acid Iv, a compound derived from Gymnema Sylvestre leaves in Streptozotocin-Diabetic Mice. J Asian Nat Prod Res 2(4):321–327

Swellam T, Miyanaga N, Onozawa M, Hattori K, Kawai K, Shimazui T, Akaza H (2003) Antineoplastic activity of honey in an experimental bladder cancer implantation model: in vivo and in vitro studies. Int J Urol 10(4):213–219

Trimurtulu G, Ohtani I, Patterson GML, Moore RE, Corbett TH, Valeriote FA, Demchik L (1994) Total structures of cryptophycins, potent antitumor depsipeptides from the blue-green alga nostoc sp. strain Gsv 224. J Am Chem Soc 116(11):4729–4737

Urdiales J, Morata P, De Castro IN, Sánchez-Jiménez F (1996) Antiproliferative effect of dehydrodidemnin B (Ddb), a depsipeptide isolated from mediterranean tunicates. Cancer Lett 102(1):31–37

Vasarri M, Leri M, Barletta E, Ramazzotti M, Marzocchini R, Degl'Innocenti D (2020) Anti-inflammatory properties of the marine plant Posidonia Oceanica (L.) Delile. J Ethnopharmacol 247:112252

Wang L, Yang R, Yuan B, Liu Y, Liu C (2015) The antiviral and antimicrobial activities of licorice, a widely-used chinese herb. Acta Pharm Sin B 5(4):310–315

Winter JM, Tang Y (2012) Synthetic biological approaches to natural product biosynthesis. Curr Opin Biotechnol 23(5):736–743

Zang Y, Zhang L, Igarashi K, Yu C (2015) The anti-obesity and anti-diabetic effects of kaempferol glycosides from unripe soybean leaves in high-fat-diet mice. J Food Func 6(3):834–841

Zhang L, Wei J, Yang Z, Chen F, Xian Q, Su P, Pan W, Zhang K, Zheng X, Du Z (2018) Distribution and diversity of twelve curcuma species in China. Nat Prod Res 32(3):327–330

Nutraceuticals and Superfoods

Mehdi Mohammadian, Maryam Salami, Maryam Moghadam, Zahra Emam-Djomeh, and Ali Akbar Moosavi-Movahedi

Abstract

Nowadays, there is an ever-increasing trend in the case of nutraceuticals and superfoods as a result of growing concerns about the effects of diet on health. Nutraceuticals are natural biologically active compounds extractable from various food sources. In contrast, a superfood is any fresh or processed food claimed to have particular health-promoting attributes and/or can decrease the risk of chronic disease further than its basic nutritional function. Different studies have shown that the nutraceuticals and superfoods have various beneficial physiological effects, and their consumption can reduce the risk for disease development or can even cure some diseases because they are rich sources of a wide range of bioactive molecules and specific nutrients. Some examples of nutraceuticals and superfoods are curcumin, pomegranate, camel milk, bioactive peptides, and walnut, which their potential health benefits and applications for the development of functional food products with health-promoting properties have been studied in the present chapter.

Keywords

Nutraceuticals · Superfoods · Functional food products · Bioactive compounds · Human health · Biological properties

1 Introduction

Nowadays, the many health benefits of certain foods have been realized by consumers and food scientists with respect to the increasing of interest on the part of consumers, researchers, and food industry into how foods or their derived bioactive compounds can help maintain the health of humans (Viuda-Martos et al. 2011). Different terms such as "nutraceutical" and "superfood" have been used to describe a compound or a food with potential health benefits beyond basic nutritional function (Sohaimy 2012). The concept of nutraceutical is a hybrid of nutrition and pharmaceutical. In fact, "nutraceuticals" is a

M. Mohammadian · M. Salami (✉) · M. Moghadam · Z. Emam-Djomeh
Department of Food Science and Engineering, University College of Agriculture & Natural Resources, University of Tehran, Karaj, Iran
e-mail: msalami@ut.ac.ir

M. Mohammadian
e-mail: m.mohamadian@ut.ac.ir

M. Moghadam
e-mail: moghadam.maryam@ut.ac.ir

Z. Emam-Djomeh
e-mail: emamj@ut.ac.ir

A. A. Moosavi-Movahedi
Institute of Biochemistry & Biophysics, University of Tehran, Tehran, Iran
e-mail: moosavi@ut.ac.ir

broad umbrella term that is employed to describe any ingredient, which is a food or part of it; providing positive effects on human health and can be applied to prevent or treat different diseases. This term was first presented by the chairperson and founder of "Foundation for Innovation in Medicine" by Mr. Stephen DeFelice in 1989 (Ali et al. 2019; Piccolella et al. 2019). The nutraceuticals are naturally found in many foods and can be extracted by different methods. These compounds can be formulated and taken in a dosage form, such as capsules, tinctures, and tablets (Sohaimy 2012). Some of the common nutraceuticals are: curcumin, lycopene, vitamins, phenolic compounds, coenzyme Q10, minerals such as calcium and magnesium, biologically active peptides form plant and animal proteins, prebiotic fibers such as inulin, polyunsaturated fatty acids, and many others (Ghaffari and Roshanravan 2020). The global market of nutraceuticals was at US$165.62 billion in 2014 and is expected to reach US$278.96 billion at the end of 2021 regarding its significant annual growth rate, which is 7.3% (Ali et al. 2019).

"Superfood" is another term using to describe food products with health-promoting properties, which are ideal candidates for strengthening and promoting the proper functioning of the human body. Unlike to nutraceuticals, superfoods are products that are consumed as foods and not in dosage form (Proestos 2018). Superfoods are defined as foods that contain some component(s) which are beneficial for health beyond traditional nutrients (Shah 2007). Superfoods are also identified as designer foods, medicinal foods, therapeutic foods, and functional foods. However, it should be noted that the term superfood is mainly used as a marketing tool, and no generally accepted definition exists (Driessche et al. 2018). After searching on the internet, it was investigated that a wide range of food products have been identified as superfoods including vegetables such as beetroots, tomatoes, spinach, and pumpkin; fruits such as pomegranates, oranges, apples, avocado, kiwi, grapefruit, and lemons; berries such as goji berries, strawberries, black raspberries, and blueberries; fish and seafood products such as mackerel, salmon, and sardines; poultry such as turkey; herbs and spices such as turmeric, garlic, chili peppers, and ginger; nuts such as walnuts, pistachio, almonds, and peanuts; grain, legumes, and beans such as lentils, black beans, oats, and soybeans; seeds such as flaxseed, hemp seed, chia seed, and quinoa; dairy products such as yogurt and kefir; and many other food products such as eggs, camel milk, green tea, dark chocolate, honey, royal jelly, coconut oil, cocoa, olive oil, fish oil, mushrooms, seaweed, nutritional yeast, fermented foods, microgreens, spirulina, and maca (Viuda-Martos et al. 2011, 2008; Driessche et al. 2018). These food products have been categorized as superfoods with respect to their well-known positive health effects on digestion, heart and cardiovascular, brain, skin and hair, weight loss, immune system, memory, and cancer prevention. In fact, the superfoods contain different biologically active compounds such as antioxidants, which have anti-cancer activities. They also have healthy fats, which can prevent heart disease, fiber, useful to prevent diabetes and digestive issues, and phytochemicals, which are responsible for colors and smells of plants having various benefits (Proestos 2018). Superfoods can be considered as the healthiest foods on the plant, attracting a lot of attention from different fields. It seems that the consumption of superfoods and nutraceutical is a worthy way to improve health. Therefore, research on nutraceuticals and superfoods appears to be essential in order to understand better different aspects of their structure, bio-functionality, and health-promoting properties. In this regard, some of the most important superfoods and nutraceuticals have been reviewed with respect to the results of recent scientific studies.

2 Some Examples of Nutraceuticals and Superfoods

The nutraceuticals and superfoods include a wide range of food products, ingredients, and compounds such as fruits, vegetables, nuts, seeds, herbs, spices, fish and seafood, dairy products, polyphenols, phytosterols, carotenoids, and curcumin which have been claimed to have health benefits. In the following sections, some of the most critical nutraceuticals and superfoods which have been thoroughly investigated by different studies will be discussed with a focus on their potential health benefits and applications for developing of novel food products aiming to improve the health of consumers.

2.1 Curcumin

Curcumin is a hydrophobic natural polyphenolic-type nutraceutical, which is the dominant pigment of the root of turmeric (*Curcuma Longa* Linn) and is widely used as a seasoning and coloring agent in the food products owing to its intense yellow color (David et al. 2015). Different biological activities have been suggested for curcumin such as antioxidant, antibacterial, anticancer, anti-inflammatory, anti-parasitic, anti-mutagenic, anti-proliferative, and antiviral activity (Joung et al. 2016; Kumar et al. 2016; Zheng et al. 2019). Moreover, curcumin can be used as a capable biologically active molecule to treat and prevent different diseases and disorders such as cardiovascular ailments, infectious disease, cancer, cystic fibrosis, Alzheimer's disease, gastric ulcer, diabetes, and psoriasis (Gutierres et al. 2012; Chang et al. 2019). The ability of curcumin to scavenge reactive oxygen and nitrogen free radicals can be considered as the main responsible for those mentioned above biological and health-elevating properties (David et al. 2015). Despite having a broad range of potential health benefits, the application and therapeutic potential of curcumin as a nutraceutical is limited by its low oral bioavailability, which is attributed to its poor solubility in aqueous media, rapid metabolism, and low chemical stability under physiological and food processing conditions (Kharat and McClements 2019; Kotha and Luthria 2019). Therefore, encapsulation in different delivery systems such as emulsions, liposomes, hydrogels, biopolymer-based particles, or complexation with food biopolymers such as proteins were used as an efficient method to overcome the above challenges for expanding the applications of curcumin in functional foods and drinks (Mohammadian et al. 2019a). Among different biopolymers which used for the encapsulation of curcumin, food proteins have attracted the more considerable attention due to their high nutritional value, excellent functional properties, amphiphilic nature, biodegradability, and biocompatibility (Chang et al. 2019). Various plant and animal proteins such as whey proteins (Mohammadian et al. 2019a, b; Li et al. 2015; Taghavi Kevij et al. 2019), casein (Kumar et al. 2016; Esmaili et al. 2011; Pan et al. 2014), egg white proteins (Chang et al. 2019), soy proteins (Tapal and Tiku 2012; Chen et al. 2015), and walnut proteins (Moghadam et al. 2020a) have been used to enhance the water solubility and bioavailability of curcumin. It was observed that the water solubility of curcumin was improved by about 812 and 1200-folds by loading into soy proteins (Tapal and Tiku 2012) and whey protein nanofibrils (Mohammadian et al. 2019a), respectively. These studies also reported that the radical scavenging capacity, reducing power, and chemical stability of curcumin were significantly improved by loading into the carriers. Moreover, it was investigated that the anti-proliferation of curcumin capsulated in casein particles against human colorectal and pancreatic cancer cells was higher than free curcumin. In fact, encapsulation enhanced the cellular uptake of curcumin, improving its anticancer activity (Pan et al. 2014). Therefore, it seems that the encapsulated curcumin can be considered as a more bioactive ingredient compared to its free form regarding the higher solubility, bioavailability, and chemical stability of the encapsulated form.

According to the numerous health benefits, curcumin was used in the formulation of products such as dairy milk (Zheng et al. 2019), yogurt (Gutierres et al. 2012; Assis et al. 2017), ice cream (Kumar et al. 2016; Borrin et al. 2018), cakes (Lim et al. 2010; Seo et al. 2010; Park et al. 2012), and beverages (David et al. 2015; Joung et al. 2016) to improve their health-promoting attributes. Therefore, the resulting curcumin-enriched foods can be considered as functional foods or superfoods.

Some of the studies used curcumin to develop functional dairy products with health-promoting properties. Curcumin-loaded dairy milks were produced by the pH-shift method (Zheng et al. 2019). The resulting curcumin-enriched milks had suitable physical and chemical stabilities under storage conditions. pH-shifting is a simple solvent-free method which is based on the high solubility of curcumin at alkaline pHs. This method was also used to encapsulate the curcumin in the walnut proteins, and the resulting curcumin-loaded samples showed a good in vitro anticancer activity against the breast cancer cell lines (Moghadam et al. 2020a). Yogurt, as a popular dairy product, was also enriched with curcumin. It was reported that the curcumin-supplemented yogurt showed good anti-diabetic activity and had the ability to improve the classical markers for experimental diabetes (Gutierres et al. 2012). The curcumin-enriched yogurt was also produced by Assis et al. (2017) and introduced as an attractive complementary therapy for diabetic complications owing to its antioxidants and antiatherogenic potentials.

Turmeric, as a food ingredient rich in curcumin, was used to enrich different types of cakes for improving their biological activity. Lim et al. (2010) produced a yellow layer cake containing turmeric powder and evaluated its antioxidant properties. They reported that the antioxidant properties of cakes, including reducing power, free radical scavenging activity, and chelating ability, were significantly improved by enriching with turmeric attributing to the presence of curcumin in the turmeric powder which has an excellent antioxidant activity. Seo et al. (2010) also produced sponge cake containing turmeric and introduced it as a functional food with different biological advantages. In another study conducted by Park et al. (2012), it was observed that the incorporation of turmeric into the wheat flour cakes significantly increased their curcumin content and antioxidant activity. Therefore, curcumin can be used as an effective nutraceutical to enrich cakes to improve their biological properties, especially antioxidant activity.

2.2 Pomegranate

Pomegranate (*Punica granatum* L.) as a superfruit is native to Iran and appreciated for its excellent health benefits from the ancient times (Mousavinejad et al. 2009). This fruit is constituted by peel, arils, and seeds in an approximate ratio of 50:40:10, respectively (Andrade et al. 2019). Pomegranate is well-known for its different biological properties such as antioxidant, antibacterial, antifungal, antiviral, and anti-inflammatory activity, as well as the ability to prevent various diseases such as obesity, diabetes, and cardiovascular disease (Vučić et al. 2019). Moreover, it was reported that the pomegranate as a rich source of phytochemicals has excellent anticancer activity against prostate, colon, oral, liver, lung, skin, thyroid, and breast cancers (Li et al. 2016; Khwairakpam et al. 2018; Bassiri-Jahromi 2018). The anticancer activity of pomegranate and its derived nutraceuticals was attributed to their ability to interference with tumor cell proliferation, cell cycle, invasion, and angiogenesis (Vučić et al. 2019). Ma et al. (2015) assessed the in vivo impact of pomegranate peel as a source of polyphenols, especially ellagic acid, gallic acid, and punicalagin on human prostate cancer PC-3 cells. They observed that the tumor volume and weight were decreased, and the cancer cell apoptosis was significantly increased in tumor-bearing nude mice administered by pomegranate peel.

The health benefits of pomegranate, its extracts and juices, have been attributed mainly to the high polyphenolic content of pomegranate, especially punicalagins, punicalins, gallagic acid, and ellagic acid (Trigueros et al. 2014). A wide range of valuable compounds and phyto-constituents have been identified in various parts of the pomegranate plant such as pomegranate juice (anthocyanins, quercetin, rutin, ellagic acid, gallic acid, catechin, glucose, ascorbic acid, caffeic acid, different minerals particularly iron, and amino acids), seed oil (punicic acid, ellagic acid, and various fatty acids and sterols), pericarp (phenolic punicalagins, gallic acid, catechin, quercetin, rutin, anthocyanidins, flavones, and flavonones), leaves (tannins including punicalin and punicafolin and flavone glycosides including luteolin and apigenin), flowers (gallic acid, ursolic acid, triterpenoids including maslinic, and asiatic acid), and roots and bark (ellagitannins including punicalin and punicalagin, and numerous piperidine alkaloids) which possessed different biological activities (Ahmadiankia 2019; Fateh et al. 2013). Therefore, pomegranate fruits, beverages, and other related food products enriched with pomegranate can be considered as superfoods owing to their immense potentials for health benefits. Accordingly, different parts of pomegranate fruit as a rich source of nutraceuticals were used to enrich various types of food products such as ice cream (Ali and Prasad 2016; Çam et al. 2013), yogurt (Trigueros et al. 2014; Nikmaram et al. 2015), bread (Bhol et al. 2016; Altunkaya et al. 2013), and cakes (Topkaya and Isik 2019) for enhancing their health benefits.

In a study carried out by Cam et al. (2013), the pomegranate by-products, including pomegranate peel extract and seed oil, were used to enrich ice cream for improving its antioxidant and antidiabetic activities. They reported that the antioxidant and antidiabetic activities of ice cream were significantly enhanced by enriching with pomegranate by-products without harming the techno-functional and sensorial attributes of the resulting product. Ali et al. (2016) investigated the effects of pomegranate seed powder addition at different levels (1–4%) on the antioxidant properties of ice cream. The results of the above study indicated that the antioxidant activity of ice cream was enhanced through the incorporation of pomegranate seed powder. The phenolic compounds from pomegranate juice were also used in the formulation of yogurt (Trigueros et al. 2014). They reported that the incorporation of pomegranate phenolic compounds into yogurt significantly improved its free radical scavenging performance due to this fact that the pomegranate juice is rich in anthocyanins and also other phenolic compounds such as ellagic acid and punicalagins which are potent antioxidants. Nikmaram et al. (2015) also used the pomegranate juice for the enrichment of yogurt drink and indicated that the antioxidant properties of drinks promoted through the supplementation with pomegranate juice. Moreover, these authors observed that the pomegranate juice showed a positive impact on the survival of *Lactobacillus casei* as a probiotic in the yogurt drink samples.

The pomegranate by-products were also employed to produce functional breads and cakes. In this regard, Altunkaya et al. (2013) enriched the wheat bread with pomegranate peel powder and reported that the antioxidant capacity of breads significantly improved by adding pomegranate peel. Moreover, they observed that the peroxide value of the bread enriched with pomegranate peel was lower compared to the control bread sample. Bhol et al. (2016) also used the pomegranate whole fruit bagasse for the preparation of functional bread and reported a high free radical scavenging activity for the resulting breads. They also observed that the mineral content of bread was increased by enriching with pomegranate whole fruit bagasse. In a study conducted by Topkaya and Isik (2019), pomegranate peel was used in the formulation of muffin cakes. The muffin cakes were prepared by substituting of wheat flour by pomegranate peel powder at levels of 5, 10, or 15%. The results showed that the enrichment of cakes by pomegranate peel powder considerably increased their nutritional value, including the content of insoluble and total dietary fibers, phenolic compounds, antioxidant properties, and the content of minerals (Mg, Ca, and K). Therefore, the cake supplemented with pomegranate peel could be considered as a rich source of biologically active compounds which have different health benefits.

2.3 Walnut

The walnut (*Juglans regia* L.) as a favorite tree nut is cultivated widely all over the world and is well-known as a rich source of various valuable compounds. Different parts of the walnut tree, including the kernel, fresh green fruit, husk, shell, skin, bark, leaves, and root, are studied to employ in food, cosmetic, and pharmaceutical industries (Moghadam et al. 2020a; Jahanban-Esfahlan et al. 2019). The walnut seed or kernel represents 30–40% of the nut weight and has excellent nutritional value owing to its abundant lipids (52–70%), proteins (up to 24% of the walnut kernel weight), carbohydrates (12–16%), fibers (1.5–2%), minerals (1.7–2%), vitamins, and phenolic compounds (Feng et al. 2019; Labuckas et al. 2008). Walnut is one of the two highest-ranked tree nuts in terms of antioxidant activity and total phenolic content. Moreover, the walnut is a good source of essential unsaturated fatty acids, tocopherols, and potent antioxidant hormone, melatonin (Grace et al. 2014). The main identified polyphenolic compounds in walnuts are pedunculagin, ellagic acid, tellimagrandin I, casuarictin, tellimagranin II, rugosin C, casuarinin, and gallic acid which have effects on memory enhancement, neurogenesis, and prevention of cell death in neurodegenerative diseases (Gorji et al. 2018). Several biological functions have been reported for the walnuts such as anti-atherogenic, antioxidant, anticancer, anti-inflammatory, and anti-mutagenic properties (Jahanbani et al. 2018). Moreover, walnuts have the ability to improve memory and cognition, attributing to their unique phytochemical composition (Grace et al. 2014).

The therapeutic effects of walnut and its bioactive components consumption have been investigated by many studies. Nagel et al. (2012) studied the effect of dietary walnuts on colorectal cancer. In this study, the human colon cancer cells (HT-29) were injected into female nude mice. After a one-week acclimation period, the mice were subjected to diets containing 19% of total energy from walnuts. They observed that the tumor growth rate and the final tumor weight were meaningfully decreased in the walnut-fed mice. These authors suggested that the consumption of walnuts can inhibit colorectal cancer growth by suppressing angiogenesis. This anticancer activity can be due to the presence of putative anti-tumorigenic compounds in walnuts such as ellagic acid, selenium, phytosterols, and dietary fibers. The effect of a walnut-rich diet on the growth of human prostate cancer cells in nude mice was also investigated by Reiter et al. (2013). They reported that the final average tumor size in the walnut-diet mice was roughly one-fourth of the average size of the prostate tumors in the animals that ate the control diet. This anticancer activity was attributed to the bioactive ingredients of walnut, including omega-3 fatty acids, phytosterols, gamma-tocopherol, carotenoids, polyphenolic compounds, ellagic acid and its derivatives, and melatonin. These phytochemicals have good antioxidant activity, which generally is beneficial in terms of cancer suppression. In another study conducted by Hardman (2014)), the potential of walnut-rich diet for cancer prevention and treatment in mice was assessed. This study reported different results including: (1) the growth rate of human breast cancers implanted in nude mice reduced by 80% as a result of subjecting to the walnut-containing diet; (2) the walnut-rich diet reduced the number of mammary gland tumors by 60% in a transgenic mouse model; (3) the decrease in mammary gland tumors was greater with whole walnuts than with a diet containing the same amount of n-3 fatty acids, suggesting that multiple bioactive components in walnuts such as n-3 fatty acids, tocopherols, β-sitosterol, and pedunculagin, additively or synergistically contribute to cancer suppression; and (4) the growth of prostate, colon, and renal cancers was slowed by walnut-rich diet through the anti-proliferative and anti-angiogenic mechanisms. In another study carried out by Soriano-Hernandez et al. (2015), it was investigated that the high consumption of walnuts decreased the risk of breast cancer by 2–3 times. However, it should be noted that this study reported that the protective effect against breast cancer was not found with low or moderate consumption of walnuts in comparison with null consumption. Jahanbani et al. (2016) also studied the antioxidant and anticancer activities of walnut protein hydrolysates. They reported that the hydrolysates had excellent radical scavenging capacity and were able to inhibit the activity of reactive oxygen species. Moreover, they studied the effect of walnut protein hydrolysates on the viability of human breast (MDA-MB231) and colon (HT-29) cancer cell lines. They reported that the walnut protein antioxidant hydrolysates were able to inhibit the growth of breast and colon cancer cells. In another study conducted by Jahanbani et al. (2018) also, it was reported that the peptide hydrolysate extracted from walnut could be used as antihypertensive agents in food formulations owing to its hypotensive effects. In a recent study by Alsuhaibani and Al-Kuraieef (2019), the impact of walnut-containing diet was investigated on streptozotocin-induced diabetes in rats. They reported that the consumption of walnuts as 2.5, 5 and 7.5% of a basal diet fed to diabetic rats significantly decreased the glycosylated hemoglobin and glucose levels and significantly increased circulating insulin in comparison with the positive controls. This antidiabetic effect was attributed to the significant components of walnut seeds, including phenols and fatty acids. Generally, the results of the above studies indicated that the walnut could be considered as a superfood regarding its various health-promoting properties and also can be used for the fortification of food formulations.

2.4 Camel Milk

Nowadays, the consumption of non-bovine milk has been increased, and new sources of milk have gained a lot of interest (Khalesi et al. (2017)). Camel milk as a non-bovine milk can be considered as a superfood owing to its high nutritional value and excellent therapeutic effects. The composition and structure of camel milk components differ from those of bovine milk and has advantages over the bovine milk such as easier digestion, higher content of Cu and Fe, high levels of vitamin C, and formation of soft curd in the human stomach which makes it suitable as an infant food (Ayyash et al. 2018). Moreover, camel milk is suitable for those who are allergic to cow milk due to the lack of β-lactoglobulin in the camel whey (Momen et al. 2019; Kamal et al. 2018). Owing to these superiorities, the camel milk-based food products such as pasteurized milk, ice cream, and cheese have been developed and sold in many countries (Ayyash et al. 2018). In addition to the nutritional benefits, different medicinal properties including antibacterial, antigenotoxic, anticytotoxic, anticancer, antioxidant, antihypertensive, antithrombotic, anti-inflammatory, and antidiabetic properties as well as curing hepatitis C infection, hypoallergenic effect, and treatment of autism have been reported for the camel milk by many in vitro and in vivo studies (Ayoub et al. 2018; Alavi et al. 2017; Salami et al. 2011) introducing the camel milk as an attractive superfood for researchers and consumers. These therapeutic properties of camel milk were attributed to its different components, such as vitamins E and C, lysozymes, lactoferrins, lactoperoxidase, and immunoglobulins (Krishnankutty et al. 2018). Most of the resent studies in the case of camel milk therapeutic properties have focused on its anticancer and antidiabetic activities.

A very few studies have been done to investigate the anticancer property of crude camel milk. In this regard, Korashy et al. (2012) assessed the effect of camel milk on the proliferation of human cancer cells using in vitro model of human hepatoma (HepG2) and human breast (MCF7) cancer cells. They observed that the proliferation of HepG2 and MCF7 cells was significantly inhibited by camel milk through the activation of caspase-3 mRNA and activity levels, and the induction of death receptors in both cell lines. Moreover, they reported that the camel milk increased the expression of oxidative stress markers, heme oxygenase-1 and reactive oxygen species production in both cells. Generally, these authors concluded that camel milk could induce apoptosis in human cancer cells by apoptotic- and oxidative-stress-mediated mechanisms. Hasson et al. (2015) also studied the in vitro apoptosis triggering in the BT-474 human breast cancer cell line by camel milk. Their result showed that camel milk could be used as a novel drug without any side effects to develop new strategies to treat breast cancer as a global concern through its apoptotic and oxidative-stress-mediated mechanisms. The anticancer activity of commercially available camel milk on human colorectal (HCT 116) and breast cancer (MCF-7) cells were also investigated by Krishnakutty et al. (2018). They reported that the camel milk considerably reduced the proliferation, viability, and migration of both the cells. The above study showed that the camel milk anti-proliferative effect on colorectal and breast cancer cells was governed by inducing autophagy.

Camel milk is traditionally has been prescribed for diabetes. The antidiabetic property of camel milk was attributed to the presence of insulin/insulin-like molecules in this milk (Ayoub et al. 2018; Alavi et al. 2017; Fallah et al. 2020). Therefore, it was suggested that camel milk consumption could be considered as an effective bio-remedy for treating diabetes (Izadi et al. 2019). Agrawal et al. (2005) studied the effect of raw milk in type 1 diabetic patients during a 52-week randomized study. They showed that the dose of insulin required maintaining long-term glycaemic control was significantly reduced in patients with type 1 diabetes resulted from the consumption of camel milk. The effect of camel milk was also assessed on the glycaemic and lipid profile of patients with type 2 diabetes by Fallah et al. (2020). They reported that the consumption of camel milk decreased the required dose of long-acting insulin in patients with type 2 diabetes and suggested that the raw camel milk consumption can be considered as an effective complementary way for glycaemic control in patients with type 2 diabetes.

2.5 Food Proteins-Originated Bioactive Peptides

Food proteins-originated biologically active peptides can be considered as a new class of nutraceuticals owing to their excellent health-promoting properties. They are short sequences of amino acids that are inactive within the sequence of the parent protein but have a positive health effect on systems of the body once released (Lafarga and Hayes 2017). Many of the in vivo bio-functional properties of dietary animal and plant proteins are related to the presence of these bioactive peptides in their sequences (Chalamaiah et al. 2018). The bioactive peptides or hydrolysates can be released from proteins by different methods, including enzymatic hydrolysis by digestive enzymes (pepsin, trypsin, and chymotrypsin) or enzymes from plants and microorganisms, chemical and physical hydrolysis, and fermentation by proteolytic starter cultures such as lactic acid bacteria (Mohammadian et al. 2017). Among the methods mentioned above, the enzymatic hydrolysis seems to be the most appropriate approach to prepare the tailor made bioactive peptides due to the large scale availability and moderate cost of enzymes as well as the high quality of the resulting peptides (Gani et al. 2015). Bioactive peptides from plant and animal sources may exert various physiological functions such as antioxidant, antimicrobial, mineral binding, antidiabetic, antihypertensive or angiotensin converting enzyme (ACE)-inhibitory, antithrombotic, immunomodulatory, anticancer, opioid, and satiating properties which are dependent on the amino acid composition and sequences of bio-peptides (Sarmadi and Ismail 2010).

Different investigations have been done to study the health-promoting characteristics of bioactive peptides released from food proteins originated from animal and plant sources. For example, Umayaparvathi et al. (2014) purified the antioxidant peptides from oyster hydrolysate and studied their anticancer activity on human colon cancer cell lines (HT-29). They observed that the hydrolysates exerted a significant cytotoxic effect of HT-29 cell lines, whereas they did not show any cytotoxic effect on normal cells. In another study conducted by Logarušić et al. (2019), the anticancer activity of hempseed protein antioxidant hydrolysates was investigated on cancer cells (HeLa). The hydrolysates showed dose-dependent anti-proliferative effects on HeLa cancer cells, which make them as efficient nutraceuticals that can be used in food and drug formulations. In a study carried out by Fritz et al. (2011), the in vitro and in vivo antihypertensive activity of a plant protein hydrolysate was investigated. They reported that the amaranth seed protein hydrolysates were able to lower blood pressure of male spontaneously hypertensive rats. The hypertensive effect of these hydrolysates can be due to the lowering of peripheral resistance. Many other studies also assessed the antioxidant activity of protein hydrolysates. For example, Mohammadian and Madadlou (2016) showed that the reducing capacity and free radical scavenging property of whey proteins were significantly improved by enzymatic hydrolysis. This increase in antioxidant activity was attributed to the exposure of amino acids that were naturally buried in the native conformation of protein, increasing of hydrogen ions availability, and concentration of carboxylic acid groups as a result of the enzymatic hydrolysis. Alavi et al. (2019) also indicated that the free radical scavenging capacity of Kilka fish proteins was increased by applying native proteases from melon attributing to high total hydrophobic amino acid content in the hydrolysates. In addition, it was recently investigated that the enzymatic hydrolysis can improve the bioactive-loading properties of the proteins. Moghadam et al. (2020b) investigated the consequence of trypsin-mediated hydrolysis on the ability of walnut proteins for loading of curcumin and quercetin as bioactive hydrophobic agents. They observed that the loading capacity of bioactives for hydrolysates was remarkably higher than the native un-hydrolyzed walnut proteins. This was attributed to the higher surface hydrophobicity of hydrolysates compared to the native counterpart. Therefore, hydrolysates can form soluble complexes with curcumin and quercetin through the formation of hydrophobic interactions. Moreover, these authors found that the loading capacity of walnut hydrolysates was improved by increasing the enzymatic hydrolysis time, which can result in the formation of shorter bioactive peptides with a higher amount of exposed hydrophobic patches. The hydrolysates of zein were also introduced as novel effective delivery systems for curcumin. The high ability of these hydrolysates to load curcumin can be due to their amphiphilic nature achieved by enzyme-mediated hydrolysis (Wang et al. 2015).

The recent studies have shown that the bioactive peptides originated from hydrolysis of food proteins can be purified and concentrated for developing novel physiologically functional foods. Accordingly, food proteins-originated biologically active peptides and hydrolysate were used to develop novel functional food products. Most of the studies regarding the food applications of bioactive peptides and hydrolysates are related to the dairy bioactive peptides, especially casein and whey protein hydrolysates. Sinha et al. (2007) used the bioactive peptides formed by enzymatic hydrolysis of whey proteins to develop a functional beverage and reported that the resulting beverages had good sensory properties and stability during storage. Whey protein hydrolysates were also used as a nutraceutical additive for the fortification of yogurt beverage, and the ACE-inhibitory activity of the resulting products was evaluated (Lim et al. 2011). The results showed that the fortified beverages maintained the antihypertensive activity. Therefore, these authors suggested that the bioactive peptides from whey proteins can be effectively used as a nutraceutical ingredient in the production of antihypertensive dairy-based superfoods. The whey protein hydrolysates with high antioxidant and ACE-inhibitory activities were also successfully employed to produce apple juice beverages by Goudarzi et al. (2015). They reported that the resulting beverages containing bioactive whey protein hydrolysates met the organoleptic requirements of a sensory panel and can be considered as a novel functional food. The antioxidant activity of whey protein hydrolysates as natural bio-functional ingredients was also determined in milk beverage system by Mann et al. (2015). They reported that the fortification of strawberry and chocolate flavored milk with whey protein antioxidant peptides significantly increased their free radical scavenging antioxidant activity. The tryptic whey protein hydrolysate at different levels (1, 2, and 3% v/milk) was also used as an additive in sweetened Indian yogurt (Chatterjee et al. 2016). They indicated that the addition of whey protein hydrolysate into the yogurt samples significantly improved their ACE-inhibitory activities due to the presence of ACE inhibitor peptides in whey protein hydrolysate. Casein-originated bioactive peptides were also used to develop different functional food products with health promoting attributes. Crowley et al. (2002) studied the application of casein hydrolysates in bakery products. The antioxidant casein peptides were also used to inhibit the lipid oxidation in beef homogenates and mechanically deboned poultry meat by Rossini et al. (2009). They investigated that the incorporation of casein peptides significantly inhibited lipid peroxidation in the above products helping to prevent the off-flavor formation in meat products and increasing shelf life. The enzymatic hydrolysates of whey and casein protein were also successfully employed to develop functional cookies (Gani et al. 2015).

In addition to the milk protein-based hydrolysates, bioactive peptides derived from other sources were also employed to develop functional healthy foods and superfoods. Hydrolysates from oyster proteins produced by protamex were used to produce a functional drink (Cho et al. 2010). The resulting hydrolysates-enriched drink showed a good antiradical activity, which makes it an appropriate candidate for being used as a healthy drink, especially for decreasing the effects of free radicals in the body. However, this drink had a low preference score, and more studies are still needed to overcome these challenges related to the commercialization of peptides-enriched drinks and beverages. The protein hydrolysates from blue whiting as an under-utilized fish released by different commercial enzymes were used for the fortification of beverages (Egerton et al. 2018). In the above study, the solubility of fish hydrolysates was evaluated in a vitamin-tea beverage as an acidic beverage with a pH value of 3.3. The findings indicated that the hydrolysates had an excellent solubility (higher than 85%) in this condition and have the potential to be used as an active ingredient in the production of functional beverage and foods. Ujiroghene et al. (2019) studied the ACE and α-glucosidase inhibitory activities of peptides from sprouted quinoa yogurt beverages, which were fermented by *Lactobacillus casei*. All of the released hydrolysates and peptides have the ability to inhibit the action of the above enzymes in a dose- and strain-dependent manner. Moreover, it was shown that the peptide fractions with the sequences of LAHMIVAGA and VAHPVF were dual function as were able to inhibit both of the ACE and α-glucosidase. Therefore, the above-mentioned quinoa-based hydrolysates and purified peptides can be considered as promising ingredients to develop superfoods with protective roles against hypertension and diabetes. Choi et al. (2019) used antioxidant hydrolysates released by single and sequential enzyme-mediated hydrolysis of wheat gluten to produce a functional chocolate beverage. The resulting functional beverages showed good functional and sensorial properties suggesting that the bioactive peptides originated from wheat proteins can be used in the formulation of antioxidant functional beverages. The hydrolysates formed by alcalase-mediated hydrolysis of amaranth proteins were employed to produce cookies with antihypertensive properties (Ontiveros et al. 2020). The efficiency of produced cookies to reduce the systolic blood pressure was investigated in spontaneously hypertensive rats. The results showed that the antihypertensive activity of the hydrolysate was not affected by the baking process of cookies, and they were effectively able to reduce the blood pressure in the tested rats. The rice bran hydrolysates were also used as natural antioxidant ingredients in the formulation of fried fish cake (Supawong et al. 2019). Enriching with these bioactive peptides drastically improved the antioxidant properties of the resulting fish cakes. Therefore, the results indicated that the bioactive hydrolysates could be used as a safe and natural alternative to synthetic antioxidants in the formulation of food products, especially those which are susceptible to oxidation. The bioactive hydrolysates produced by hydrolysis of salmon proteins using alcalase and papain were used to fortify the whole wheat cracker (Idowu et al. 2019). The analysis showed a better nutritional profile for fortified crackers compared to the control sample without the fortification. Moreover, it was investigated that the physical, textural, and sensorial properties of crackers were affected by enriching with protein hydrolysates. The enriched crackers can be consumed as superfoods owing to their improved nutritional values. The shrimp protein hydrolysate powder was also used to produce functional biscuits (Sinthusamran et al. 2019). These hydrolysates were produced by the action of alcalase for two h. It was shown that the fortification of biscuits with shrimp protein hydrolysates at a level of 5% of four substitutions could improve their nutritive value and acceptability. The fortification also can modify the rheological and textural properties of the final product. The hydrolysates from food proteins were also used as fat replacer to produce low-fat functional foods. In this regard, the hydrolysates from soy proteins (Chen et al. 2019) and camel milk caseins (Hajian et al. 2020) were used to develop low-fat functional ice creams. The resulting ice creams had good sensorial.

3 Conclusion

Nutraceuticals and superfoods enriched in the bioactive compounds represent a unique group of healthcare products. The tendency to find new ways of shielding health as well as the consumer demand for healthy and health-enhancing functional foods resulted in the continuous spread of superfoods. It is well-known the stable and meticulous consumption of nutraceuticals and superfoods in a balanced diet can improve human health and also can prevent chronic diseases. The literature review suggested that the consumption of nutraceuticals such as curcumin, pomegranate, biologically active peptides, camel milk, and walnut, as investigated in this study, can result in the overall health improvement and the treatment of certain diseases. Despite having many health-promoting properties, few studies have been conducted on superfoods (especially on their commercialization) as well as the incorporation of different nutraceutical into the food products, and there are still many challenges in these areas. Therefore, more well-conducted studies are needed to address these challenges attributed to the claimed biological properties of superfoods.

References

Agrawal R, Beniwal R, Sharma S, Kochar D, Tuteja F, Ghorui S, Sahani M (2005) Effect of raw camel milk in type 1 diabetic patients: 1 year randomised study. J Camel Pract Res 12(1):27

Ahmadiankia N (2019) Molecular targets of pomegranate (Punica Granatum) in preventing cancer metastasis. Iran J Basic Med Sci 22(9):977

Alavi F, Salami M, Emam-Djomeh Z, Mohammadian M (2017) Nutraceutical properties of camel milk. In: Nutrients in dairy and their implications on health and disease. Elsevier, pp 451–468

Alavi F, Jamshidian M, Rezaei K (2019) Applying native proteases from melon to hydrolyze kilka fish proteins (clupeonella cultriventris caspia) compared to commercial enzyme alcalase. Food Chem 277:314–322

Ali MN, Prasad SG, Singh M (2016) Functional, antioxidant and sensory qualities of ice-cream from pomegranate seed powder. Asian J Chem 28(9):2013

Ali A, Ahmad U, Akhtar J, Khan MM (2019) Engineered nano scale formulation strategies to augment efficiency of nutraceuticals. J Func Foods 62:103554

Alsuhaibani AM, Al-Kuraieef AN (2019) Effect of phenolic compounds and fatty acid contents of walnut seeds on streptozotocin-induced diabetes in rats. J Food Measure Charac 13(1):499–505

Altunkaya A, Hedegaard RV, Brimer L, Gökmen V, Skibsted LH (2013) Antioxidant capacity versus chemical safety of wheat bread enriched with pomegranate peel powder. Food Func 4(5):722–727

Andrade MA, Lima V, Silva AS, Vilarinho F, Castilho MC, Khwaldia K, Ramos F (2019) Pomegranate and grape by-products and their active compounds: are they a valuable source for food applications? Trends Food Sci Technol 86:68–84

Assis RP, Arcaro CA, Gutierres VO, Oliveira JO, Costa PI, Baviera AM, Brunetti IL (2017) Combined effects of curcumin and lycopene or bixin in yoghurt on inhibition of Ldl oxidation and increases in Hdl and paraoxonase levels in streptozotocin-diabetic rats. Int J Mol Sci 18(4):332

Ayoub MA, Palakkott AR, Ashraf A, Iratni R (2018) The molecular basis of the anti-diabetic properties of camel milk. Diabetes Res Clin Pract 146:305–312

Ayyash M, Al-Dhaheri AS, Al Mahadin S, Kizhakkayil J, Abushelaibi A (2018) In vitro investigation of anticancer, antihypertensive, antidiabetic, and antioxidant activities of camel milk fermented with camel milk probiotic: a comparative study with fermented bovine milk. J Dairy Sci 101(2):900–911

Bassiri-Jahromi S (2018) Punica granatum (pomegranate) activity in health promotion and cancer prevention. Oncol Rev 12(1)

Bhol S, Lanka D, Bosco SJD (2016) Quality characteristics and antioxidant properties of breads incorporated with pomegranate whole fruit bagasse. J Food Sci Technol 53(3):1717–1721

Borrin TR, Georges EL, Brito-Oliveira TC, Moraes IC, Pinho SC (2018) Technological and sensory evaluation of pineapple ice creams incorporating curcumin-loaded nanoemulsions obtained by the emulsion inversion point method. Int J Dairy Technol 71(2):491–500

Çam M, Erdoğan F, Aslan D, Dinç M (2013) Enrichment of functional properties of ice cream with pomegranate by-products. J Food Sci 78(10):C1543–C1550

Chalamaiah M, Yu W, Wu J (2018) Immunomodulatory and anticancer protein hydrolysates (peptides) from food proteins: a review. Food Chem 245:205–222

Chang C, Meikle TG, Su Y, Wang X, Dekiwadia C, Drummond CJ, Conn CE, Yang Y (2019) Encapsulation in egg white protein nanoparticles protects antioxidant activity of curcumin. Food Chem 280:65–72

Chatterjee A, Kanawjia S, Khetra Y (2016) Properties of sweetened indian yogurt (mishti dohi) as affected by added tryptic whey protein hydrolysate. J Food Sci Technol 53(1):824–831

Chen F-P, Li B-S, Tang C-H (2015) Nanocomplexation of soy protein isolate with curcumin: influence of ultrasonic treatment. Food Res Int 75:157–165

Chen W, Liang G, Li X, He Z, Zeng M, Gao D, Qin F, Goff HD, Chen J (2019) Effects of soy proteins and hydrolysates on fat globule coalescence and meltdown properties of ice cream. Food Hydrocolloids 94:279–286

Cho K, Baik M, Choi Y, Hahm Y, Kim B (2010) Manufacture of the functional drink using hydrolysate from oyster and other extracts. J Food Qual 33:1–13

Choi YLT, He Y, Hwang KT (2019) Chemical characteristics and antioxidant properties of wheat gluten hydrolysates produced by single and sequential enzymatic hydrolyses using commercial proteases and their application in beverage system. J Food Measure Char 13:745–754

Crowley P, O'brien C, Slattery H, Chapman D, Arendt E, Stanton C (2002) Functional properties of casein hydrolysates in bakery applications. Eur Food Res Technol 215(2):131–137

David S, Zagury Y, Livney YD (2015) Soy β-conglycinin—curcumin nanocomplexes for enrichment of clear beverages. Food Biophys 10(2):195–206

Egerton S, Culloty S, Whooley J, Stanton C, Ross RP (2018) Characterization of protein hydrolysates from blue whiting (micromesistius poutassou) and their application in beverage fortification. Food Chem 245:698–706

El Sohaimy S (2012) Functional foods and nutraceuticals-modern approach to food science. World Appl Sci J 20(5):691–708

Esmaili M, Ghaffari SM, Moosavi-Movahedi Z, Atri MS, Sharifizadeh A, Farhadi M, Yousefi R, Chobert J-M, Haertlé T, Moosavi-Movahedi AA (2011) Beta casein-micelle as a nano vehicle for solubility enhancement of curcumin; food industry application. LWT-Food Sci Technol 44(10):2166–2172

Fallah Z, Ejtahed H-S, Mirmiran P, Naslaji AN, Movahedi AM, Azizi F (2020) Effect of camel milk on glycaemic control and lipid profile of patients with type 2 diabetes: randomised controlled clinical trial. Int Dairy J 101:104568

Fateh MV, Ahmed S, Ali M, Bandyopadhyay S (2013) A Review on the medicinal importance of pomegranate. J Pharm Sci 3(4):23–25

Feng L, Peng F, Wang X, Li M, Lei H, Xu H (2019) Identification and characterization of antioxidative peptides derived from simulated in vitro gastrointestinal digestion of walnut meal proteins. Food Res Int 116:518–526

Fritz M, Vecchi B, Rinaldi G, Añón MC (2011) Amaranth seed protein hydrolysates have in vivo and in vitro antihypertensive activity. Food Chem 126(3):878–884

Gani A, Broadway A, Ahmad M, Ashwar BA, Wani AA, Wani SM, Masoodi F, Khatkar BS (2015) Effect of whey and casein protein hydrolysates on rheological, textural and sensory properties of cookies. J Food Sci Technol 52(9):5718–5726

Ghaffari S, Roshanravan N (2020) The role of nutraceuticals in prevention and treatment of hypertension: an updated review of the literature. Food Res Int 128:108749

Gorji N, Moeini R, Memariani Z (2018) Almond, hazelnut and walnut, three nuts for neuroprotection in Alzheimer's disease: a neuropharmacological review of their bioactive constituents. Pharmacol Res 129:115–127

Goudarzi M, Madadlou A, Mousavi ME, Emam-Djomeh Z (2015) Formulation of apple juice beverages containing whey protein isolate or whey protein hydrolysate based on sensory and physicochemical analysis. Int J Dairy Technol 68(1):70–78

Grace MH, Warlick CW, Neff SA, Lila MA (2014) Efficient preparative isolation and identification of walnut bioactive components using high-speed counter-current chromatography and Lc-Esi-It-Tof-Ms. Food Chem 158:229–238

Gutierres VO, Pinheiro CM, Assis RP, Vendramini RC, Pepato MT, Brunetti IL (2012) Curcumin-supplemented yoghurt improves physiological and biochemical markers of experimental diabetes. Br J Nutr 108(3):440–448

Hajian N, Salami M, Mohammadian M, Moghadam M, Emam-Djomeh Z (2020) Production of low-fat camel milk functional ice creams fortified with camel milk casein and its antioxidant hydrolysates. Appl Food Biotechnol 7(2):95–102

Hardman WE (2014) Walnuts have potential for cancer prevention and treatment in mice. J Nutrition 144(4):555S-560S

Hasson S, Al-Busaidi JZ, Al-Qarni Z, Rajapakse S, Al-Bahlani S, Idris MA, Sallam TA (2015) In vitro apoptosis triggering in the Bt-474 human breast cancer cell line by lyophilised camel's milk. Asian Pacific J Cancer Prevent 16(15):6651–6661

Idowu AT, Benjakul S, Sinthusamran S, Pongsetkul J, Sae-Leaw T, Sookchoo P (2019) Whole wheat cracker fortified with biocalcium and protein hydrolysate powders from salmon frame: characteristics and nutritional value. Food Qual Saf 3(3):191–199

Izadi A, Khedmat L, Mojtahedi SY (2019) Nutritional and therapeutic perspectives of camel milk and its protein hydrolysates: a review on versatile biofunctional properties. J Func Foods 60:103441

Jahanban-Esfahlan A, Ostadrahimi A, Tabibiazar M, Amarowicz R (2019) A comparative review on the extraction, antioxidant content and antioxidant potential of different parts of walnut (Juglans Regia L.) fruit and tree. Molecules 24(11):2133

Jahanbani R, Ghaffari SM, Salami M, Vahdati K, Sepehri H, Sarvestani NN, Sheibani N, Moosavi-Movahedi AA (2016) Antioxidant and anticancer activities of walnut (Juglans Regia L.) protein hydrolysates using different proteases. Plant Foods Human Nutrition 71(4):402–409

Jahanbani R, Ghaffari M, Vahdati K, Salami M, Khalesi M, Sheibani N, Moosavi-Movahedi AA (2018) Kinetics study of protein hydrolysis and inhibition of angiotensin converting enzyme by peptides hydrolysate extracted from walnut. Int J Pept Res Ther 24(1):77–85

Joung HJ, Choi MJ, Kim JT, Park SH, Park HJ, Shin GH (2016) Development of food-grade curcumin nanoemulsion and its potential application to food beverage system: antioxidant property and in vitro digestion. J Food Sci 81(3):N745–N753

Kamal H, Jafar S, Mudgil P, Murali C, Amin A, Maqsood S (2018) Inhibitory properties of camel whey protein hydrolysates toward liver cancer cells, dipeptidyl peptidase-Iv, and inflammation. J Dairy Sci 101(10):8711–8720

Khalesi M, Salami M, Moslehishad M, Winterburn J, Moosavi-Movahedi AA (2017) Biomolecular content of camel milk: a traditional superfood towards future healthcare industry. Trends Food Sci Technol 62:49–58

Kharat M, McClements DJ (2019) Recent advances in colloidal delivery systems for nutraceuticals: a case study-delivery by design of curcumin. J Colloid Interf Sci 557:506–518

Khwairakpam AD, Bordoloi D, Thakur KK, Monisha J, Arfuso F, Sethi G, Mishra S, Kumar AP, Kunnumakkara AB (2018) Possible use of punica granatum (pomegranate) in cancer therapy. Pharmacol Res 133:53–64

Korashy HM, Maayah ZH, Abd-Allah AR, El-Kadi AO, Alhaider AA (2012) Camel milk triggers apoptotic signaling pathways in human hepatoma Hepg2 and breast cancer Mcf7 cell lines through transcriptional mechanism. J Biomed Biotechnol

Kotha RR, Luthria DL (2019) Curcumin: biological, pharmaceutical, nutraceutical, and analytical aspects. Molecules 24(16):2930

Krishnankutty R, Iskandarani A, Therachiyil L, Uddin S, Azizi F, Kulinski M, Bhat AA, Mohammad RM (2018) Anticancer activity of camel milk via induction of autophagic death in human colorectal and breast cancer cells. Asian Pacific J Cancer Prevent APJCP 19(12):3501

Kumar DD, Mann B, Pothuraju R, Sharma R, Bajaj R (2016) Formulation and characterization of nanoencapsulated curcumin using sodium caseinate and its incorporation in ice cream. Food Func 7(1):417–424

Labuckas DO, Maestri DM, Perello M, Martínez ML, Lamarque AL (2008) Phenolics from walnut (Juglans Regia L.) kernels: antioxidant activity and interactions with proteins. Food Chem 107(2):607–612

Lafarga T, Hayes M (2017) Bioactive protein hydrolysates in the functional food ingredient industry: overcoming current challenges. Food Rev Int 33(3):217–246

Li M, Cui J, Ngadi MO, Ma Y (2015) Absorption mechanism of whey-protein-delivered curcumin using Caco-2 cell monolayers. Food Chem 180:48–54

Li Y, Ye T, Yang F, Hu M, Liang L, He H, Li Z, Zeng A, Li Y, Yao Y (2016) Punica Granatum (pomegranate) peel extract exerts potent antitumor and anti-metastasis activity in thyroid cancer. RSC Adv 6(87):84523–84535

Lim HS, Ghafoor K, Park SH, Hwang SY, Park J (2010) Quality and antioxidant properties of yellow layer cake containing Korean turmeric (Curcuma Longa L.) powder. J Food Nutrition Res 49(3)

Lim S-M, Lee N-K, Park K-K, Yoon YC, Paik H-D (2011) Ace-inhibitory effect and physicochemical characteristics of yogurt beverage fortified with whey protein hydrolysates. Korean J Food Sci Animal Res 31:886–892

Logarušić M, Slivac I, Radošević K, Bagović M, Redovniković IR, Srček VG (2019) Hempseed protein hydrolysates' effects on the proliferation and induced oxidative stress in normal and cancer cell lines. Mol Biol Rep 46(6):6079–6085

Ma G-Z, Wang C-M, Li L, Ding N, Gao X-L (2015) Effect of pomegranate peel polyphenols on human prostate cancer Pc-3 cells in vivo. Food Sci Biotechnol 24(5):1887–1892

Mann B, Kumari A, Kumar R, Sharma R, Prajapati K, Mahboob S, Athira S (2015) Antioxidant activity of whey protein hydrolysates in milk beverage system. J Food Sci Technol 52(6):3235–3241

Moghadam M, Salami M, Mohammadian M, Delphi L, Sepehri H, Emam-Djomeh Z, Moosavi-Movahedi AA (2020a) Walnut protein-curcumin complexes: fabrication, structural characterization, antioxidant properties, and in vitro anticancer activity. J Food Measure Char 14(2):876–885

Moghadam M, Salami M, Mohammadian M, Emam-Djomeh Z, Jahanbani R, Moosavi-Movahedi AA (2020) Physicochemical and bio-functional properties of walnut proteins as affected by trypsin-mediated hydrolysis. Food Biosci 100611

Mohammadian M, Madadlou A (2016) Characterization of fibrillated antioxidant whey protein hydrolysate and comparison with fibrillated protein solution. Food Hydrocolloids 52:221–230

Mohammadian M, Salami M, Emam-Djomeh Z, Alavi F (2017) Nutraceutical properties of dairy bioactive peptides. In: Dairy in human health and disease across the lifespan. Elsevier, pp 325–342

Mohammadian M, Salami M, Momen S, Alavi F, Emam-Djomeh Z, Moosavi-Movahedi AA (2019a) Enhancing the aqueous solubility of curcumin at acidic condition through the complexation with whey protein nanofibrils. Food Hydrocol 87:902–914

Mohammadian M, Salami M, Momen S, Alavi F, Emam-Djomeh Z (2019b) Fabrication of curcumin-loaded whey protein microgels: structural properties, antioxidant activity, and in vitro release behavior. LWT-Food Sci Technol 103:94–100

Momen S, Salami M, Alavi F, Emam-Djomeh Z, Moosavi-Movahedi AA (2019) The techno-functional properties of camel whey protein compared to bovine whey protein for fabrication a model high protein emulsion. LWT-Food Sci Technol 101:543–550

Mousavinejad G, Emam-Djomeh Z, Rezaei K, Khodaparast MHH (2009) Identification and quantification of phenolic compounds and their effects on antioxidant activity in pomegranate juices of eight Iranian cultivars. Food Chem 115(4):1274–1278

Nagel JM, Brinkoetter M, Magkos F, Liu X, Chamberland JP, Shah S, Zhou J, Blackburn G, Mantzoros CS (2012) Dietary walnuts inhibit colorectal cancer growth in mice by suppressing angiogenesis. Nutrition 28(1):67–75

Nikmaram P, Mousavi SM, Emam-Djomeh Z, Kiani H, Razavi SH (2015) Evaluation and prediction of metabolite production, antioxidant activities, and survival of lactobacillus casei 431 in a pomegranate juice supplemented yogurt drink using support vector regression. Food Sci Biotechnol 24(6):2105–2112

Obaroakpo JU, Liu L, Zhang S, Lu J, Pang X, Lv J (2019) A-glucosidase and ace dual inhibitory protein hydrolysates and peptide fractions of sprouted quinoa yoghurt beverages inoculated with lactobacillus casei. Food Chem 299:124985

Ontiveros N, López-Teros V, de Jesús V-J, Islas-Rubio AR, Cárdenas-Torres FI, Cuevas-Rodríguez E-O, Reyes-Moreno C, Granda-Restrepo DM, Lopera-Cardona S, Ramírez-Torres GI (2020) Amaranth-hydrolyzate enriched cookies reduce the systolic blood pressure in spontaneously hypertensive rats. J Func Foods 64:103613

Pan K, Luo Y, Gan Y, Baek SJ, Zhong Q (2014) Ph-driven encapsulation of curcumin in self-assembled casein nanoparticles for enhanced dispersibility and bioactivity. Soft Matter 10(35):6820–6830

Park SH, Lim HS, Hwang S-Y (2012) Evaluation of antioxidant, rheological, physical and sensorial properties of wheat flour dough and cake containing turmeric powder. Food Sci Technol Int 18(5):435–443

Piccolella S, Crescente G, Candela L, Pacifico S (2019) Nutraceutical polyphenols: new analytical challenges and opportunities. J Pharm Biomed Anal 175:112774

Proestos C (2018) Superfoods: recent data on their role in the prevention of diseases. Curr Res Nutrition Food Sci J 6(3):576–593

Reiter RJ, Tan D-X, Manchester LC, Korkmaz A, Fuentes-Broto L, Hardman WE, Rosales-Corral SA, Qi W (2013) A walnut-enriched diet reduces the growth of Lncap human prostate cancer xenografts in nude mice. Cancer Invest 31(6):365–373

Rossini K, Norena CP, Cladera-Olivera F, Brandelli A (2009) Casein peptides with inhibitory activity on lipid oxidation in beef homogenates and mechanically deboned poultry meat. LWT Food Sci Technol 42(4):862–867

Salami M, Moosavi-Movahedi AA, Moosavi-Movahedi F, Ehsani MR, Yousefi R, Farhadi M, Niasari-Naslaji A, Saboury AA, Chobert J-M, Haertlé T (2011) Biological activity of camel milk casein following enzymatic digestion. J Dairy Res 78(4):471

Sarmadi BH, Ismail A (2010) Antioxidative peptides from food proteins: a review. Peptides 31(10):1949–1956

Seo MJ, Park JE, Jang MS (2010) Optimization of sponge cake added with turmeric (Curcuma Longa L.) powder using mixture design. Food Sci Biotechnol 19(3):617–625

Shah NP (2007) Functional cultures and health benefits. Int Dairy J 17(11):1262–1277

Shinha R, Radha C, Prakash J, Kaul P (2007) Whey protein hydrolysate: functional properties, nutritional qualities, nutrional quality and utilization in beverage formulation. Food Chem 101:1484–1491

Sinthusamran S, Benjakul S, Kijroongrojana K, Prodpran T (2019) Chemical, physical, rheological and sensory properties of biscuit fortified with protein hydrolysate from cephalothorax of pacific white shrimp. J Food Sci Technol 56(3):1145–1154

Soriano-Hernandez AD, Madrigal-Perez DG, Galvan-Salazar HR, Arreola-Cruz A, Briseño-Gomez L, Guzmán-Esquivel J, Dobrovinskaya O, Lara-Esqueda A, Rodríguez-Sanchez IP, Baltazar-Rodriguez LM (2015) The protective effect of peanut, walnut, and almond consumption on the development of breast cancer. Gynecol Obstet Invest 80(2):89–92

Supawong S, Park JW, Thawornchinsombut S (2019) Effect of rice bran hydrolysates on physicochemical and antioxidative characteristics of fried fish cakes during repeated freeze-thaw cycles. Food Biosci 32:100471

Taghavi Kevij H, Mohammadian M, Salami M (2019) Complexation of curcumin with whey protein isolate for enhancing its aqueous solubility through a solvent-free Ph-driven approach. J Food Process Preserv 43(12):e14227

Tapal A, Tiku PK (2012) Complexation of curcumin with soy protein isolate and its implications on solubility and stability of curcumin. Food Chem 130(4):960–965

Topkaya C, Isik F (2019) Effects of pomegranate peel supplementation on chemical, physical, and nutritional properties of muffin cakes. J Food Process Preserv 43(6):e13868

Trigueros L, Wojdyło A, Sendra E (2014) Antioxidant activity and protein–polyphenol interactions in a pomegranate (Punica Granatum L.) yogurt. J Agric Food Chem 62(27):6417–6425

Umayaparvathi S, Arumugam M, Meenakshi S, Dräger G, Kirschning A, Balasubramanian T (2014) Purification and characterization of antioxidant peptides from oyster (saccostrea cucullata) hydrolysate and the anticancer activity of hydrolysate on human colon cancer cell lines. Int J Pept Res Ther 20(2):231–243

van den Driessche JJ, Plat J, Mensink RP (2018) Effects of superfoods on risk factors of metabolic syndrome: a systematic review of human intervention trials. Food Func 9(4):1944–1966

Viuda-Martos M, Ruiz-Navajas Y, Fernández-López J, Pérez-Álvarez J (2008) Functional properties of honey, propolis, and royal jelly. J Food Sci 73(9):R117–R124

Viuda-Martos M, Ruiz-Navajas Y, Fernández-López J, Pérez-Alvarez JA (2011) Spices as functional foods. Crit Rev Food Sci Nutritions 51(1):13–28

Vučić V, Grabež M, Trchounian A, Arsić A (2019) Composition and potential health benefits of pomegranate: a review. Curr Pharm Des 25(16):1817–1827

Wang Y-H, Wang J-M, Yang X-Q, Guo J, Lin Y (2015) Amphiphilic zein hydrolysate as a novel nano-delivery vehicle for curcumin. Food Func 6(8):2636–2645

Zheng B, Lin H, Zhang X, McClements DJ (2019) Fabrication of curcumin-loaded dairy milks using the ph-shift method: formation, stability, and bioaccessibility. J Agric Food Chem 67(44):12245–12254

Spices as Traditional Remedies: Scientifically Proven Benefits

Mona Miran, Maryam Salami, and Zahra Emam-Djomeh

Abstract

Spices have been added to foods for centuries as flavors, preservatives, and colors and have also been used in traditional medicine in various countries to treat many diseases. Spices play an important role in human health and can be considered as the first functional foods. Although the amount of spices consumed is very low compared to many other foods, the role of spices in the daily diet should not be underestimated due to their health properties. Saffron, ginger, cinnamon, and turmeric are four globally common spices that have been widely used owing to well-known medical benefits in different traditional medicine systems, including Ayurveda, traditional Chinese, and Persian medicine since ancient times. Some general or specific health benefits of these spices include anti-inflammatory, antioxidant, antimicrobial, anti-diabetic, and antihypertensive activities, which have potential protective properties against some ailments such as cancer, type 2 diabetes, neurodegenerative and cardiovascular diseases. Recent scientific studies on the therapeutic properties of these common spices have been reviewed in this chapter.

Keywords

Spices · Traditional medicine · Saffron · Ginger · Cinnamon · Turmeric · Therapeutic properties

1 Introduction

Spices and herbs have historically been utilized as flavors, preservatives, and therapeutic agents to fortify food. They have been used to increase food acceptability and improve their health. Herbs and spices have also been utilized for centuries by different cultures as food additives worldwide, to increase the organoleptic properties as well as shelf life by reducing or eliminating food-borne pathogens as preservatives (El-Sayed and Youssef 2019). Several spices are applied to prevent spoilage in pickles, bread, and meat products. The first scientific experiment regarding the preservative effect of spices was carried out in the 1880s, which demonstrated cinnamon oil has antibacterial properties against *Bacillus anthracisspores* El-Sayed and Youssef 2019; De and De 2019). Studies done over the

M. Miran · M. Salami · Z. Emam-Djomeh (✉)
Department of Food Science and Engineering, University College of Agriculture & Natural Resources, University of Tehran, Karaj, Iran
e-mail: emamj@ut.ac.ir

M. Miran
e-mail: mona.miran@ut.ac.ir

M. Salami
e-mail: msalami@ut.ac.ir

last decades validate the inhibition of the growth of gram-negative and gram-positive foodborne bacteria, mold, and yeast by spices such as cinnamon, turmeric, thyme, garlic, cloves and onions (De and De 2019).

Spices and herbs are low-priced products, but they have been worth as much as gold and jewelry for centuries (El-Sayed and Youssef 2019; De and De 2019). Besides culinary use for taste, they also have been used as medicines, cosmetics, perfumes, soap producing, and pesticides. Natural yellow and red color made from saffron and turmeric were utilized as colorants. Spices have been one of the most precious commercial goods in the middle ages and ancient times (De and De 2019).

Due to the well-known medical benefits of spices and herbs, they have been utilized for treating various ailments since ancient times (Vázquez-Fresno et al. 2019). Herbs and spices have been used for hundreds of years in different forms of traditional medicine such as Persian, Chinese, Greek, ancient Rome, Ayurveda, Sino-Tibetan, and Unani systems (Akaberi et al. 2019). Spices are heavily involved in the treatment of significant body disorders in Ayurveda. They are formally identified as a medicine in many countries such as China, India, Europe, and the United States. Spices and herbs are applied as antiseptics, carminatives, or masking drugs. In most cases, homeopathic medicine has used spices as one of the most critical ingredients (De and De 2019).

Spices play a key role in people's health and disease and might be regarded as the first functional food. Daily use of spices at low doses over the long term shows beneficial effects beyond their role in the transfer of flavor and aroma to food (De and De 2019). Numerous studies of spices have recognized their customary role in the drug. Some of the beneficial effects on human health through the impact of herbs and spices include anti-inflammatory, antioxidant, immunemodulatory, anti-proliferative, anti-hypercholesterolemic, analgesic, anti-pollutant, anti-obesity and anti-mutagenic properties in addition to protection against cardiovascular disease, arthritis, diabetes, neurodegeneration and some types of cancers comprising liver, stomach, breast, lung, cervix, prostate and colorectum (El-Sayed and Youssef 2019; De and De 2019; Vázquez-Fresno et al. 2019). Therefore, spices might be the primary source of therapeutic agents forthcoming (De and De 2019). Researchers have been able to isolate bioactive compounds from herbs and spices using modern scientific methods that can be used to produce drugs to treat various diseases (De and De 2019).

Spices can come from many different plants, including parts of plants, for instance, buds, barks, roots, seeds, and flowers. Volatile oils, non-volatile oils, and some resins give the spices a taste. Spices flavor a combination of phenols, alcohols, organic acids, esters, alkaloids, and sulfur (Table 1). Spices also contain common herbal ingredients like fiber, carbohydrates, tannins, protein, vitamins, and minerals (De and De 2019).

Around 86 varieties of spices are grown in various regions in the world (De and De 2019). This chapter is focused on four globally common spices, including saffron, ginger, cinnamon and turmeric.

2 Saffron

Saffron (*Crocus sativus* L.), the world's most precious spice, is grown in various countries such as Iran, Turkey, Greece, India, Spain, Morocco, and Italy with Middle East origin (Vázquez-Fresno et al. 2019; Melnyk et al. 2010). Saffron, also known as golden spice or Red Gold, is the dried stigmas of the saffron flower, which is the Iridaceae (Iris) family member (Melnyk et al. 2010). For producing one pound of saffron, approximately 75,000 crocus blossoms of the blue-purple saffron flower are needed. To protect volatile compounds, stigmas should be hand-picked (Melnyk et al. 2010).

Well-drained sand soils and warm subtropical climate are the most favorable conditions for saffron planting (Akaberi et al. 2019). Saffron is well adapted to extreme environmental conditions and requires low water and fertilizer. Therefore it has been considered one of the

Table 1 Characteristics and bioactive functions of four globally common spices

Name	Botanical name	Part of plants	Bioactive constituents	Bioactive function	References
Cinnamon	*Cinnamomum zeylanicum Blume*	Bark	Cinnamaldehyde, eugenol, linalool, ethyl cinnamate, methyl chavicol, beta-caryophyllene	Anti-inflammatory and antioxidant activity, Decrease triglycerides and cholesterol in the blood	El-Sayed and Youssef (2019), De and De (2019)
Ginger	*Zingiber officinale Roscoe*	Rhizome	Gingerols, galanolactone, 6-shogaol, gingerdione,	Strong anti-inflammatory, Pain killer, Nausea treatment	El-Sayed and Youssef (2019), De and De (2019)
Saffron	*Crocus Sativus*	Stigma	Safranal, crocin, picrocrocin, crocetin, quercetin, zeaxanthin, kaempferol, numerous α-carotene, and β-carotene, lycopene	Antibacterial, anti-inflammatory, antioxidant, antitumor, anti-apoptotic, antidepressant, anticonvulsant, hypolipidemic and hypotensive properties, memory enhancer, insulin resistance prevention, Neuroprotective Treatment of diseases including respiratory, gastrointestinal, cardiovascular, many types of cancers, Ocular, Urogenital, Alzheimer's, psychiatric, insomnia, fatigue and anxiety	Vázquez-Fresno et al. (2019), Akaberi et al. (2019), Melnyk et al. (2010), Boskabady et al. (2019), Ghaffari and Roshanravan (2019), Hosseini et al. (2018), Moshiri et al. (2015)
Turmeric	*Curcuma longa Linn*	Rhizome	Curcuminoids (curcumin and demethoxycurcumin)	Powerful anti-inflammatory, Strong antioxidant, Combat Alzheimer's	El-Sayed and Youssef (2019), De and De (2019)

sustainable agriculture and low-input farming systems (Ghanbari et al. 2019). The most important factors which influence the taste and flavor of saffron are harvesting and drying processes (Akaberi et al. 2019).

Iran is the largest producer of this golden spice. Saffron is famous for its impressive traditional applications (Akaberi et al. 2019). It is traditionally utilized as a fragrant, seasoning, flavoring, and coloring agent (Melnyk et al. 2010; Ghanbari et al. 2019). By far, the most popular use of saffron is as a food additive for cooking purposes. Saffron is well known in traditional medical systems around the world, and many reports highlight its ethnic medical applications. Saffron has been used for healing or culinary purposes in Iran for several centuries. In ancient Iranian textbooks, scientists such as Ibn Sina and Razi have described the medicinal properties of saffron (Akaberi et al. 2019). In Iranian traditional medicine, saffron has received much attention due to its many therapeutic properties, including sedative agent, improving the infectious wounds and uterus disorders, strengthening the liver and stomach (Rezaee-Khorasany et al. 2019). As can be seen in Traditional Medicine textbooks, Iranian physicians have prescribed saffron commonly in a single drug or combination with other spices or herbs (Akaberi et al. 2019). In Traditional and modern data, it has extensively been used for healing the respiratory, gastrointestinal, cardiovascular, insulin resistance, Alzheimer's, psychiatric, insomnia, depression, fatigue and anxiety in addition to most cancers (Akaberi et al. 2019; Melnyk et al. 2010).

The cardiovascular effects of saffron are due to (a) Anti-inflammatory, antioxidant, and anti-apoptotic properties (b) Hypolipidemic and hypotensive activities (Ghaffari and Roshanravan 2019). Moreover, it has been used as an antitumor, antidepressant, and anticonvulsant agent. It has the potential to enhance memory, immune, and radical scavenging (Hosseini et al. 2018; Moshiri et al. 2015). However, more clinical trials are needed to verify the therapeutic properties of the golden spice (Akaberi et al. 2019).

More than 150 volatile and non-volatile components exist in golden spice. The major compounds present in saffron's volatile oil are terpenes, terpene alcohols, and their esters, which safranal is the main volatile components (70%) (Vázquez-Fresno et al. 2019; Akaberi et al. 2019; Boskabady et al. 2019). The main non-volatile components present in saffron are crocins, picrocrocin, crocetin, and flavonoids, such as quercetin and kaempferol (Akaberi et al. 2019; Boskabady et al. 2019) (Table 1). Different health advantages of saffron are owing to its antioxidant potential and bioactive compounds (Melnyk et al. 2010; Ghanbari et al. 2019). Various phytochemicals commonly found in saffron, including crocin, crocetin, picrocrocin, and safranal, are the most studied bioactives in several in vitro and in vivo studies (Melnyk et al. 2010). Besides the four bioactives mentioned above, saffron contains minerals, essential oils, and tiny amounts of riboflavin and thiamine (Shahi et al. 2016; Garavand et al. 2019). Crocin, picrocrocin, and safranal respectively result in the color, bitterness, and aroma of the saffron (Zhang et al. 2019).

Crocin, a water-soluble carotenoid, includes the crocetin and gentiobiose, which has strong free-radical scavenging property and various medicinal effects, containing anti-Schizophrenia, anti-Alzheimer's, memory boosters, hypolipidemic, antioxidant, anticancer, and antiatherosclerotic impact (Garavand et al. 2019; Zhang et al. 2019). Picrocrocin displayed anti-cancer and anti-proliferate activities. Two unstable, volatile constituents, including safranal and isophorone, are derived from picrocrocin. These components have anti-convulsant and anti-depressant activities (Garavand et al. 2019).

Clinical findings indicate that saffron is a safe and beneficial herb (Shahi et al. 2016). Research results showed that saffron and its constituents at a smaller concentration or medicinal doses do not lead to any harmful effects on the body (Ghaffari and Roshanravan 2019). It should be considered that doses used in the investigations that reported side effects are remarkably higher than the amount of saffron used in daily dietary intakes (Shahi et al. 2016). Regarding lethal dose (LD_{50}) values of saffron, 20 g/kg has been determined as lethal dose, 5 g/kg as toxic, and 1/5 g/day as safe (Bukhari et al. 2018). It is worth noting that previous reports of toxicity of saffron have observed in the case of gestation when the continuous dosage is over 10 g stimulates uterine and abortion (Ghaffari and Roshanravan 2019).

In the food industry, saffron is used as a natural food flavoring without restriction based on the FDA rules. The stigma of yellow saffron should be yellow, and the highest external organic constituents, only 10%. Volatiles and moisture content of dried saffron should not exceed 14%. The highest soluble ash and total ash content should not exceed 1%. Grinding saffron into powder is the best way to utilize it. To obtain the most beneficial properties of saffron and release the most flavor and color, it should be steeped into

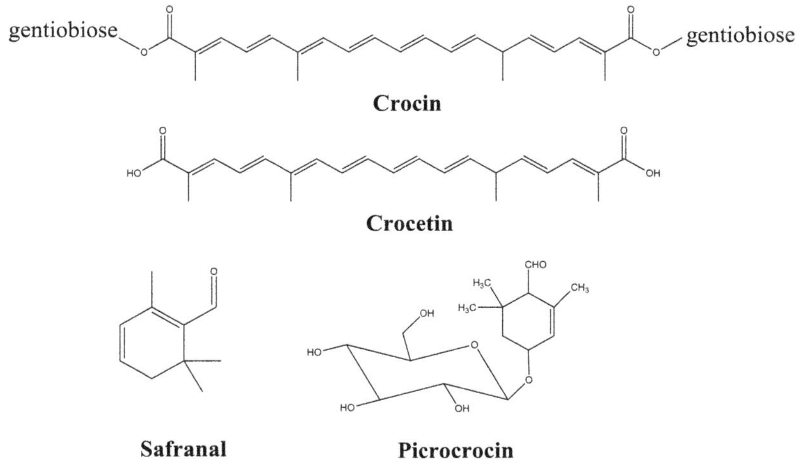

Fig. 1 Chemical structures of crocin, crocetin, picrocrocin, and safranal

boiling or hot water and avoid direct heating as it may reduce its properties (Ghaffari and Roshanravan 2019) (Fig. 1; Table 2).Please check and confirm if the inserted citations of Figs. 1–4 and Tables 2–5 are correct. If not, please suggest an alternate citations.Yes, they are correct

The extract from the cold-pressed saffron floral by-products in terms of in vitro antioxidant properties were investigated using the FRAP test and DPPH assay, and two models of lipid oxidation including activity in protection against Cu^{2+}-mediated degradation of the liposomal unsaturated fatty acids and preventing cholesterol degradation. On the other hand, in cancer Caco-2 cells, the cytotoxic activity of saffron extracts was evaluated using the MTT assay. Significant antioxidant activity in numerous in vitro systems of oxidative stress was obtained. Moreover, in colon cancer cells, a moderate impact on cell viability was observed (Tuberoso et al. 2016).

Saffron is considered to be precious in the prevention/treatment of age-related oxidative stress and diseases. Papandreou et al. observed that saffron significantly improved learning and memory, higher total brain antioxidant activity, decreased lipid peroxidation products, and decreased caspase-3 activity in mice. Meanwhile, a significant reduction in salt- and detergent-soluble acetylcholinesterase activity was observed only in adult mice (Papandreou et al. 2011).

Table 2 Important components of saffron's stigma with antioxidant capacity (Akaberi et al. 2019; Ghaffari and Roshanravan 2019; Zhang et al. 2019)

Family	Name	Point	Contribute to
Carotenoids	Crocin	Glucosyl esters of crocetin The major compound of saffron Water-soluble carotenoid	Color
	Crocetin		
	α-carotene		
	β-carotene		
	Zeaxanthin		
Flavonoids	Kaempferol		
	Quercetin		
Monoterpene aldehydes	Picocrocin		Bitterness
	Safranal	60–70% of volatile components	Aroma

Chronic stress has been shown to impair spatial learning and memory. In a study, the effect of saffron on learning and memory impairment, as well as the induction of oxidative stress in the hippocampus, were investigated. Rats were exposed to chronic restraint stress (6 h/day) with an injection of crocin or saffron extract for three weeks. Ghadrdoost et al. resulted that crocin and saffron could prevent learning and memory loss in addition to the damage to oxidative stress in the hippocampus due to chronic stress (Ghadrdoost et al. 2011).

Linardaki et al. investigated the probable reverse effects of saffron against established aluminum-toxicity. Exerted neurotoxic effects and metal accumulation in mice brain tissues was observed in a long-term administration of a relatively high dose of $AlCl_3$ through consuming of drinking water as confirmed by metal-induced inhibition of cholinesterase, decreased learning and memory capacity, the production of oxidative damage and changes of monoamine oxidase. Besides, short-term consumption of saffron extract had a positive effect on mouse brain oxidative stress, monoamine oxidase activity, and antioxidant status markers that were impaired by aluminum. According to the obtained findings, the biochemical changes support further investigation of the possibility of saffron as neuroprotective agents (Linardaki et al. 2013).

Asadollahi et al., in a randomized clinical trial, confirmed the short and long-term protective properties of saffron's aqueous extract as a neuroprotective natural product on ischemic stroke in humans during a four-day hospital stay and the three-month follow-up period (Asadollahi et al. 2019).

Shahmansouri et al. surveyed the influence of saffron on 40 patients who were suffering from mild to moderate depression with prior history of performing percutaneous coronary intervention (PCI) in the randomized, double-blind parallel-group for six weeks. The result showed the same antidepressant efficacy compared with fluoxetine (Shahmansouri et al. 2014).

Lopresti et al. examined the effect of the saffron extract on the treatment of mild-to-moderate depressive and anxiety symptoms in young people (aged from 12 to 16 years) for the first time. Sixty-eight participants have completed the randomized, double-blind, placebo-controlled study. The findings showed that the administration of saffron extract over two months helped to improve depressive and anxiety symptoms in adolescents with mild to moderate symptoms. And these advantageous effects were confirmed by parental observances. However, more significant improvements were informed by adolescents rather than parents (Lopresti et al. 2018).

Anti-obesity benefits of ethanolic extract of crocin and saffron were observed in the animal model (rats) in a study. Crocin showed a higher reduction level of total cholesterol and triacylglycerol of plasma. At the same time, saffron extract displayed significant improvement in low-density lipoprotein to high-density lipoprotein levels as the atherogenic index. Meanwhile, saffron extract appeared to reduce appetite considerably and food consumption (Mashmoul et al. 2014). Effect of saffron on lipid profile, antioxidant, and glycemic status in overweight/obese individuals with prediabetes was investigated with a randomized, double-blind, placebo-controlled trial method for eight weeks. The findings demonstrated that saffron supplementation could enhance glycemic index and antioxidant activity. However, no beneficial effect was found on anthropometric parameters and lipid profile (Karimi-Nazari et al. 2019).

Considering the therapeutic ability of saffron in diabetes treatment, Kang et al., demonstrated that saffron strongly enhanced glucose uptake and increased insulin sensitivity in muscle cells via multi-pathway mechanisms. Hypoglycemic action mechanism of saffron by examining its signaling pathways related to glucose metabolism in C_2C_{12} skeletal muscle cells was surveyed. Saffron plays an essential role in the glucose metabolism of differentiated C_2C_{12} skeletal muscle cells. Saffron-induced glucose uptake is directly associated with the activation of AMPK (AMP-activated protein kinase)/ACC (acetyl-CoA carboxylase) and MAPKs (mitogen-activated protein kinases) pathways. Saffron also enhances insulin sensitivity associated with basal glucose translocation of GLUT4 through both insulin-dependent (PI 3-kinase / Akt and mTOR) and insulin-independent (AMPK/ACC and MAPKs) pathways (Kang et al. 2012).

Effect of the aqueous saffron extract on diabetic rats induced with streptozotocin for the immunomodulatory effects was investigated by Samarghandian et al. Authors stated that saffron extract significantly decreased total lipids, triglycerides, cholesterol levels, blood glucose, nitric oxide, malondialdehyde and increased catalase, superoxide dismutase activities and glutathione level in the saffron-treated diabetic groups, in a dose-dependent manner. Saffron-treated diabetic rats were found to inhibit the expression of inflammatory cytokines in the abdominal aorta. As a result, the utilization of saffron to treat diabetes mellitus and its vascular complications was confirmed (Samarghandian et al. 2017).

In numerous experimental models of inflammation, oxidative stress, and cancer, saffron is known to be an active protective agent. Menghini et al. demonstrated protective effects exerted by saffron stigmas and byproducts (tepals + anther) extracts, in in vitro and ex vivo models of inflammation and oxidative stress. The antioxidant activity was surveyed through the assessment of reactive oxygen level and lactate dehydrogenase activity on mouse myoblast and human colon cancer cell lines. Saffron stigmas aqueous extract was the most useful in decreasing hydrogen peroxide-induced oxidative stress in both cell lines and in vitro assays and were rich in phenolic content. Both water extracts reduced lipopolysaccharide-induced malondialdehyde levels in rat colon specimens. Besides saffron stigmas and tepals + anther extract treatment on α-amylase, cholinesterases, and α-glucosidase activity was evaluated in vitro. Both extracts showed to be enzyme inhibitory agents (Menghini et al. 2018).

Protective activities of saffron extract, essential oil, crocin and safranal on bovine aortic endothelial cells against oxidative injury were investigated by Rahiman et al., According to the obtained data, anti-apoptotic and antioxidant properties of saffron and its significant compounds are mediated via mitogen-activated protein kinase signaling pathways. They may be of therapeutic potential to treat cardiovascular disease and endothelial dysfunction (Rahiman et al. 2018).

In a double-blinded parallel-group randomized test, 66 patients with Irritable Bowel Syndrome participated for six weeks. The result showed that saffron might be a useful treatment for Irritable Bowel Syndrome with no remarkable difference with fluoxetine with similar anxiolytic and antidepressive properties (Najafabadi et al. 2019).

Alcohol detoxification has been another critical feature of saffron in traditional medicine. Rezaee-Khorasany et al. demonstrated that aqueous extract of saffron has protective effects against ethanol-induced renal toxicity and hepatotoxicity in rat liver and kidney via anti-inflammatory, anti-apoptosis and antioxidant properties through reducing the levels of caspase-3, caspase-8 and caspase-9 (Rezaee-Khorasany et al. 2019).

One of the essential points regarding the growing pharmaceutical usage of saffron is the probable interactions between its bioactive compounds and the activity of the enzymes involved in the biotransformation of medicines that are used clinically. The activity of phase I and II enzymes involved in xenobiotic metabolism may be affected by aqueous herbal extracts. Begas et al. studied the effects of usage of saffron infusion on the in vivo activity of xenobiotic-metabolizing enzymes in humans. It was observed that short-term usage of saffron infusion could not lead to remarkable interactions of herb-drug under the CYP2A6, XO, and NAT2 enzyme activities, except for possible interactions with xenobiotics metabolized by CYP1A2 in males (Begas et al. 2019).

3 Ginger

Ginger (*Zingiber officinale Roscoe*) is a spice belonging to the *Zingiberaceae* family derived from the root or rhizome of the ginger plant, which is a tropical plant (Vázquez-Fresno et al. 2019). This plant is native to Southeast Asia (supposed to be originated from India). Its commercial cultivation is not limited to Southeast Asia and is also grown in other tropical and subtropical countries of Africa and South America (Arablou and Aryaeian 2018; Krüger et al. 2018). It is widely cultivated in India, China, Africa, Jamaica, Mexico, and Hawaii (Murthy and Gautam 2015).

Volatile oils (1–3% by weight of fresh ginger) and non-volatile oleoresin from ginger rhizomes are responsible for pungency, scent, aroma and flavor characteristics of ginger, about 25% of the components in each segment are responsible for the pungent taste (Vázquez-Fresno et al. 2019; Krüger et al. 2018). Various types of active compounds in ginger, including (6-, 8- and 10-gingerols), shogaols (6-, 8- and 10-shogaols) have been identified (Vázquez-Fresno et al. 2019). These phenolic components are mainly gingerols and, to a lesser extent, shogaols (Krüger et al. 2018). The other components of ginger include 6-paradol, zingerone, zerumbone, and dehydrozingerone (Choi et al. 2018). The essential pungent compounds in the fresh ginger rhizome are gingerols (especially 6-gingerol), with a ratio of 10: 1 6-gingerol to 6-shogaol. But when the ginger is dried, the amount of shogaols increases significantly, and the ratio of 6-gingerol to 6-shogaol increases to 1:1 (Vázquez-Fresno et al. 2019). As a result, 6-shogaol is mainly responsible for the rise in pungent taste in ginger during storage and in dried products (Vázquez-Fresno et al. 2019; Krüger et al. 2018). Furthermore, 6-paradol has a biotransformed metabolite of 6-shogaol, which is a non-pungent compound (Choi et al. 2017) (Fig. 2).

Ginger has long been utilized extensively as an old culinary additive as hot, aromatic spice. This popular spice has been used worldwide in foods, desserts, and drinks. Ginger, as a popular medicine, has been utilized in the prevention and treatment of many diseases for centuries. It has also been used as a dietary supplement (De and De 2019; Arablou and Aryaeian 2018).

Ginger has been utilized in a traditional ethnomedicinal system like Ayurveda and Traditional Chinese medicine. Ginger has long been used to treat a wide variety of diseases such as diarrhea, nausea, stomachache, arthritis, toothache, gingivitis, and respiratory infections in traditional medicine (Jafarzadeh and Nemati 2018).

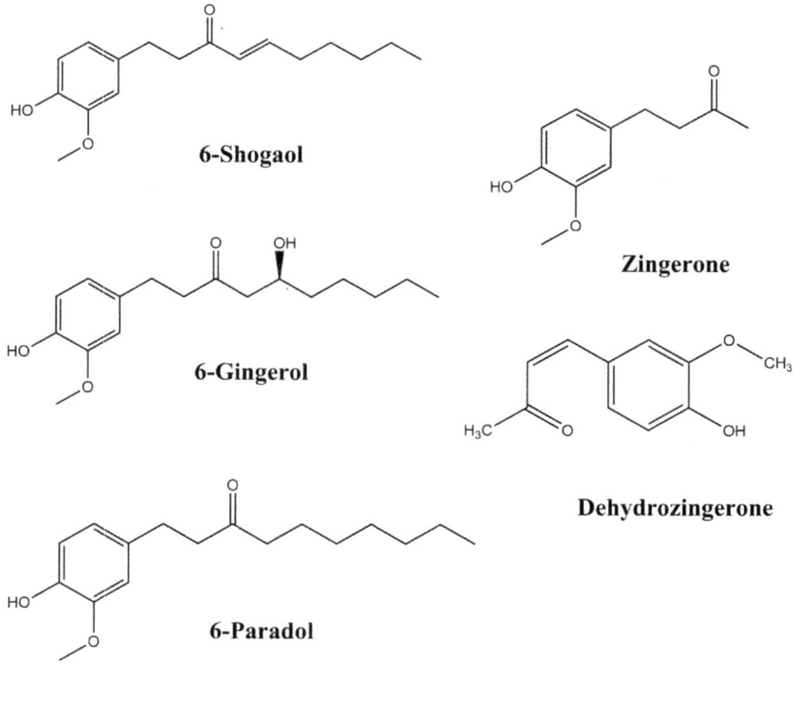

Fig. 2 Chemical structures of some ginger-derived compounds

Ginger has long been utilized as a pain killer for a variety of aches and pains. For example, an ointment that has been prepared by rubbing dried ginger with a little water on a grinding stone should be placed on the forehead to relieve the headache. Besides, a few drops of ginger juice can be used to relieve earache. It also reduces toothache when used on the gum (De and De 2019).

Useful properties of ginger that have been proven in in vitro and in vivo studies include antibacterial, antifungal, anti-inflammatory, antioxidant, cancer preventive, antipyretic, antilipidemic, anti-tumorigenic, acetylcholinesterase inhibitory, anticoagulation, antiangiogenic, as well as positive effects on blood pressure, blood clotting, and the gastrointestinal tract (De and De 2019; Arablou and Aryaeian 2018; Krüger et al. 2018).

Ginger essential oils and oleoresin as decontaminating agents have been given special attention in the food industry, which is Generally Recognized as Safe. The growth of many microbes is inhibited by ginger. The phytochemicals in the essential oil and oleoresin inhibit bacterial growth to varying degrees against foodborne and food-spoilage pathogenic bacteria (De and De 2019; Murthy and Gautam 2015). Murthy et al. extracted ginger oleoresin using acetone and analyzed by high-performance liquid chromatography, which showed gingerol as a major component. It showed remarkable antioxidative, antimicrobial properties. Using ginger oleoresin as a natural preservative in sugarcane juice was powerful in inhibiting microbial proliferation, which provides food safety and nutritional properties (Murthy and Gautam 2015).

In an overview of systematic reviews by Li et al., was demonstrated that ginger, as a promising efficacy herbal medicine, is useful for vomiting and nausea, pain and metabolic syndrome (Li et al. 2019a).

Tóth et al. assessed systematically the effectiveness of ginger on postoperative vomiting and nausea, based on placebo-controlled clinical trials. In this meta-analysis review, they concluded that ginger is safe and well-tolerated. The severity of postoperative nausea and vomiting is reduced by ginger and may also decrease the incidence of postoperative vomiting and nausea. They suggested that ginger may be a favorable alternative to antiemetic medications to reduce postoperative nausea and vomiting (Tóth et al. 2018) (Table 3).

To treat several inflammatory diseases, ginger has been used. In some experimental and clinical studies, anti-inflammatory, antioxidative, and immunomodulatory properties of ginger and its several components have been proven (Jafarzadeh and Nemati 2018).

In inflammatory bowel disease, colitis is a regular pathological lesion. In a study, improvement of 2,4,6-trinitrobenzene sulphonic acid-induced colitis in mice via ginger extract and zingerone was observed in a dose-dependent manner through modulation of nuclear factor-κB activity and interleukin-1β signaling pathway. Hsiang et al. have demonstrated that ginger may be utilized as a dietary supplement to prevent and treat patients with inflammatory bowel disease (Hsiang et al. 2013).

Table 3 Traditional and modern medicinal applications of ginger

Traditional medicine	Modern application	References
• Useful for nausea and vomiting • Treat cough • Stop bleeding • Useful for asthma • Detoxify toxins • Pain killer such as toothache, earache, headache, muscle pain	• Treat vomiting • Prevent cancer • Treat metabolic dysfunction such as diabetes • Treat Vascular disorders such as hypertension • Treat bone disorders such as rheumatoid arthritis	De and De (2019), Choi et al. (2018), Jafarzadeh and Nemati (2018)

Oxidative stress and inflammation are processes that conducive to various pathologies. In a study, Toma et al. stated that ginger extract reduces vascular cell adhesion molecule-1, monocyte adhesion, and chemoattractant protein-1. The results indicated new mechanisms of applying anti-inflammatory action by ginger extract and its gingerol-related compounds in tumor necrosis factor α-exposed cultured human endothelial cells. The beneficial effects of the ginger extract were more significant than 6-gingerol and 6-shogaol, respectively. Therefore, ginger can improve a wide range of disorders in addition to atherosclerosis (Toma et al. 2018).

Ginger also has the potential to reduce the symptoms of some neurological ailments, including epilepsy, Parkinson's disease, migraines, and Alzheimer's disease (Choi et al. 2018; Jafarzadeh and Nemati 2018).

Ho et al., examined the inhibitory properties of ginger extract and seven gingerol-related compounds on neuroinflammation using a lipopolysaccharide-activated BV2 microglial culture model. 6-gingerol and 10-gingerol were the most abundant compounds in fresh ginger extract, respectively. The pure ginger extract showed remarkable anti-inflammatory capacity, mainly due to 10-gingerol. They stated that due to potent anti-neuroinflammatory power, ginger and gingerol-related components are suitable dietary adjuvants for neurodegenerative diseases (Ho et al. 2013a).

Regular neuropathological conditions of the central nervous system, such as neuroinflammation, oxidative stress, and protein misfolding, commonly characterize Age-related neurological disorders. Ginger and its components have therapeutic potential in Age-related neurological diseases. Ginger can be utilized for the treatment of them by targeting different ligand sites. In a review, Choi et al. illustrated that ginger and its compounds, including 6-gingerol, zingerone, 6-paradol, 6-shogaol, and dehydrozingerone are efficient in improving pathological conditions and neurological symptoms of Age-related neurological disorders via cell survival signaling molecules or modulating cell death (Choi et al. 2018).

Biotransformation of 6-shogaol to 6-paradol, which has anti-inflammatory, anti-oxidative, and anti-cancer properties was surveyed by Choi, J. W., et al. Furthermore, fermented ginger extract as a valuable food ingredient and a neuroprotective agent was evaluated against neurotoxicity induced by amyloid-beta in primary hippocampal neurons of rats. They concluded fermentation of 6-shogaol-enriched ginger extracts could be a useful method for the formation of 6-pradol and also, the fermented ginger extract has a neuroprotective effect (Choi et al. 2017).

Ginger and its components have the potential for the treatment of Multiple sclerosis (MS) due to its anti-inflammatory, antioxidant, and immunomodulatory activities. Ginger and its active constituents improve clinical, immunological, and inflammatory factors in Experimental autoimmune encephalomyelitis mice (Jafarzadeh and Nemati 2018).

Systematic review and meta-analysis of randomized controlled trials were surveyed by Maharlouei et al. The result stated that ginger intake reduced body weight, hip ratio, waist-to-hip ratio, fasting glucose and homeostasis model assessment of insulin resistance, and increased high-density lipoprotein cholesterol, but did not affect insulin, body mass index, triglycerides, low-density lipoprotein cholesterol, and total cholesterol levels (Maharlouei et al. 2019).

Ginger has a robust angiostatic potential that can be used to control obesity. In a review by Sarkar and Thirumurugan, the role of ginger in angiogenesis and adipogenesis has been discussed. According to some in vitro and in vivo studies, ginger has the most useful anti-obesity activity. 6-gingerol and 6-shogaol are its active compounds. The anti-obesity mechanism is due to increase in energy consumption and thermogenesis by reducing the expression of lipogenesis and adipogenesis related genes, increasing beta-oxidation enzymes, as well as enhancing physical function by switching between muscle fibers (Sarkar and Thirumurugan 2019). In another study by Oh et al., the effects of ginger extract on the metabolism of high-density lipoprotein-cholesterol and muscle mitochondrial biogenesis in rats were investigated. The results of this study showed the protective effect of ginger extract against obesity-induced metabolic disorders. It could have beneficial effects on obesity by increasing muscle mitochondrial biogenesis and serum high-density lipoprotein-cholesterol level (Oh et al. 2017) (Table 4).

The ginger extract might be considered for protective effects against AFB1-induced oxidative stress and hepatotoxicity. Human hepatoma cells were protected from AFB1 by pretreatment with ginger extract due to inhibition of reactive oxygen species generation, DNA damage, and cell death. On the other hand, the protective effects of ginger extract against AFB1 induced hepatotoxicity were observed with rat model experiments because of the up-regulation of the Nrf2/HO-1 pathway and ameliorating antioxidants enzymes levels (Vipin et al. 2017). The protective effects of ginger and its phytochemicals against a wide range of toxins such as pesticides, heavy metals, environmental pollutants, drugs, radiation, bacterial and fungal toxins in both in vitro and in vivo models were reviewed by Alsherbiny et al., Its protective mechanisms may be due to its radical scavenging, antioxidant properties, and regulation of apoptotic and inflammatory responses. The protective function of the phytochemicals of ginger is accomplished through various mechanisms and cell signaling pathways. The importance of ginger compounds in cancer treatment regime not only as a radioprotective agent for healthy cells but also because of its improving effect on the toxicity of chemotherapy. Meanwhile, ginger and its components due to its protective effects can have benefits for humans or animals exposed to toxic agents, smokers, or elderly patients taking several different medications (Alsherbiny et al. 2019).

One of the main causes of atherosclerosis and, subsequently, cardiovascular disease is elevated blood lipid levels (Pourmasoumi et al. 2018). Ginger may be considered a lipid-lowering agent, especially in diabetic patients due to its useful antioxidants (shogaols and gingerols) (Arablou and Aryaeian 2018). Pourmasoumi et al., in a systematic review and meta-analysis of clinical trials, demonstrated that ginger had a suitable effect on triacylglycerol and low-density lipoprotein cholesterol. Meanwhile, based on the results, consuming less than 2 g per day of ginger had a more significant impact on lowering total cholesterol and triglyceride glycerol (Pourmasoumi et al. 2018).

Ginger has a protective effect in diabetes due to the reduction of oxidative stress, hepatic, and renal damage (Shanmugam et al. 2011; Taghavi et al. 2020). The result of ginger dose–response and evaluation of probable protective effects of dietary ginger on oxidative stress and streptozotocin-induced genotoxicity on diabetic rats fed for one month were investigated. Ginger protected against streptozotocin-induced diabetes through lipid and protein oxidation, modulation of antioxidant enzymes, and genotoxicity. The results indicated that a diet containing small

Table 4 Protective effects of ginger against natural, chemical, and radiation-induced toxicities

Toxicities			Organs toxicities	Protective effects	Reference
Natural	Chemical	Radiation			
Bacterial Toxins Mycotoxins	Fungicides, herbicides, insecticides & pesticides, Heavy metals, Drug-induced toxicity, Recreational drugs Miscellaneous	γ-Radiation Ultraviolet	• Non-organ directed noxiousness (carcinogenesis, endocrine disruption & teratogenicity) • Single or multiple organ-directed noxiousness on Kidney, liver, heart, brain & reproductive system	Alleviation of the toxic effect such as apoptosis, inflammation, oxidative stress	Alsherbiny et al. (2019)

amounts of ginger is useful in antioxidant and antigenotoxic effects by inhibiting streptozotocin-induced clastogenic activity (Kota et al. 2012). Similarly, in another study, the therapeutic protective effect of ginger on lipid peroxidative condition and the tissue antioxidant defense system in streptozotocin-induced diabetic rats were investigated by Shanmugam et al. In this study, they compared the antioxidant property of ginger with glibenclamide, a hypoglycaemic medicine. The diabetic rats showed lower activities of catalase, superoxide dismutase, glutathione reductase, and glutathione peroxidase, and decreased glutathione content and a higher level of malondialdehyde in hepatic and renal tissues as compared with normal rats. Remarkable antioxidant activities and dose-dependent hypoglycaemic were observed as a result of one month of ginger supplementation in diabetic rats (Shanmugam et al. 2011).

4 Cinnamon

Cinnamon is a common bark spice which belongs to genus *Cinnamomum*, Lauraceae family obtained from the inner bark of around 250 species, (Vázquez-Fresno et al. 2019) four of which are utilized to obtain the spice including Indonesian cinnamon (*Cinnamomum burmannii*), Cassia cinnamon or Chinese cinnamon (*Cinnamomum cassia* or *Cinnamomum aromaticum*), Ceylon cinnamon (*Cinnamomum verum* or *Cinnamomum zeylanicum*) and Vietnamese cinnamon (*Cinnamomum loureiroi*) (Ribeiro-Santos et al. 2017; Kawatra and Rajagopalan 2015; Thomas and Kuruvilla 2012). Cinnamon, a tropical evergreen tree, is native to Indonesia, China, Sri Lanka and Vietnam (Ribeiro-Santos et al. 2017) which are major producers and exporters of the spice besides Madagascar, India, Myanmar, and Bangladesh which are the other major ones (Vázquez-Fresno et al. 2019; Ribeiro-Santos et al. 2017).

The name cinnamon means sweet wood derived from a Greek word (Ribeiro-Santos et al. 2017; Thomas and Kuruvilla 2012).

The cinnamon flavor is mainly due to cinnamaldehyde (up to 90%), which is the aromatic essence and responsible for the sweet taste of cinnamon. The overall flavor and aroma are as a result of the contribution of more than eighty components which have been identified in different parts of cinnamon, including cinnamyl acetate, cinnamyl alcohol, eugenol, cinnamic acid, linalool, cinnamon, and various coumarins (Vázquez-Fresno et al. 2019; Ribeiro-Santos et al. 2017; Huang et al. 2019). Cinnamon contains many other components such as polyphenols, dietary fiber, minerals such as calcium, iron, and manganese (De and De 2019). The concentration of phytochemicals varies in different parts of the plant. From different parts of the plant, volatile oil can be obtained with the same array of hydrocarbons in different degrees (Jayaprakasha and Rao 2011) and can be divided into monoterpenes, phenylpropenes, and sesquiterpenes (Ribeiro-Santos et al. 2017) (Fig. 3; Table 5).

Different methods of extraction are used to recover non-volatile and volatile cinnamon compounds. The most common extraction methods include steam distillation, solvent extraction, hydrodistillation, and Soxhlet. Other methods of extraction include pressurized liquid extraction, supercritical fluids, microwave, and ultrasound extraction (Ribeiro-Santos et al. 2017).

Essential parameters for high-quality spices production include cultivation methods, ripening stage, and climatic conditions. Factors affecting the phytochemical content of aromatic plants include harvesting season, drying method, the process used to reduce particle size. Drying is a crucial step in the production process of cinnamon that inhibits biochemical changes and prevents microbial growth (Ribeiro-Santos et al. 2017).

Cinnamon, a seasoning spice, has been utilized for many centuries in cooking preparations as a condiment and flavoring material by various cultures in the human diet around the world (Lv et al. 2012) as a result of its delicate aroma, sweet and spicy flavor, it is commonly consumed in

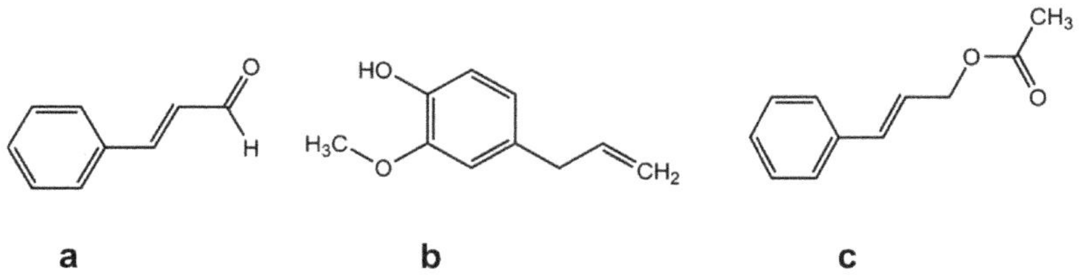

Fig. 3 Structures of the major constituents in cinnamon. **a** Cinnamaldehyde, **b** Eugenol, **c** Cinnamyl acetate (*Source* https://chem.nlm.nih.gov/chemidplus/)

Table 5 Major constituents of different parts of Cinnamon

Major constituents	Part of plant	References
Camphor	Root	Ribeiro-Santos et al. (2017), Jayaprakasha and Rao (2011)
Cinnamaldehyde	Bark	Ribeiro-Santos et al. (2017), Jayaprakasha and Rao (2011)
Eugenol	Leaf	Ribeiro-Santos et al. (2017), Jayaprakasha and Rao (2011)
Trans-cinnamyl acetate	Fruits and flowers	Ribeiro-Santos et al. (2017), Jayaprakasha and Rao (2011)

flavorings of sauces, meat, beverages, and baked goods. Ground, whole, oil, or extract form of cinnamon, obtained from bark or leaves, can be added to food. Through drying the central part of the bark, this spice is produced and is marketed as powder or sticks (Ribeiro-Santos et al. 2017).

In addition to its use for culinary purposes, it can also be used in pharmaceuticals, perfumes, incense, cosmetics, soap, dental preparations as a flavoring agent, pesticides, and insecticides (Vázquez-Fresno et al. 2019; Ribeiro-Santos et al. 2017).

Cinnamon was used in Egypt about 3000 BC to embalm mummies, and because of its flavoring properties (Ribeiro-Santos et al. 2017; Kawatra and Rajagopalan 2015; Thomas and Kuruvilla 2012). It has traditionally been utilized owing to its antibacterial, astringent and antispasmodic nature. However, it also has other properties, including treatment of impotence, Cough, diarrhea, gastrointestinal disease, colonic diseases, liver problems, neuralgia, eye inflammation, frigidity, rheumatism, vaginitis, toothaches, oral infections, acne, gallstones and to heal wounds (Ribeiro-Santos et al. 2017; Barceloux 2008). For example, the ancient Romans used cinnamon to treat digestive and respiratory ailments and to prevent the smell of the dead body. Also, in Ayurvedic medicine, cinnamon has been used as a remedy in the treatment of respiratory, gynecological, and gastrointestinal diseases for over 6000 years (Ribeiro-Santos et al. 2017). Cinnamon powder has long been utilized in traditional Chinese medicine and Ayurvedic medicines as an anti-diabetic drug (Cheng et al. 2012).

Cinnamon has a long history of its therapeutic potential. Various parts of the cinnamon tree, containing bark, fruits, leaves, roots, and flowers, have biological functions (Ribeiro-Santos et al. 2017). Consumption of Cinnamon has several health benefits, including antimicrobial, anti-inflammatory, insecticidal, antioxidant, anti-allergenic, anti-ulcerogenic, anti-pyretic, anesthetic activities, anti-tumor properties (Angiogenesis inhibitor), and anticancer effects (De and De 2019; Ribeiro-Santos et al. 2017; Huang et al. 2019; Lv et al. 2012; Ho et al. 2013b). A wide range of biological activities of cinnamon and its potential applications are due to a variety of chemical compounds of the plant, plant extract, and essential oil (Ribeiro-Santos et al. 2017). Cinnamon is a valuable source for fighting frequent epidemics containing diabetes, obesity, and cardiovascular diseases (Cheng et al. 2012). The glucose-lowering and anti-diabetic properties of cinnamon are well known (Vázquez-Fresno et al. 2019). Cinnamon is used to treating chronic bronchitis, dyspepsia, neurological disorders, infectious diseases, blood circulation issues (Ribeiro-Santos et al. 2017; Lv et al. 2012; Ho et al. 2013b).

Cinnamon has a variety of antimicrobial ingredients. Antimicrobial activity of cinnamon can be utilized to preserve food. This spice effectively inhibits the growth of Gram-negative and Gram-positive bacteria. Several studies have been done on the antibacterial and antifungal properties of volatile oil from cinnamon. Cinnamon oil has significant bacteriostatic and fungistatic activities against microorganisms, including *Bacillus subtilis*, *Pseudomonas fluorescens*, *Pseudomonas aeruginosa*, *Vibrio parahaemolyticus*, *Clostridium botulinum*, *Listeria monocytogenes*, *Salmonella typhimurium*, *Staphylococcus aureus*, *Escherichia coli*, *Aspergillus parasiticus* and *Aspergillus flavus* (El-Sayed and Youssef 2019; De and De 2019; Huang et al. 2019). In a study by Huang et al., The antimicrobial property of cinnamon oil against spoilage of microorganisms, including *Shewanella putrefaciens*, *Aeromonas veronii*, and *Pseudomonas jessenii* was surveyed. As a result, *Shewanella putrefaciens* was found to be more effective in particular. Cinnamaldehyde was identified as one of the main active compounds in cinnamon oil (Huang et al. 2019).

The influences of cinnamon extract or cinnamon powder on symptoms of diabetes have been evaluated in several clinical trials with mixed results. Several cinnamon compounds, including cinnamaldehyde, cinnamic acid, and proanthocyanidin, have been shown to ameliorate glucose balance in vivo through bioactivities in cellular pathways (Qin et al. 2010). A significantly higher level of lowering blood glucose was observed in human trials when aqueous extracts of cinnamon were used. A meta-analysis of randomized placebo-controlled clinical trials with the extracts that evaluated fasting blood sugar revealed notable overall effects on lowering fasting blood sugar (Davis and Yokoyama 2011). Glucose intake and glycogen synthesis in adipocytes were invigorated by aqueous cinnamon extracts (Cheng et al. 2012). The insulin-like and hypoglycemic effects of cinnamon extract might help to improve type 2 diabetes. Nighty percent of people who have diabetes suffer from type 2 diabetes mellitus. In a study by Cheng et al., The effect of cinnamon extract on the short-term improvement of glucose metabolism in vitro and in vivo was investigated. The cinnamon extract significantly reduced fasting blood glucose in dietary-induced obese hyperglycemic mice. Dose-dependent prevention of hepatic glucose production by the cinnamon extract was demonstrated. Besides, the extract reduced the expression of two major regulators of hepatic gluconeogenesis, glucose-6-phosphatase, and phosphoenolpyruvate carboxykinase. As a result, cinnamon-enriched food matrices or aqueous cinnamon extract can induce glucose homeostasis (Cheng et al. 2012). In a review by Santos and da Silva administration of cinnamon and its hypoglycemic effect in clinical trials was investigated. It was concluded that in patients with type 2 diabetes mellitus, the fasting blood glucose was decreased, although serum insulin reduced in few studies. Considering the treatment of type 2 diabetes mellitus and other states of glycemic impairment, around 1–6 g of cinnamon, mostly powder form of cinnamon, appears to be effective (Santos and Silva 2018). On the other study, the effect of cinnamon supplementation on glycemic status and anthropometric indices in type 2 diabetic patients was evaluated in a systematical review by Namazi et al. Cinnamon without altering other glycemic parameters, and anthropometric indices can decrease serum glucose levels. There may be other mechanisms involved other than raising serum levels of insulin, losing weight, and decrease in insulin resistance following cinnamon administration in anti-diabetic effects of cinnamon. Nevertheless, since the findings are highly heterogenic, it should be explained with great caution and higher quality randomized clinical trials that are needed (Namazi et al. 2019).

The hypolipidemic effects of cinnamon on humans and laboratory animals are described (Lopes et al. 2018). Cinnamon is a possible triglyceride reductant in direct contact with blood serum. The results of a study by Salehi et al. indicated that cinnamon as a unique serum-contact biosorbent was effective in reducing serum triglycerides in human blood. They demonstrated that adsorption on cinnamon was endothermic and physical. It may be potential for application in extracorporeal blood perfusion therapy (Salehi et al. 2019). Cinnamon has controversial lipid-lowering potential. In a review by Santos and da Silva administration of cinnamon and its lipid-lowering effect in clinical trials was surveyed. It was declared that *C. zeylanicum/verum* and *C. cassia/aromaticum* are two species that most surveyed. Cinnamon consumption has been stated to decrease fat mass and increase serum antioxidants, although the researches had not utilized accurate methods. Hence more controlled clinical trials are required (Santos and Silva 2018).

In a study, the expression of the small intestinal epithelial gene, which is involved in lipid metabolism and immunity, was investigated. The result showed that cinnamon increased some genes expression and affected lipid absorption and immunity in the small intestinal epithelium. Moreover, the microbial changes were analyzed in the small and large intestines of mice that had consumed cinnamon water extract. It was concluded that cinnamon affected microbial composition in the intestines (Kim et al. 2018).

Hypothyroidism is often associated with hyperlipidemia. In a study by Lopez et al., the influences of chronic consumption of cinnamon on lipid metabolism in hypothyroid rats were investigated. The results showed that in animal models with metabolic diseases, chronic cinnamon ingestion has not been able to modify changes in the lipid metabolism, and might even lead to increased disturbances. They concluded that the normal concentration of thyroid hormones is a determining factor for the beneficial properties of cinnamon (Lopes et al. 2018).

Asians who usually consume spices suffer from a much lower rate of neurodegenerative diseases than Westerners. Thus spices may be functional foods against neurodegenerative diseases (Ho et al. 2013b). Cinnamon has anti-inflammatory and neuroprotective properties and may be used in the future as a dietary supplement against neurodegenerative diseases. Cinnamon and its main phytochemicals, cinnamaldehyde, have inhibitory capacities to prevent microglia-mediated neuroinflammation (Ho et al. 2013b). In a study by Ho et al., it was observed that cinnamon extract reduced the production and expression of nitric oxide remarkably, interleukin-6, interleukin-1β, and tumor necrosis factor in lipopolysaccharide-activated BV2microglia. The most responsible mechanism for inhibition was blocking of nuclear factor-κB activation. Furthermore, cinnamaldehyde primarily has a strong anti-neuroinflammatory capacity in cinnamon (Ho et al. 2013b). In another study by Khorvash et al., the impact of cinnamon on migraine was investigated. The frequency, severity, and duration of migraine attacks significantly were reduced in migraine patients by Cinnamon, which may be useful in a clinical setting to alleviate pain and other migraine complications (Khorvash et al. 2019).

The pathogenesis of numerous diseases is caused by oxidative stress. Cinnamon is utilized to treat oxidative stress-related diseases. Intracellular antioxidant capacity was improved by Cinnamon. It seems cinnamon's function in inhibiting oxidative stress-related diseases is due to the presence of cinnamaldehyde and its analogs. In addition to cinnamaldehyde and its analogs, flavonol $(-)-(2R,3R)-5,7$-dimethoxy-$3',4'$-methylenedioxy-flavan-3-ol and lignan pinoresinol are two compounds which are against oxidative stress-related diseases (Li et al. 2019b).

Cinnamon can potentially be utilized as a source of bioactive phytochemicals to improve health. The phenolic profile of cinnamon and peppermint and their anti-inflammatory, antioxidant, and anti-proliferative activities were investigated in a study by Lv et al. In both spices gallic acid, catechin, (-)-epigallocatechin gallate, vanillic acid, syringic acid, and ρ-coumaric acid were identified. Cinnamon and peppermint extracts showed potent anti-inflammatory and anti-proliferative activities. Cinnamon was more effective in preventing IL-1β and COX-2 expression, while peppermint exhibited a higher inhibitory property on IL-6 and MCP-1 (Lv et al. 2012).

Information on the influences of cinnamon supplementation on obesity measurements is inconsistent. A systematic review and meta-analysis of 12 randomized controlled trials involving 786 participants by Mousavi et al. surveyed the impact of cinnamon intake on obesity measurements in adults. Cinnamon supplementation has a significant effect on obesity measurements, which can be recommended as a weight-reducing supplement to control obesity. The findings showed that cinnamon supplementation could significantly reduce body mass index, body weight, waist circumference, and fat mass. Further effects on body weight were observed in individuals less than 50 years old with baseline body mass index over 30 kg/m^2. Cinnamon intake at doses over 2 g/day significantly reduced fat mass when administered for over 12 weeks (Mousavi et al. 2020).

Cinnamon bark and residues are the potential substrates to improve the functionality of yogurt. Tang et al. successfully boosted the antioxidant activity of yogurt with extracts of cinnamon bark and twigs residue. It was observed that even after in vitro digestion, the antioxidant activity of cinnamon bark yogurt remained the highest. It was demonstrated that complex protein–phenolic interaction influenced the antioxidant activity of the yogurt (Tang et al. 2019) (Fig. 4).

Cinnamon supplementation might have anti-inflammatory effects by reducing high serum sensitivity-C-reactive protein levels. In a systematic review and meta-analysis of randomized controlled trials, the impact of cinnamon on serum C-reactive protein levels which is commonly identified as an inflammatory marker, in 285 participants was determined by Vallianou et al., Cinnamon supplementation improves serum C-reactive protein levels, especially in a chronic condition where C-reactive protein levels are elevated. The effect was noticeable when high basal sensitivity- C-reactive protein levels were over 3 mg/L, in trials with over 12 weeks duration, and at doses of 1500 mg/day (Vallianou et al. 2019).

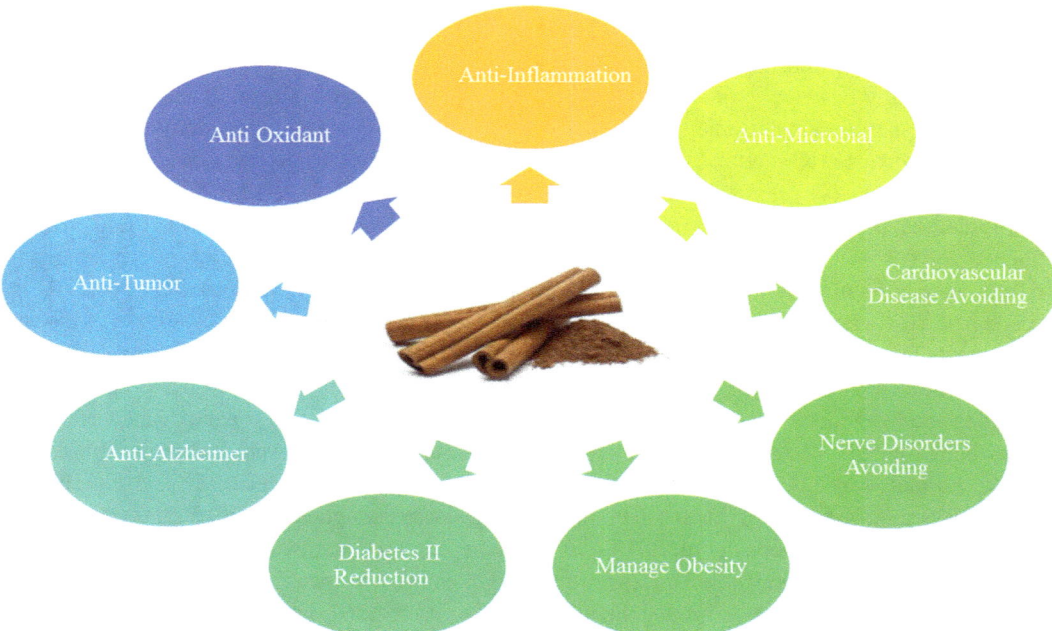

Fig. 4 Effects of cinnamon on some diseases

5 Turmeric

Turmeric (*Curcuma longa*), a member of the ginger family (*Zingiberaceae*), is a spice derived from the rhizome of the turmeric plant which is mainly cultivated in tropical regions such as India. This perennial plant is native to Southeast Asia with yellow flowers and broad leaves (Vázquez-Fresno et al. 2019; Srinivasan 2019; Martin et al. 2012; Zhou et al. 2019).

The main phytochemical components of turmeric are two secondary metabolites, which include curcuminoids and essential oils. Among the curcuminoids, curcumin (diferuloylmethane), demethoxycurcumin, and bisdemethoxycurcumin are the major constituents. There are more than 40 identifiable components in turmeric oils. The most important constituents in essential oils include aromatic-turmerone (17–26%), α-turmerone (30–32%) and β-turmerone (15–18%) (Vázquez-Fresno et al. 2019; Zhou et al. 2019). Curcumin (1,7-bis (4-hydroxy-3-methoxyphenyl)1,6-heptadiene -3,5-dione), a natural polyphenolic compound, is responsible for the yellow color of the spice (Srinivasan 2019; Alavi et al. 2018). Curcuminoids and various sesquiterpenes of turmeric or the extract of turmeric have been well known to possess several biological properties, e.g., antioxidant, anticancer or antitumor, anti-inflammatory, anti-proliferative, hepatoprotective, anti-allergy properties, choleretic, chemosensitizing, antiviral, cardioprotective, lipid-modifying, antiatherogenic and antibacterial effects (Alavi et al. 2018; Singh et al. 2019; Mohammadian et al. 2019; Hadi et al. 2019) and also has medicinal effects on diseases such as diabetes, atherosclerosis, and Alzheimer's (Zhou et al. 2019; Alavi et al. 2018) although low absorption, poor water dispersibility, rapid metabolism and systemic elimination of curcumin leads to low oral bioavailability and also restrict its applications in food products (Vázquez-Fresno et al. 2019; Alavi et al. 2018; Mohammadian et al. 2019).

Turmeric has been utilized as a spice in culinary, flavoring agent, coloring agent, and preservative, condiment, dyestuff, medicine, cosmetic since time immemorial (Vázquez-Fresno et al. 2019; Martin et al. 2012; Zhou et al. 2019). Turmeric has been suggested as a tonic, stomachic, carminative, according to Ayurveda (Li et al. 2018). Turmeric has been considered an appetizer, antibacterial, antiseptic, diuretic, antitumor, antispasmodic, and cardiovascular protectant for many years (Srinivasan 2019). It has been widely used as an ethnomedicine in Ayurvedic, homeopathic and Traditional Chinese medicine for its properties in the prevention and treatment of many diseases for centuries including wounds healing, respiratory disorders such as coughing, colds, asthma, relieving edema or swelling, pain-relieving, healing of itching and skin diseases such as leprosy, indigestion, urinary disorders, blood anemia, eliminating blood stasis and stimulating menstrual discharge, in liver diseases such as jaundice, dysmenorrhea, and amenorrhea (De and De 2019; Srinivasan 2019; Martin et al. 2012; Zhou et al. 2019).

Turmeric is used as an antimicrobial and antiseptic agent (De and De 2019). The antibacterial activity of turmeric against various bacteria such as *Salmonella paratyphi*, *Mycobacterium tuberculosis*, and *Trichophyton gypseum* has been investigated. Extracts and oils have an antibacterial role against Gram-positive (*Staphylococcus epidermidis*, *Streptococcus aureus*) and Gram-negative (*Escherichia coli*, *Pseudomonas aeruginosa*, *Salmonella typhimurium*) pathogens (Singh et al. 2019).

The antifungal activities of turmeric essential oil were investigated in vitro and in vivo. Hu et al. suggested that turmeric essential oils are potent fungicide and can be used to control fungal contamination in foods. The effect of turmeric essential oils was studied in vitro and in vivo on *Aspergillus flavus*. Its ability to disrupt plasma membrane integrity and mitochondrial dysfunction, including metabolic stagnation, involves in the inhibitory behavior of fungal growth. Mycotoxin gene expression in the aflatoxin biosynthesis pathway can be regulated by turmeric essential oils. Besides, the highly antifungal effect of the essential oils of turmeric on maize samples was observed during storage (Hu et al. 2017).

The antioxidant properties of turmeric and curcumin have been under consideration for decades, and most studies have focused on their anti-carcinogenic activity (Srinivasan 2019). Harmful mutagens can be protected by turmeric, which is one of the few spices with this ability (De and De 2019). The anticancer activity of turmeric has been investigated in breast, lung, ovarian, colorectal, prostate cancers, leukemia, and multiple myelomas. Lipid peroxidation can be reduced through curcumin antioxidant effect (Singh et al. 2019). Experimental research shows that both tumor initiation and promotion can be suppressed by curcumin (Srinivasan 2019).

The expression of cancer-related marker genes can be modified by curcuminoids. Moreover, turmeric is a chemoprotective agent (Singh et al. 2019). In a study by Zhou et al., the anticancer influences of curcuminoids were evaluated based on the natural proportion in turmeric using chemical markers knockout method and metabolomics. The activity of turmeric crude extract was comparative with curcuminoids, curcumin, and bisdemethoxycurcumin. Curcuminoids are the essential anticancer agent of turmeric. The results showed that the anticancer effects of turmeric against A549 lung cancer cells might be based on the "multi-compounds and multitarget" method (Zhou et al. 2019). The antioxidant functionality of the product by adding turmeric powder has been stated in only a few experiments. In another study by Lim and Han, several amounts of turmeric powder were added to fried rice snack, Yukawa, and the oxidative property was reported. With the addition of turmeric powder, oxidative deterioration was remarkably inhibited, and more turmeric powder in Yukawa resulted in more free radical scavenging activity (Lim and Han 2016).

Arun and Nalini examined the effects of turmeric or curcumin on diabetes mellitus in a rat model. They used alloxan to induce diabetes. Blood sugar, hemoglobin, and glycosylated hemoglobin were significantly decreased after usage of turmeric or curcumin in diabetic rats. It also reduced oxidative stress. Besides, the activity of sorbitol dehydrogenase (catalyzing the conversion of sorbitol to fructose) in treatment with turmeric or curcumin was significantly reduced (Arun and Nalini 2002). In a study by Lekshmi et al., The effect of volatile oils obtained from fresh and dried turmeric on inhibition of a-glucosidase was investigated in vitro. As a result, it was found that the volatile oil from turmeric was a potent inhibitor of a-glucosidase and a-amylase, which was dose-dependent. Glucosidase was inhibited more effectively than the acarbose (reference standard drug) by turmeric's volatile oils. As the rhizome dried, there was a significant increase in the inhibitory potential of glucosidase (Lekshmi et al. 2012). The efficacy of turmeric as a metformin (an oral anti-diabetic drug) adjuvant in the treatment of diabetes in 60 patients for four weeks was evaluated by Selvi et al. Turmeric supplement (2 g) as a metformin adjuvant in type 2 diabetes mellitus had a beneficial effect on oxidative stress, inflammation, and blood glucose. The results suggested that turmeric had a synergistic effect with metformin in people with diabetes in lowering fasting blood glucose. Turmeric helps maintain normoglycemic status, improves redox imbalance, and prevents further complications (Selvi et al. 2015). Curcumin is the major bioactive compounds in turmeric with anti-diabetic characteristics. Its Potential mechanism is due to improved functions of β-cells (Bi et al. 2017).

The role of curcumin/turmeric in regulating blood pressure has been investigated in some clinical trials. Some reported that curcumin/turmeric consumption reduced blood pressure levels, while others reported no significant change. In a systematic review and meta-analysis of randomized trials, controlled trials by Hadi et al. Curcumin/Turmeric supplementation, as a potential adjuvant antihypertensive drug, has a favorable effect on blood pressure when administered 12 weeks or more. Besides, the high antioxidant capacity of curcumin/turmeric has made it a viable option for enhancing cardiovascular dysfunction along with other conventional therapies (Hadi et al. 2019).

Cardiac derangement caused by chemotherapy is an essential concern regarding chemotherapy. Cyclophosphamide is a chemotherapeutic agent that induces acute cardiotoxicity through its toxic metabolite (acrolein). In a study by Komolafe et al., the impact of oral usage of turmeric ethanol extract on cyclophosphamide-induced acute cardiotoxicity in rat left ventricular myocardium. As a result, it was observed that cyclophosphamide-induced myocardial alterations of the left heart were notably ameliorated by turmeric extract (Komolafe et al. 2020).

Turmeric is efficient as a hypocholesterolemic agent under different hypercholesterolemia/hyperlipidemia conditions (De and De 2019). Anti-hyperlipidemia and antioxidant properties of turmeric oil were investigated in a study on hyperlipidemic rats induced by a high-fat diet. Turmeric oil increased high-density lipoprotein cholesterol and significantly reduced triglycerides, low-density lipoprotein cholesterol, total serum cholesterol, and free fatty acid. Also, to suppress oxidative reactions, the activities of glutathione peroxidase and superoxide dismutase were significantly elevated, and maleic dialdehyde activity was reduced. Besides, the histological morphology examination showed that turmeric oil prevented liver tissue damage caused by a high-fat diet. Turmeric oil can, therefore, protect against cardiovascular disease (Ling et al. 2012). Increased lipolysis and decreased lipid accumulation were observed in 3T3L1 cells following administration of 20 μg/ml turmeric methanol extract. The mRNA expression of adipose triglyceride lipase, which triggers glycerol degradation and the hormone-sensitive lipase, an enzyme that initiates lipolysis, increased and led to increased glycerol release. Hormone-sensitive lipase and adipose triglyceride lipase are essential for lipolysis in adipose tissues (Lee and Jun 2009).

In one study, fermented turmeric extract was made in equal proportions by mixing brown sugar and turmeric, and its effect was investigated. This mixed turmeric extract reduced LDL, cholesterol, leptin, adiponectin, and aspartate aminotransferase levels, which was able to reduce diet-induced obesity (Yang et al. 2011). The anti-obesity mechanism of curcumin is due to damages to neovascularization by targeting HIF1α, VEGF, and NF-κB (Sarkar and Thirumurugan 2019).

Turmeric has traditionally been used as an anti-inflammatory medicine (Srinivasan 2019). The molecular effects of turmeric and curcumin have been demonstrated in the role of anti-inflammatory therapy. The effect of turmeric/curcumin intake on the diet of rats for three weeks was investigated by Martin et al. Turmeric was found to increase the levels of iNOS, IL-8, IL-6, and COX-2, so it was concluded that turmeric had a higher bioavailability or more significant effect on pro-inflammatory genes than curcumin. Because of the significant bioavailability differences, the need for more chemo preventative research trials should be considered in the setting of upper gastrointestinal cancers (Martin et al. 2012). Curcumin has the most anti-inflammatory property on animals. Still, there are other compounds in turmeric that have been observed to have anti-inflammatory effects in animals such as curdione, cyclocurcumin, furanodiene, turmerin, and turmerone. Turmeric extract or curcumin or curcuminoids may appear to have anti-inflammatory effects in patients with chronic inflammatory diseases. A systematic review of randomized controlled trials on the impact of oral turmeric or curcumin/curcuminoid bioactive compounds (administration time between 4 and 16 weeks) and meta-analysis on inflammatory markers in patients with a wide range of pro-inflammatory diseases was surveyed by White et al. Chronic diseases including metabolic syndrome, cardiovascular diseases, rheumatoid arthritis and advanced chronic kidney disease with hemodialysis were studied. They reported that turmeric or curcumin did not significantly reduce levels of TNF alpha, IL-1 beta, IL-6, CRP, and hsCRP compared to control. There was no difference between curcumin and turmeric consumption. Several additional trials evaluating the impact on CRP and hsCRP should be sufficient for the analysis, if consistent with the results of previous research. However, the presence of heterogeneity needs to be further investigated (White et al. 2019).

The anti-metastatic and anti-tumor activities of turmeric extract on both the orthotopic mouse model and colorectal cancer cells were demonstrated through the regulation of several targets.

Inhibiting colony formation, cytotoxic effect, decreasing cellular motility, migration, and epithelial-mesenchymal transitions were showed by turmeric extract through the regulation of several pathways in murine colorectal cancer cells. Turmeric extract at 200 mg/kg reduced colon tumor burden and inhibited lung and liver metastasis in vivo. Treatment with turmeric extract caused immunity to be enhanced by T-cell stimulation, altered tumor microenvironment, exerted anti-metastatic properties. As a result, the usage of turmeric extract as a chemotherapeutic or chemopreventive agent was suggested for patients with metastatic colorectal cancer (Li et al. 2018).

Different doses of curcumin/saffron and curcumin have been investigated to reduce the symptoms of depression and anxiety in individuals with significant depressive disorder. In one research, one hundred and twenty-three individuals whose suffering from major depressive disorder were studied in a randomized, double-blind, placebo-controlled study for three months by Lopresti and Drummond. The findings showed the anxiolytic and antidepressant properties of curcumin in patients with main depressive disorder, although no remarkable difference in efficiency was observed between low and high doses. Adding saffron to low-dose curcumin did not increase the effectiveness of the treatment. Curcumin has also been shown to be highly efficient in treating individuals with atypical depression compared to other people who suffer from depression, although more studies are needed (Lopresti and Drummond 2017).

6 Conclusion

Spices have been used in both cooking and traditional medicine for centuries. There have been extensive studies of the healing properties of spices and their active ingredients in recent decades, confirming their traditional role in the treatment of certain diseases. As research on the bioactive constituents of spices continues, many of their applications in ancient therapies have been identified. Studies have shown that long-term use of spices can have beneficial effects on health. Saffron, ginger, cinnamon, and turmeric are four spices widely used in different countries and have many health benefits. Either traditional or experimental evidence demonstrates the probable medicinal effects of them and their constituents on many types of diseases. Antioxidant, anticancer, anti-inflammatory, antimicrobial properties of these spices can be mentioned. Also, these spices have little or no side effects, so they may be one of the main sources of cheap medicines that come from inexpensive sources in the near future and contribute to the future of human health. However, more experimental evidence and clinical trials are required before the introduction of them as treatment of diseases.

References

Akaberi M, Boghrati Z, Amiri MS, Emami SA (2019) Saffron: the golden spice. In: Science of spices and culinary herbs-latest laboratory, pre-clinical, and clinical studies, vol 1, pp 1–29

Alavi F, Emam-Djomeh Z, Yarmand MS, Salami M, Momen S, Moosavi-Movahedi AA (2018) Cold gelation of curcumin loaded whey protein aggregates mixed with K-carrageenan: impact of gel microstructure on the gastrointestinal fate of curcumin. Food Hydrocolloids 85:267–280

Alsherbiny MA, Abd-Elsalam WH, Taher E, Fares M, Torres A, Chang D, Li CG (2019) Ameliorative and protective effects of ginger and its main constituents against natural, chemical and radiation-induced toxicities: a comprehensive review. Food Chem Toxicol 123:72–97

Arablou T, Aryaeian N (2018) The effect of ginger (*Zingiber officinale*) as an ancient medicinal plant on improving blood lipids. J Herbal Med 12:11–15

Arun N, Nalini N (2002) Efficacy of turmeric on blood sugar and polyol pathway in diabetic albino rats. Plant Foods Hum Nutr 57(1):41–52

Asadollahi M, Nikdokht P, Hatef B, Sadr SS, Sahraei H, Assarzadegan F, Jahromi GP (2019) Protective properties of the aqueous extract of saffron (*Crocus sativus* L.) in ischemic stroke, randomized clinical trial. J Ethnopharmacol 238:111833

Barceloux DG (2008) Medical toxicology of natural substances: foods, fungi, medicinal herbs, plants, and venomous animals. Wiley

Begas E, Bounitsi M, Kilindris T, Kouvaras E, Makaritsis K, Kouretas D, Asprodini EK (2019) Effects of short-term saffron (*Crocus sativus* L.) intake on the in vivo activities of xenobiotic metabolizing enzymes in healthy volunteers. Food Chem Toxicol 130:32–43

Bi X, Lim J, Henry CJ (2017) Spices in the management of diabetes mellitus. Food Chem 217:281–293

Boskabady MH, Gholamnezhad Z, Ghorani V, Saadat S (2019) The effect of crocus sativus (saffron) on the respiratory system: traditional and experimental evidence. In: Science of spices and culinary herbs-latest laboratory, pre-clinical, and clinical studies, vol 1, pp 30–54

Bukhari SI, Manzoor M, Dhar M (2018) A comprehensive review of the pharmacological potential of *Crocus sativus* and its bioactive apocarotenoids. Biomed Pharmacother 98:733–745

Cheng DM, Kuhn P, Poulev A, Rojo LE, Lila MA, Raskin I (2012) In vivo and in vitro antidiabetic effects of aqueous cinnamon extract and cinnamon polyphenol-enhanced food matrix. Food Chem 135 (4):2994–3002

Choi JW, Park H-Y, Oh MS, Yoo HH, Lee S-H, Ha SK (2017) Neuroprotective effect of 6-paradol enriched ginger extract by fermentation using schizosaccharomyces pombe. J Funct Foods 31:304–310

Choi JG, Kim SY, Jeong M, Oh MS (2018) Pharmacotherapeutic potential of ginger and its compounds in age-related neurological disorders. Pharmacol Ther 182:56–69

Davis PA, Yokoyama W (2011) Cinnamon intake lowers fasting blood glucose: meta-analysis. J Med Food 14 (9):884–889

De AK, De M (2019) Functional and therapeutic applications of some important spices. In: The role of functional food security in global health. Elsevier, pp 499–510

El-Sayed SM, Youssef AM (2019) Potential application of herbs and spices and their effects in functional dairy products. Heliyon 5(6):e01989

Garavand F, Rahaee S, Vahedikia N, Jafari SM (2019) Different techniques for extraction and micro/nanoencapsulation of saffron bioactive ingredients. Trends Food Sci Technol 89:26–44

Ghadrdoost B, Vafaei AA, Rashidy-Pour A, Hajisoltani R, Bandegi AR, Motamedi F, Haghighi S, Sameni HR, Pahlvan S (2011) Protective effects of saffron extract and its active constituent crocin against oxidative stress and spatial learning and memory deficits induced by chronic stress in rats. Eur J Pharmacol 667(1–3):222–229

Ghaffari S, Roshanravan N (2019) Saffron; an updated review on biological properties with special focus on cardiovascular effects. Biomed Pharmacother 109:21–27

Ghanbari J, Khajoei-Nejad G, van Ruth SM, Aghighi S (2019) The possibility for improvement of flowering, corm properties, bioactive compounds, and antioxidant activity in saffron (*Crocus sativus* L.) by different nutritional regimes. Ind Crops Prod 135:301–310

Hadi A, Pourmasoumi M, Ghaedi E, Sahebkar A (2019) The effect of curcumin/turmeric on blood pressure modulation: a systematic review and meta-analysis. Pharmacol Res 104505

Ho S-C, Chang K-S, Chang P-W (2013b) Inhibition of neuroinflammation by cinnamon and its main components. Food Chem 138(4):2275–2282

Ho S-C, Chang K-S, Lin C-C (2013a) Anti-neuroinflammatory capacity of fresh ginger is attributed mainly to 10-gingerol. Food Chem 141(3):3183–3191

Hosseini SI, Farrokhi N, Shokri K, Khani MR, Shokri B (2018) Cold low pressure O_2 plasma treatment of *Crocus sativus*: an efficient way to eliminate toxicogenic fungi with minor effect on molecular and cellular properties of saffron. Food Chem 257:310–315

Hsiang C-Y, Lo H-Y, Huang H-C, Li C-C, Wu S-L, Ho T-Y (2013) Ginger extract and zingerone ameliorated trinitrobenzene sulphonic acid-induced colitis in mice via modulation of nuclear factor-κb activity and interleukin-1β signalling pathway. Food Chem 136 (1):170–177

Hu Y, Zhang J, Kong W, Zhao G, Yang M (2017) Mechanisms of antifungal and anti-aflatoxigenic properties of essential oil derived from turmeric (*Curcuma longa* L.) on aspergillus flavus. Food Chem 220:1–8

Huang Z, Jia S, Zhang L, Liu X, Luo Y (2019) Inhibitory effects and membrane damage caused to fish spoilage bacteria by cinnamon bark (*Cinnamomum tamala*) oil. LWT 112:108195

Jafarzadeh A, Nemati M (2018) Therapeutic potentials of ginger for treatment of multiple sclerosis: a review with emphasis on its immunomodulatory, anti-inflammatory and anti-oxidative properties. J Neuroimmunol 324:54–75

Jayaprakasha G, Rao LJM (2011) Chemistry, biogenesis, and biological activities of *Cinnamomum zeylanicum*. Crit Rev Food Sci Nutr 51(6):547–562

Kang C, Lee H, Jung E-S, Seyedian R, Jo M, Kim J, Kim J-S, Kim E (2012) Saffron (*Crocus sativus* L.) increases glucose uptake and insulin sensitivity in muscle cells via multipathway mechanisms. Food Chem 135(4):2350–2358

Karimi-Nazari E, Nadjarzadeh A, Masoumi R, Marzban A, Mohajeri SA, Ramezani-Jolfaie N, Salehi-Abargouei A (2019) Effect of saffron (Crocus sativus L.) on lipid profile, glycemic indices and antioxidant status among overweight/obese prediabetic individuals: a double-blinded randomized controlled trial. Clin Nutr ESPEN 34:130–136

Kawatra P, Rajagopalan R (2015) Cinnamon: mystic powers of a minute ingredient. Pharmacognosy Res 7 (Suppl 1):S1

Khorvash F, Askari G, Zarei A (2019) The effect of cinnamon on migraine treatment and blood levels of Cgrp and Il-6: a double-blinded randomized controlled clinical trial. J Neurol Sci 405:106–107

Kim J-I, Lee J-H, Song Y, Kim Y-T, Lee Y-H, Kang H (2018) Oral consumption of cinnamon enhances the expression of immunity and lipid absorption genes in the small intestinal epithelium and alters the gut microbiota in normal mice. J Funct Foods 49:96–104

Komolafe O, Arayombo B, Abiodun A, Saka O, Abijo A, Ojo S, Fakunle O (2020) Immunohistochemical and histological evaluations of cyclophosphamide-induced acute cardiotoxicity in wistar rats: the role of turmeric extract (Curcuma). Morphologie

Kota N, Panpatil VV, Kaleb R, Varanasi B, Polasa K (2012) Dose-dependent effect in the inhibition of oxidative stress and anticlastogenic potential of ginger in Stz induced diabetic rats. Food Chem 135(4):2954–2959

Krüger S, Bergin A, Morlock G (2018) Effect-directed analysis of ginger (*Zingiber officinale*) and its food products, and quantification of bioactive compounds via high-performance thin-layer chromatography and mass spectrometry. Food Chem 243:258–268

Lee J, Jun W (2009) Methanolic extract of turmeric (*Curcuma longa* L.) enhanced the lipolysis by up-regulation of lipase MRNA expression in differentiated 3t3-L1 adipocytes. Food Sci Biotechnol 18(6):1500–1504

Lekshmi P, Arimboor R, Indulekha P, Nirmala Menon A (2012) Turmeric (*Curcuma longa* L.) volatile oil inhibits key enzymes linked to type 2 diabetes. Int J Food Sci Nutr 63(7):832–834

Li M, Yue GG-L, Tsui SK-W, Fung K-P, Bik-San Lau C (2018) Turmeric extract, with absorbable curcumin, has potent anti-metastatic effect in vitro and in vivo. Phytomedicine 46:131–141

Li A-L, Li G-H, Li Y-R, Wu X-Y, Ren D-M, Lou H-X, Wang X-N, Shen T (2019b) Lignan and flavonoid support the prevention of cinnamon against oxidative stress related diseases. Phytomedicine 53:143–153

Li H, Liu Y, Luo D, Ma Y, Zhang J, Li M, Yao L, Shi X, Liu X, Yang K (2019) Ginger for health care: an overview of systematic reviews. Complement Therapies Med

Lim S-T, Han J-A (2016) Improvement in antioxidant functionality and shelf life of Yukwa (fried rice snack) by turmeric (*Curcuma longa* L.) powder addition. Food Chem 199:590–596

Linardaki ZI, Orkoula MG, Kokkosis AG, Lamari FN, Margarity M (2013) Investigation of the neuroprotective action of saffron (*Crocus sativus* L.) in aluminum-exposed adult mice through behavioral and neurobiochemical assessment. Food Chem Toxicol 52:163–170

Ling J, Wei B, Lv G, Ji H, Li S (2012) Antihyperlipidaemic and antioxidant effects of turmeric oil in hyperlipidaemic rats. Food Chem 130(2):229–235

Lopes BP, Gaique TG, Souza LL, Paula GSM, Kluck GE, Atella GC, Pazos-Moura CC, Oliveira KJ (2018) Beneficial effects of cinnamon on hepatic lipid metabolism are impaired in hypothyroid rats. J Funct Foods 50:210–215

Lopresti AL, Drummond PD (2017) Efficacy of curcumin, and a saffron/curcumin combination for the treatment of major depression: a randomised, double-blind, placebo-controlled study. J Affect Disord 207:188–196

Lopresti AL, Drummond PD, Inarejos-García AM, Prodanov M (2018) Affron®, a standardised extract from saffron (Crocus sativus L.) for the treatment of youth anxiety and depressive symptoms: a randomised, double-blind placebo-controlled study. J Affect Disord 232:349–357

Lv J, Huang H, Yu L, Whent M, Niu Y, Shi H, Wang TT, Luthria D, Charles D, Yu LL (2012) Phenolic composition and nutraceutical properties of organic and conventional cinnamon and peppermint. Food Chem 132(3):1442–1450

Maharlouei N, Tabrizi R, Lankarani KB, Rezaianzadeh A, Akbari M, Kolahdooz F, Rahimi M, Keneshlou F, Asemi Z (2019) The effects of ginger intake on weight loss and metabolic profiles among overweight and obese subjects: a systematic review and meta-analysis of randomized controlled trials. Crit Rev Food Sci Nutr 59(11):1753–1766

Martin RC, Aiyer HS, Malik D, Li Y (2012) Effect on pro-inflammatory and antioxidant genes and bioavailable distribution of whole turmeric vs curcumin: similar root but different effects. Food Chem Toxicol 50(2):227–231

Mashmoul M, Azlan A, Yusof BNM, Khaza'ai H, Mohtarrudin N, Boroushaki MT (2014) Effects of saffron extract and crocin on anthropometrical, nutritional and lipid profile parameters of rats fed a high fat diet. J Funct Foods 8:180–187

Melnyk JP, Wang S, Marcone MF (2010) Chemical and biological properties of the world's most expensive spice: saffron. Food Res Int 43(8):1981–1989

Menghini L, Leporini L, Vecchiotti G, Locatelli M, Carradori S, Ferrante C, Zengin G, Recinella L, Chiavaroli A, Leone S (2018) *Crocus sativus* L. stigmas and by products: qualitative fingerprint, antioxidant potentials and enzyme inhibitory activities. Food Res Int 109:91–98

Mohammadian M, Salami M, Momen S, Alavi F, Emam-Djomeh Z (2019) Fabrication of curcumin-loaded whey protein microgels: structural properties, antioxidant activity, and in vitro release behavior. LWT-Food Sci Technol 103:94–100

Moshiri M, Vahabzadeh M, Hosseinzadeh H (2015) Clinical applications of saffron (*Crocus sativus*) and its constituents: a review. Drug Res 65(06):287–295

Mousavi SM, Rahmani J, Kord-Varkaneh H, Sheikhi A, Larijani B, Esmaillzadeh A (2020) Cinnamon supplementation positively affects obesity: a systematic review and dose-response meta-analysis of randomized controlled trials. Clin Nutr 39(1):123–133

Murthy PS, Gautam R (2015) Ginger oleoresin chemical composition, bioactivity and application as biopreservatives. J Food Process Preserv 39(6):1905–1912

Najafabadi BT, Ghamari K, Ranjbari TK, Noorbala AA, Daryani NE, Vanaki E, Akhondzadeh S (2019) Therapeutic effects of saffron (*Crocus sativus*) versus fluoxetine on irritable bowel syndrome: a double-blind randomized clinical trial. Adv Integrat Med 6(4):167–173

Namazi N, Khodamoradi K, Khamechi SP, Heshmati J, Ayati MH, Larijani B (2019) The impact of cinnamon on anthropometric indices and glycemic status in patients with type 2 diabetes: a systematic review and meta-analysis of clinical trials. Complement Ther Med 43:92–101

Oh S, Lee M-S, Jung S, Kim S, Park H, Park S, Kim S-Y, Kim C-T, Jo Y-H, Kim I-H (2017) Ginger extract increases muscle mitochondrial biogenesis and serum hdl-cholesterol level in high-fat diet-fed rats. J Funct Foods 29:193–200

Papandreou MA, Tsachaki M, Efthimiopoulos S, Cordopatis P, Lamari FN, Margarity M (2011) Memory enhancing effects of saffron in aged mice are correlated with antioxidant protection. Behav Brain Res 219(2):197–204

Pourmasoumi M, Hadi A, Rafie N, Najafgholizadeh A, Mohammadi H, Rouhani MH (2018) The effect of ginger supplementation on lipid profile: a systematic review and meta-analysis of clinical trials. Phytomedicine 43:28–36

Qin B, Panickar KS, Anderson RA (2010) Cinnamon: potential role in the prevention of insulin resistance, metabolic syndrome, and type 2 diabetes. J Diabetes Sci Technol 4(3):685–693

Rahiman N, Akaberi M, Sahebkar A, Emami SA, Tayarani-Najaran Z (2018) Protective effects of saffron and its active components against oxidative stress and apoptosis in endothelial cells. Microvasc Res 118:82–89

Rezaee-Khorasany A, Razavi BM, Taghiabadi E, Yazdi AT, Hosseinzadeh H (2019) Effect of saffron (stigma of *Crocus sativus* L.) aqueous extract on ethanol toxicity in rats: a biochemical, histopathological and molecular study. J Ethnopharmacol 237:286–299

Ribeiro-Santos R, Andrade M, Madella D, Martinazzo AP, Moura LdAG, de Melo NR, Sanches-Silva A (2017) Revisiting an ancient spice with medicinal purposes: cinnamon. Trends Food Sci Technol 62:154–169

Salehi E, Gavari N, Chehrei A, Amani S, Amani N, Zaghi K (2019) Efficient separation of triglyceride from blood serum using cinnamon as a novel biosorbent: adsorption thermodynamics, kinetics, isothermal and process optimization using response surface methodology. Process Biochem 77:122–136

Samarghandian S, Azimi-Nezhad M, Farkhondeh T (2017) Immunomodulatory and antioxidant effects of saffron aqueous extract (*Crocus sativus* L.) on streptozotocin-induced diabetes in rats. Indian Heart J 69 (2):151–159

Santos HO, da Silva GA (2018) To what extent does cinnamon administration improve the glycemic and lipid profiles? Clin Nutr ESPEN 27:1–9

Sarkar P, Thirumurugan K (2019) Modulatory functions of bioactive fruits, vegetables and spices in adipogenesis and angiogenesis. J Funct Foods 53:318–336

Selvi NMK, Sridhar M, Swaminathan R, Sripradha R (2015) Efficacy of turmeric as adjuvant therapy in type 2 diabetic patients. Indian J Clin Biochem 30(2):180–186

Shahi T, Assadpour E, Jafari SM (2016) Main chemical compounds and pharmacological activities of stigmas and tepals of 'red gold'; saffron. Trends Food Sci Technol 58:69–78

Shahmansouri N, Farokhnia M, Abbasi S-H, Kassaian SE, Tafti A-AN, Gougol A, Yekehtaz H, Forghani S, Mahmoodian M, Saroukhani S (2014) A randomized, double-blind, clinical trial comparing the efficacy and safety of *Crocus sativus* L. with fluoxetine for improving mild to moderate depression in post percutaneous coronary intervention patients. J Affect Disord 155:216–222

Shanmugam KR, Mallikarjuna K, Nishanth K, Kuo CH, Reddy KS (2011) Protective effect of dietary ginger on antioxidant enzymes and oxidative damage in experimental diabetic rat tissues. Food Chem 124(4):1436–1442

Singh DB, Maurya AK, Rai D (2019) Antibacterial and anticancer activities of turmeric and its active ingredient curcumin, and mechanism of action. In: Science of spices and culinary herbs-latest laboratory, preclinical, and clinical studies, vol 1, pp 74–103

Srinivasan K (2019) Nutraceutical activities of turmeric (*Curcuma longa*) and its bioactive constituent curcumin. In: Science of spices and culinary herbs-latest laboratory, pre-clinical, and clinical studies, vol 1, pp 55–73

Taghavi F, Poursasan N, Moosavi-Movahedi AA (2020) Ginger: natural pharmacy. University of Tehran Press

Tang P-l, Hao E-w, Deng J-g, Hou X-t, Zhang Z-h, Xie J-l (2019) Boost anti-oxidant activity of yogurt with extract and hydrolysate of cinnamon residues. Chin Herbal Med 11(4):417–422

Thomas J, Kuruvilla K (2012) Cinnamon. In: Handbook of herbs and spices. Elsevier, pp 182–196

Toma L, Raileanu M, Deleanu M, Stancu CS, Sima AV (2018) Novel molecular mechanisms by which ginger extract reduces the inflammatory stress in Tnfα-activated human endothelial cells; decrease of ninjurin-1, Tnfr1 and nadph oxidase subunits expression. J Funct Foods 48:654–664

Tóth B, Lantos T, Hegyi P, Viola R, Vasas A, Benkő R, Gyöngyi Z, Vincze Á, Csécsei P, Mikó A (2018) Ginger (Zingiber officinale): an alternative for the prevention of postoperative nausea and vomiting. A meta-analysis. Phytomedicine 50:8–18

Tuberoso CI, Rosa A, Montoro P, Fenu MA, Pizza C (2016) Antioxidant activity, cytotoxic activity and metabolic profiling of juices obtained from saffron (*Crocus sativus* L.) floral by-products. Food Chem 199:18–27

Vallianou N, Tsang C, Taghizadeh M, Davoodvandi A, Jafarnejad S (2019) Effect of cinnamon (*Cinnamomum zeylanicum*) supplementation on serum C-reactive protein concentrations: a meta-analysis and systematic review. Complement Ther Med 42:271–278

Vázquez-Fresno R, Rosana ARR, Sajed T, Onookome-Okome T, Wishart NA, Wishart DS (2019) Herbs and spices-biomarkers of intake based on human intervention studies–a systematic review. Genes Nutr 14 (1):18–45

Vipin A, Rao R, Kurrey NK, KA AA, Venkateswaran G (2017) Protective effects of phenolics rich extract of ginger against aflatoxin B1-induced oxidative stress and hepatotoxicity. Biomed Pharmacother 91:415–424

White CM, Pasupuleti V, Roman YM, Li Y, Hernandez AV (2019) Oral turmeric/curcumin effects on inflammatory markers in chronic inflammatory diseases: a systematic review and meta-analysis of randomized controlled trials. Pharmacol Res 104280

Yang C-Y, Cho M-J, Lee C-H (2011) Effects of fermented turmeric extracts on the obesity in rats fed a high-fat diet. J Animal Sci Technol 53(1):75–81

Zhang A, Shen Y, Cen M, Hong X, Shao Q, Chen Y, Zheng B (2019) Polysaccharide and crocin contents, and antioxidant activity of saffron from different origins. Ind Crops Prod 133:111–117

Zhou J-L, Zheng J-Y, Cheng X-Q, Xin G-Z, Wang S-L, Xie T (2019) Chemical markers' knockout coupled with Uhplc-Hrms-based metabolomics reveals anticancer integration effects of the curcuminoids of turmeric (*Curcuma longa* L.) on lung cancer cell line. J Pharm Biomed Anal 175:112738

Halal Products and Healthy Lifestyle

Elnaz Hosseini, Mahdie Rahban, and Ali Akbar Moosavi-Movahedi

Abstract

The consumption of halal products includes foods, pharmaceuticals, personal care products, and cosmetics are increasing around the world. The leading causes of the strong demand for halal products are known favorable properties of these products like health, safety, and cleanliness. Several studies show that halal slaughtering affects the chemical and biochemical components such as iron, heme and glucose levels in the blood, as well as physical properties such as color and water holding capacity of the meat and its antimicrobial properties. Different parameters can affect the microbial growth in meat include the physiological condition of the animal at the time of slaughtering, spreading of microorganisms during slaughter, and storage condition. In this chapter, scientific studies on halal products' properties from microbial spoilage, lipid, and protein oxidation points of view were reviewed. Also, digestion, antioxidation, and aggregation of halal proteins are considered. Finally, to inform and assure consumers about safe and hygienic products, some detection methods of non-halal ingredients to protect the accuracy of halal products explained.

Keywords

Halal · Safety · Cosmetic · Meat · Lipid and protein oxidation · Microbial spoilage

1 Introduction

Religions and lifestyles are the main factors affecting consumer's attitudes in different societies (Karahalil 2020; Bonne and Verbeke 2008). The total number of Muslims is estimated at 1.8 billion population (Abdul-Talib and Abd-Razak 2013). The consumption of halal products is one of the essential Muslim religious rules. The halal word means lawful or permissible (Riaz and Chaudry 2003), and the halal conformity and control represent a formal performance by standardization of rules and processes as the divine legal code as halal. Studies show a plentiful desire for both Muslim and non-Muslim consumers on halal products because of some known favorable properties of these products such as healthy, safe, hygiene and cleanliness (Mathew 2014). Halal has become quite popular in the

E. Hosseini · M. Rahban ·
A. A. Moosavi-Movahedi (✉)
Institute of Biochemistry and Biophysics (IBB), University of Tehran, Tehran, Iran
e-mail: moosavi@ut.ac.ir

E. Hosseini
e-mail: hosseinielnaz@ut.ac.ir

M. Rahban
e-mail: mrohban@ut.ac.ir

Western product industry in the past decades, as part of the Middle East and Southeast Asia products are exported from the West. The global food market with improvement in the production technology, transportation, brand identify, and franchising is offering more processed foods to the consumers than before and in this way, different companies, from the biggest one to the smallest are trying to satisfy consumers all around the world by producing halal foods. However, these companies' challenge is having insufficient information about halal and mandated requirements. Therefore, it is necessary to understand the rules to produce safe, halal foods (Riaz and Chaudry 2003). Several certification bodies in Europe, Australia, New Zealand, USA, Southeast Asia and China were established to enhance the information about the halal dietary rules and their requirements and standards. These organizations' purpose is scientific research about health and nutrition aspects of foods, which has caused the creation of a good market for halal foods as healthy, organic and environmentally friendly foods (Latif et al. 2014). Based on the economic estimates, in the past few years, the global halal market has recorded a broad increment, and it was reached a value of 2.3 trillion $ in mid-2010 (Abdul-Talib and Abd-Razak 2013).

Today, consumers are faced with a wide range of products and resources, which might be doubtful. To inform and assure consumers about safe and hygienic products, the producers and marketers have been forced to acquire the halal license as a source of awareness. Complete nutrition labels, for instance, are mandatory for vegetables, fruits, and common starchy staples, and a selection of healthy food in markets must be provided. An essential factor for products to be trusted as healthy, safe, and hygiene is the halal label (Ambali and Bakar 2014).

The critical point here is that the halal concept does not restrict food but also includes pharmaceuticals, technology, personal care products, and cosmetics, etc. It also involves personal behavior and interaction with society. The below items describe Halal products.

2 Halal Food

Like other industries, the food industry responds to consumers' expectations and desires and their diverse selections between different regions, religions, and cultures. People around the world are becoming aware of foods, health, and nutrition. They are interested in eating foods that are low in cholesterol, calorie, sodium and fat (Riaz and Chaudry 2003). The determination of halal foods relies upon its nature and its processing. There are essential categories of foods such as dairy products and meat products to characterize this issue: from the halal animals are halal. For example, since pork is prohibited, any products made with this animal are non-halal.

2.1 Halal Dairy Products

As one of the oldest industries, the dairy industry produces different products, from fresh milk to frozen desserts and ice cream. The date of origin of cheese in the human diet referred to 5000 years ago. Although the milk and dairy industry is well known in all their aspects, dairy products' halal issue needs to be considered. Muslims are recommended to drink milk, a palatable and nutritious drink full of minerals, protein, and vitamins. As there are many dairy products from minimally processed (cream and fresh milk) to highly processed (dessert, sauce, and dressing), the halal issue will differ from products to products. Different additive types can be added to milk in the dairy industry for different purposes, shelf life and stability enhancement. Polysorbate, as an additive, is highly used for fortifying milk in the United States. Vitamins D and A are mixed with polysorbate as an emulsifier to be able to solubilize in the milk. This additive can have different sources, such as animal fats or plant oils. To make halal fortified milk, the polysorbate must be prepared from halal sources such as plants. Gelatin is another additive that is generally used as a thickener in flavored milk, such as milk chocolate. Chocolate ingredients include milk, emulsifiers, gelatin and preservatives. Alcohol may be used to make chocolates during the processing step but may not be listed as an ingredient, resulting in producing non-halal-chocolate. To label these kinds of dairies as halal, the gelatin and other additives should be prepared from halal sources or other plant gums (Riaz and Chaudry 2003; Lubis et al. 2016). Gelatin, which is found in the animal body's connective tissue, is a fibrous protein with high-molecular-weight and produced by collagen's thermal hydrolysis (the main structural protein of the animal body). Gelatin is widely found in fish, birds and mammals. In some cases, due to its surface behavior, gelatin has a vital role in formulating and processing food (e.g., gelling). Foaming, setting index, emulsifying, and water holding capacity are other functional properties of gelatin. It is widely used in the production of food, pharmaceutical products, cosmetics and photography. Several researchers and scientists have warned that gelatin from pig skin is used in most food products despite increased demand for halal food. Gelatin from halal animals like fish, cow, chicken, and turkey can be a good substitute (Rakhmanova et al. 2018). Halal gelatin has broad usage in food, pharmaceutical, and photographic industries, as well as biomaterial-based packaging and as edible films. Depending on the preparation method and the used ingredients, there are wide varieties of cheese types. In some types such as cottage that acid is used in its processing, there is no problem regarding the halal issue. In other types such as cheddar, Colby, and mozzarella enzymes and microbial (bacteria, molds, and yeasts), cultures are used in the processing. As the microorganisms are fed from cultures, which are generally halal, there is no problem in using them; however, about the enzymes, we should make sure that they have a halal source. In this regard, the usage of transgenic enzymes is preferred. Some sources of enzymes from animal stomachs may be Haram or doubtful and lead to halal products' major problems. Enzymes sources from the fermentation process of microorganisms are considered to be halal if raw materials used in the growth medium are from halal sources. Enzyme derived from genetically modified (GM) microorganisms (recombinant DNA) should not be from Haram (e.g., pig genes) or doubtful sources (Riaz and Chaudry 2003; Ermis 2017). Chymosin, as a common enzyme in cheese processing, can be made from two different sources. The first one is bovine rennet that it is labeled as halal; it must be obtained from calves that have been slaughtered based on the halal method. The second one is the microbially produced chymosin. It can be produced using genes from camel, calf, goat, etc., from GM microorganisms. Microbial chymosin has been included in 70–80% of total chymosin production recently. In its production process, the bovine (or another acceptable animal) rennet gene is transferred to a good microorganism. When the microorganism grows on a medium which ingredient is halal, and it was not fed by haram ingredients before, the produced enzyme is accepted as a halal product. The enzymes with a pig source and those obtained from calves that are not slaughtered through the halal method are Haram. Islamic Foods and Nutrition Council of America (IFANCA) accepts to be used flavoring factors with a limit of the ethanol residue of 0.5% in the ingredient (Karahalil 2020; Riaz and Chaudry 2003). Butter flavor, such as many other flavors in the dairy industry, is obtained through flavor compound concentration and then enzyme modification. The used enzymes in this process should be prepared from halal sources. Production of transgenic enzymes such as lipase can create a good market for manufactures. The incorporation of animal flesh into cheese is permitted whenever the animal ingredients are halal. Some types of dairy products, including whey and its derivatives, are commonly used as ingredients in other products' production because of their low cost. It is important to use the halal (dairy) ingredient to make a functional food as halal (Riaz and Chaudry 2003).

2.2 Halal Meat

A balanced diet requires the consumption of meat as a concentrated source of proteins and energy. Meat and its product are valuable for the essential amino acids that humans are unable to synthesize them as well as micronutrients, minerals, vitamin B, and particularly iron. Meat is a significant source of nutritional iron because of its hemoproteins, including myoglobin and hemoglobin. The amount of hemoproteins content of meat depends on the bleeding of the carcass as well as the vascular bed in the muscles (Sante-Lhoutellier et al. 2007; Sabow et al. 2015a).

For meat to be considered as halal, there is a consensus that animals must be of a halal species, such as sheep and poultry; more importantly, it must be slaughtered in the halal method.

Some parameters can be recognizable in halal and non-halal products of meat. These parameters include color, eating qualities like chewiness, juiciness, and tenderness. Moreover, critical parameters during manufacturing, such as protein solubility and the solubilized proteins' ability to bind water and fat, are different in halal and non-halal meat (Farouk et al. 2014). These parameters can be different in halal and non-halal products.

3 Halal Slaughtering

The first step in meat processing is Slaughtering. It means killing an animal to produce meat. Slaughtering methods worldwide include hanging, stunning (by gas or electricity), and the halal method (Addeen et al. 2014). Several studies have shown that different type of slaughtering methods was influenced on post-mortem quality, chemical and biochemical composition such as iron, heme and glucose levels in the blood, as well as physical properties such as color and water holding capacity of the meat and its antimicrobial properties (Sattari et al. 2015), which will be explained in more details in the following sections. At the time of slaughtering, the animal must be healthy and in good condition. The animal blood must be allowed to completely drain off, causing the brain function to stop irreversibly. Consumption of blood is Haram, probably since the blood remaining on the carcass may lead to spoilage (and change the meat's palpability) (Fuseini et al. 2017). Slaughtering methods can be correlated to the composition and post-mortem quality of meat, which is affected by the amount of blood loss. A suitable slaughtering method causes the most possible amount of blood loss. The halal method is performed by cutting the carotid arteries, jugular veins, esophagus and the trachea by ensuring maximal blood drainage. It has been investigated that the maximum blood loss, which is achieved by halal slaughtering, has a favorable effect on the quality of poultry meat. The existence of residual blood in the corpse during the inadequate blood drainage causes a decrease in the meat's shelf life and quality. This fact is due to hemoglobin, which is a vital component of blood and intensifies lipid oxidation. It has been observed that the meat produced by common and non-halal slaughtering methods has a higher amount of cooking loss than halal products. Cooking loss is the degree of shrinkage of meat during cooking, and it is another criterion for evaluating water holding capacity after heating. Denaturation of proteins decreases their water holding capacity and lead to more cooking loss. Higher drip loss in non-halal samples has also been correlated to loss of important flavor and protein compounds, which subsequently reduces meat quality. A study on the water holding capacity of red meat shows the contributing factors to drip loss can be stressful and different slaughtering methods. Drip loss is a process involving the transfer of water from raw meat proteins to the extracellular space. It concluded that the stress of the non-halal slaughtering method had caused the glycogen reserve in the muscle to deplete and led to high cooking loss and drip loss in non-halal meat samples (Addeen et al. 2014; Ahmed et al. 2018). Another study has compared the effect of meat quality properties in halal slaughtering (HS) and anesthesia pre-slaughter with anesthesia induction of propofol and halothane injection. This data shows that there is a sharp increase in drip loss in goats of anesthesia pre-slaughter. It has been represented that fast muscle pH decline in anesthesia pre-slaughter meat compared to halal slaughtering meat can increase drip loss (Sabow et al. 2015b).

For the first time, a study with a physiological approach was conducted to compare gas stunning

(GS) slaughter and halal slaughtering (HS) methods in terms of the welfare of animals. The investigated welfare indicators for both GS and HS in the sticking blood were considerably better than their basal values taken at the farm. Both slaughter methods were shown to cause hyperglycemia, hypercalcemia, lymphocytopenia, lactic acidemia, leukocytosis, and a rise in hematocrit and enzyme activities. A remarkable fact was observing a five and a ten times accretion in adrenaline among HS and GS animals, respectively. It was seven times higher in the sticking blood than basal values for the former and twelve times for noradrenaline. GS presented more lightness and cooking loss and lower glycogen than HS. Although they may not automatically compromise animal welfare, such alterations in these biochemical and hematological parameters in rabbits show an intensive stress response from animals to encounter this position (Nakyinsige et al. 2014a).

One study has conducted the effect of position of neck cutting on time to physical collapse of cattle as an indirect symptom of early stages of the onset of unconsciousness, any delay between the cut the neck and the onset of unconsciousness could result in stress and pain related in suffering. High neck cut (HNC) in comparison to the conventional low neck cut (LNC) was shown to significantly shorten the time to loss of posture in halal slaughtered cattle. Therefore, HNC could decrease the time to lose consciousness during slaughter and reduce the compromise to animal welfare (Gibson et al. 2015).

4 Digestion of Halal Meat

Nutritional value depends not only on the amino acid composition of any food but also on protein digestibility. Protein for entering the bloodstream should be converted to small peptides and amino acids. Protease enzymes in the digestive tract can break proteins towards passing through the small intestinal wall. This digestive process depends on the physicochemical state of proteins. Meat proteins during processing and storage may be subjected to the unfolding of their tertiary structure and protein aggregation. A basic understanding of food protein digestibility associated with protein alterations can help produce food products by improving nutritional characteristics. The digestion of meat is essential, like other protein-based products. It should be noted that the accumulation of partially hydrolyzed or non-hydrolyzed proteins in the large intestine can have a causal role in colon cancer. Potentially mutagenic products in colonic flora are proteins that escape assimilation in the small intestine. Therefore, these products are extensively fermented and leading to the formation of altered products (Sante-Lhoutellier et al. 2007; Gatellier and Santé-Lhoutellier 2009; Peram et al. 2013). Besides the essential amino acid of meat, it is well established that meat is a significant source of nutritional iron because of its hemoprotein, myoglobin (Mb), and hemoglobin (Hb). Small intestine lumen with the predominantly alkaline conditions can efficiently absorb heme iron compared to dietary inorganic iron.

Besides, heme iron has more bioavailability compared with Non-heme iron in this condition (West and Oates 2008). Hence, meat digestibility and release of heme are essential in providing the body's iron requirement. Previous studies of our group about the effect of the slaughtering method on protein digestion exhibited that the extent of halal meat's hydrolysis was preferable to non-halal meat under heating. In this work, during the protein hydrolysis examination, myoglobin was used as an indicator, and its physicochemical characterization was examined. These results showed that myoglobin in the halal meat was hydrolyzed into smaller polypeptide chains compare with the non-halal myoglobin. During the heating, water molecules between fibrous proteins were lost, and these proteins contracted subsequently; these alterations disturbed the function of digestive enzymes. Studies showed that contraction between fibrous proteins in non-halal meat is more considerable than halal meat and makes them inaccessible to protease activity. Cooking loss in halal samples was lower than in non-halal samples. Cooking loss is a result of shrinkage of muscle fibers and connective tissues by heating. During the heating, thermal denaturation of meat proteins occurs. This denaturation appears in the secondary structure of proteins. Therefore, aggregation in β-sheet structures increases and α-helices content decline (Hosseini et al. 2019).

5 Microbiological Spoilage

Meat quality affecting both antemortem and postmortem factors. Antemortem factors include the species of the animal, age, sex, muscle groups, genetic pattern, and nourishment. The postmortem factor is generally the refrigerated storage (called aging) (Sabow et al. 2016a). The slaughtering method, including halal slaughtering, is considered an antemortem factor and an important meat quality parameter. Different parameters can affect the microbial growth in meat include the physiological condition of the animal at the time of slaughtering, spreading of microorganisms during slaughter, and storage condition (Sabow et al. 2016b). Humans' protection from food-borne diseases is necessary by monitoring the microbial conditions of meat and its products. The micro bacteria of poultry travel from the first place of production to the production lines and spread even more by further contamination. Slaughterhouses, operators' hands, equipment and clothing, water and air are possible origins of the heterogeneous micro bacteria in raw meat (Ibrahim et al. 2014).

Both producers and consumers are highly concerned with microbial safety and quality of meat. Malpractices in processing, handling, cooking, or post-cooking storage of the meat products lead to contamination of poultry meat with pathogens, a crucial concern for public health; meat and other food products analyzed by different microbial methods (Mead 2004).

The amount of blood that remains inside the carcass is one of the most decisive factors in the corpse's contamination and decomposition rates. Blood is an excellent medium for microbial growth due to its high nutritive value. The slaughtering method affects the amount of blood bled. The slaughtering methods on mesophilic bacteria counts (MBC) and psychrophilic bacteria counts (PBC) in cooked chicken patties during refrigerator storage were investigated. In all samples, MBC and PBC increased concurrently with storage duration. The bacteria counts in halal samples were lower in the same storage duration than other slaughtering methods (Addeen et al. 2017).

Microbial detection methods were performed to analyze chicken meat and sausage obtained from halal slaughtering and non-halal slaughtering. According to Table 1, the halal meat and halal meat sausage samples were not contaminated with either Coliform, *E. coli* or Salmonella. In contrast, the non-halal meat samples contained all three species of bacteria (Ibrahim et al. 2014).

Results of a study on the effects of conscious halal slaughtering and halal slaughtering after minimum anesthesia showed the only microorganism increased after 24 h of storage at 4 °C was the lactic acid bacteria in the anesthesia cases. However, no difference was observed in bleeding performance and the quality of goat meat slaughtered by each of the above methods (Sabow et al. 2015a).

One study evaluated the chemical alterations and microbial quality of broiler chicken meat obtained by halal slaughtering and the non-halal methods during refrigerated storage. The results

Table 1 Microbial load of halal and Non-halal poultry meat (c.f.u/g) Sample

Sample	Coliforms (c.f.u./g)	E. coli (c.f.u./g)	Salmonella (c.f.u./g)
HM	Nil	Nil	Nil
NHM	3.0×10^3	4.0×10^4	4.3×10^4
HMS	Nil	Nil	Nil
NHMS	15.0×10^5	23.3×10^4	15.0×10^4

HMS halal meat sausage, *NHMS* non-halal meat sausage

showed that, during the storage time, total viable count bacteria and lactic acid bacteria count were significantly more in non-halal samples than the halal samples. According to all results, halal slaughtering by neck cutting following the Islamic law is the better choice method to achieve the most blood drainage amount and further meat quality leading to longer shelf life for chicken meat products during refrigerated storage (Ahmed et al. 2018).

In an experiment in New Zealand, 80 male rabbits were selected and put into two groups of 40 animals, and then the amount of blood bleeding and meat stability during storage was measured. One group was subjected to halal slaughter (HS) without stunning, and the other gas stun-kill (GK). Meat stability during storage is evaluated by microbial analysis and measuring lipid oxidation concerning thiobarbituric acid reactive substances (TBARS). The results showed considerably more blood loss in the HS method than the GK method. On the third day of slaughtering, amounts of pseudomonas aeruginosa and *E. coli* bacteria were higher in the meat obtained from the GK group. However, thermosphacta and total aerobic count of bacteria in any of the slaughter methods were the same. After the fifth and seventh days of post-mortem, considerably more bacterial proliferation was observed in the GK group than in the HS group. The results suggest that the quality and shelf-life of meat are affected by the method of slaughtering. Therefore, the HS without a stunning method results from more blood loss may be more efficient than the GK method. This study affirms that in terms of premier meat quality, slaughtering relevant to the halal law can be a favorable alternative to conventional methods. However, it is necessary to have animal welfare in mind while carrying out the slaughtering procedure (Nakyinsige et al. 2014b). Another study was conducted on the effect of pre-slaughter electrical stunning and slaughter without stunning on the efficiency bleeding performance and shelf-life of chevon throughout a 14 days post-mortem aging. Four slaughtering methods randomly performed on 32 crossbred Boer bucks, namely: slaughter without stunning (SWS); low frequency head-only electrical stunning (LFHO; 1 A for 3 s at a frequency of 50 Hz); low frequency head-to-back electrical stunning (LFHB; 1 A for 3 s at a frequency of 50 Hz); and high-frequency head-to-back electrical stunning (HFHB; 1 A for 3 s at a frequency of 850 Hz). Compared to LFHB, goats slaughtered by SWS, LFHO, and HFHB methods lost more blood and retained less hemoglobin in their muscles. On the seventh and fourteenth days of post-mortem, TBARS values were higher in the meat acquired from LFHB than other methods. After the third day of post-mortem, LFHB meat contained more bacterial counts than SWS, LFHO, and HFHB. This study concludes that lower lipid oxidative stability and microbial quality of aging chevron from LFHB may result from lower bleed-out in this method (Sabow et al. 2016b).

One study showed that the slaughtering method (Halal vs. Classical slaughter) has no effects on the superficial pattern of microorganisms concerning the particular microbial markers of the digestive or respiratory tract. This study utilized traditional microbiological procedures and 16S rRNA metagenomics (Korsak et al. 2017).

6 Lipid and Protein Oxidation

In addition to microbial spoilage, other leading causes of deterioration of meat in terms of sensory, functional, and nutritional values are lipid and protein oxidation. Metabolic and other processes produce reactive oxidative species like hydroxyl, peroxide, superoxide, and nitric oxide radicals; they have the ability to interact with lipids and proteins at times of meat maturation and storage. Undesirable qualities such as unpleasant taste and smell, protein deterioration, discoloration, shorter shelf-life, and association of toxic compounds are all results of lipid oxidation and can be dangerous for consumers' health. Some chemical transformations emerge during protein oxidation, leading to biological modifications like protein solubility, protein aggregation, and fragmentation that affect meat quality. Moreover, chemical changes may have adverse effects on meat color and softness and also decrease the water holding capacity of meat (Sabow et al. 2016a,b). Meat products expose more oxidative reactions during storage and processes like cooking, mincing, and salt addition, that create more radical oxygen species (ROS). ROS may cause oxidation of protein and alters their backbone and side chains. Therefore, the primary, secondary, and tertiary structure of proteins transforms. The alteration of the typical structure of proteins makes them prone to be aggregated, and finally, protein malfunctionality occurs. It can be concluded that, in addition to more common microbial spoilage and lipid oxidation, protein oxidation can be a deteriorating agent in meat (Taghavi et al. 2017; Nakyinsige et al. 2015). Color is the primary indicator of meat quality. Lipid oxidation and protein (myoglobin) oxidation contribute to meat discoloration (Lubis et al. 2016). In addition, lipid oxidation produces by-products and contains cytotoxic and genotoxic properties in meat, and then it can be dangerous to human health (Rakhmanova et al. 2018). In the commercial gas stunning (GS) slaughtering method, the accumulation of CO_2 might have adverse effects on meat quality. The effects of the GS method, specifically CO_2 concentration on meat color and lipid peroxidation, were studied in broilers stored at 4° for a long time. The results showed that the GS slaughtering method had adverse effects on the breast meat color and, both 40% and 79% CO_2, suppressed gene expression in the antioxidant pathway. On the other hand, oxidative stress and lipid peroxidation of the stored meat was higher in the GS with 40% CO_2 than other groups (Xu et al. 2018).

The results of a study on halal-slaughtered chicken meat suggested that, compared to other slaughtering methods, halal meat contained less heme and non-heme iron and coincided with lower lipid oxidation. The main cause of deterioration and lower quality in chicken meat is lipid oxidation induced by iron from heme and microbial proliferation. Therefore, chicken meat obtained from the halal slaughtering method has better quality and more oxidative stability during storage (Addeen et al. 2014).

A comparison between halal slaughtering without stunning with three electrical stunning slaughtering methods showed more hemoglobin concentration, which contained residual blood in the carcasses. Heme pigment is a pro-oxidative factor in the muscles. Radical oxygen species (ROS) can modify muscle proteins in such a way to lower their function and, consequently, the quality of meat. An excellent promoter of lipid oxidation hemoglobin consists of 4 polypeptide chains, each comprising one heme group with an iron atom inside a porphyrin ring. If the porphyrin ring is damaged, Heme molecules might breakdown, and the iron atom released. Therefore, in long storage of the time of this process may stimulate lipid oxidation in the muscle. Also, blood as a generator of lipid oxidation is capable of producing superoxide, hydrogen peroxide, and hydroxyl radicals. Therefore, blood loss is insufficient in the slaughtering method, and a greater lipid oxidation rate occurs. In this study, no difference in protein oxidation was found in any slaughtering method (Sabow et al. 2016b).

7 Antioxidant Effects

Radical oxygen species (ROS) might lead to uncontrolled oxidative stresses, which cause some diseases such as cancer, diabetes, and diabetes-related complications. In nuerodegeative diseases, including Alzheimer's and Parkinson's, oxidative-stress mechanisms can impair the neuronal proteins and result in plaques formation (Arasteh et al. 2014). Antioxidant materials can use for the treatment of many human diseases such as different types of atherosclerosis, cardiovascular diseases, inflammatory injuries, and neurodegenerative diseases by reducing ROS in cells. Hence, natural antioxidants can consider as a type of preventive medicine (Barzegar and Moosavi-Movahedi 2011). Antioxidant properties have now been attributed to a number of proteins, amino acids and peptides (Xu et al. 2016; Collins

2005). For example, consumption of camel milk produces the bioactive peptides from the digestion of camel milk proteins and act as natural antioxidants and Angiotensin Converting Enzyme (ACE)-inhibitors (reduction of blood pressure) (Salami et al. 2011).

A value-added product that obtains from animal and plant proteins through hydrolysis is protein hydrolysate. For example, gelatin hydrolysates have attracted much attention from researchers because of a potent antioxidant and have applicable functional properties. Many researchers have shown that fish gelatin hydrolysates have excellent functional capabilities. Hydrolysis is performed by treatments with acids, alkalis, enzymes and fermentation. Different types of enzymes are utilized for enhancing functional and antioxidant properties and preparing protein hydrolysates. These enzymes include bromelain, alcalase, nutrase, flavourzyme, trypsin, pepsin, and papain (Razali et al. 2015).

Myofibrillar proteins contain amino acids and can deactivate metal ions oxidative activity, making meat protein a favorable source for antioxidant peptides. Another source of antioxidants in meat products is hydrolysates, which are produced through protease treatment. The antioxidant activity of halal meat proteins and non-halal meat proteins investigate by our group researchers. Hydrolysates peptides produced by digestion of meat proteins in halal samples exhibited more antioxidant activities than non-halal hydrolysates (Hosseini et al. 2019) significantly. Another aspect of our study was measuring the amount of aggregation of the protein. The data on transmission electron microscopy (TEM) and dynamic light scattering (DLS) show more protein aggregation of the non-halal sample than the halal sample.

Gelatin polymer is biodegradable and has antioxidant properties, therefore attracted attention from all around the world. Although gelatin can be produced from several sources, there has been an increasing interest in gelatin obtained from fish as other sources are either dangerous (e.g., cattle with mad cow disease) or unacceptable (non-halal). Other superior properties of fish gelatin include the presence of biologically active peptides that have antioxidant effects against the like of linoleic acid. Further, to produce antioxidant peptides with high radical scavenging properties, the fish gelatin hydrolyzes with papain. Hydrolysates of fish gelatin induce immunity against ultraviolet A and can act as functional food substances that have protective effects on biological systems and food oxidation. Conclusively gelatin obtained from pigs can be easily replaced by fish gelatin, which acts as an antioxidant driver. Another alternative source of gelatin that can be a halal substitute for porcine gelatin is gelatin isolated from the poultry waste, which shows properties of metal chelating and radical scavenging (Rakhmanova et al. 2018).

The skin of the Pacific cod produced gelatin, which was hydrolyzed with pepsin and created two bioactive peptides of GASSGMPG (662 Da) and LAYA (436 Da). These bioactive peptides inhibited the Angiotensin-I-converting enzyme (ACE). ACE is a peptic dipeptide hydrolase that plays a significant role in regulating blood pressure and controls hypertension and type-2 diabetes. Also, adding it to functional food appeared to lower blood pressure and cardiovascular disease (CVD) (Ngo et al. 2016). Studies show that gelatin obtained from cuttlefish donate an atom to peroxyl radicals of linoleic acid, causing stopping the β-carotene bleaching. All gelatins, probability, have electron or hydrogen donor peptides, react with free radical and dismiss the radical chain reaction, and finally convert the free radical to the more stable product. However, recent investigations show that fish gelatin (being odorless) is superior to poultry gelatin because poultry waste is difficult to manage. Therefore, porcine gelatin can be substituted by better alternatives in terms of gelling, oxidation-inhibiting, and function (Rakhmanova et al. 2018).

8 Halal Cosmetics

Today, a rising trend is observed in using beauty and personal care products to improve personal hygiene and beauty, delay the skin's aging process, and protect against pollutants and ultraviolet light. Cosmetic and beauty products refer to the materials produced to contact different external parts of the human body or the oral cavity and teeth. As these types of products are used daily by consumers, the cosmetics industry must inevitably offer available safe and cheap products. The ingredients used in cosmetics should be authentic and acceptable. Therefore, the domain of the halal issue expands to personal care and cosmetics products. Many people do not have a comprehensive view of the halal issue and think it is only associated with animals slaughtering. Hence, they do not care about the cosmetics they use and their ingredients. Halal cosmetics products mean that the products must be free from Haram (unlawful) ingredients such as alcohol, by-products of porcine, blood, carrion, human body parts, and derivatives. The use of lard because of its low price and availability is usually applied instead of oil is not permitted. Religious people only permit the usage of halal products in these products. Therefore, any person involved in the production of cosmetics must know the halal issue and ingredients. By the growth of awareness in this regard, halal care products and cosmetics will be bought by not only Muslims but also other people if accessible (Hashim and Mat Hashim 2013; Sugibayashi et al. 2019).

8.1 Halal Cosmetics Ingredients

As the beauty industry has paid more attention to halal cosmetics production and in this regard, it is necessary to check the sources, quality, and purity of the used ingredients and make sure that they are halal. Ingredients in halal cosmetic products are permitted based on the defined standards. Halal ingredients include water, soil, chemicals, microorganisms, plants, aquatic and halal land animals. All the plants and their derivatives can be used as halal ingredients without any concern. However, the plants processed in toxic methods or provided with unhygienic or haram ingredients cannot be allowed to use. The land animals are permitted to be used as ingredients, but animals like pigs and those that are not halal-slaughtered are not allowed. Also, their derivatives, such as the placenta and collagen, are not halal. All the aquatic animals and the animals that live in the water are halal except those that are toxic and hazardous. However, amphibious animals like frogs, crocodiles, and turtle are Haram and cannot be used to produce halal products. Incorporation of ingredients with human sources like cysteine and placenta are not allowed. As an ingredient of halal products, alcohol (primarily ethanol) is an issue of controversy. Some standards permit the use of industrial alcohol. Hence, halal cosmetic products having the halal logo must be identified as an indicator of safety, cleanliness, purity, and quality (Hashim and Mat Hashim 2013; Sugibayashi et al. 2019).

9 Detection of Halal Products

Nowadays, halal products' trade is considered an effective economic program by most Muslim and even non-Muslim countries (Tabatabaee et al. 2012). In terms of food product quality control, a significant ethical concern for consumers is unintentional or fraudulent meat blending from various animal sources. Moreover, the halal product means that sources, enzyme derivatives, flavor enhancers, and even the water used during food processing must be from halal and purified sources (Shariff and Mona 2013). A sensitive mass spectrometric approach to discover the trace amount of contamination in pork meat and horse meat is used and demonstrate the specificity of the identified biomarker peptides against lamb, chicken, and beef (Bargen et al. 2013). To facilitate the detection of pork, beef, buffalo, chicken, goat, quail, and rabbit meat PCR–RFLP, PCR-restriction fragment length polymorphism, the method developed. PCR–RFLP was performed based on the analysis of the cyt b gene of mitochondrial DNA and could be detected in different animal DNA. Therefore, PCR- RFLP is an easy and practical method to trace meat

Table 2 Modern biological approaches in halal food analysis

Protein-based analysis methods	DNA-based analysis methods
Immunoassay	PCR
Aptamers	Isothermal amplification
Isoelectric focusing	Analysis of alcohol in food products
Chromatography and mass spectrometry	Analysis of porcine protein and DNA using commercially available products
Mass spectrometry soft ionization techniques	
Fourier transform infrared spectroscopic and chemometrics	

fraudulent and halal authentication Because of its potential to distinguish species present in mixed meat (Murugaiah et al. 2009).

It is essential to assure consumers of cosmetic and self-care products' status by detecting any non-halal ingredient. Recently, to help religious authorities, extensive examination techniques have been promoted to ensure halal compliance and the absence of no non-halal material. Discovering methods for detection of alcohol, fat, oils, and gelatin in cosmetics include fourier transform infrared (FTIR) spectroscopy, gas chromatography-mass spectrometry (GCMS), and comprehensive two-dimensional gas chromatography hyphenated with time-of-flight mass spectrometry (GCxGC-TOF–MS). These methods also are utilized for traditional cosmetics and self-care products that require halal certification (Hashim and Mat Hashim 2013). Gelatin hydrolysates have a long history of cosmetic products like anti-aging creams, lipsticks, and hair care products. Owing to their ability to promote firmness, elasticity, and moisture are essential ingredients for skincare products. Also, hair care products, they improve hair gloss and softness. Fourier transform infrared (FTIR), in combination with attenuated total reflectance (ATR), is a method to classify and characterize unknown gelatin into the species of origin (Hashim et al. 2010). Also, a conventional technique to identify the animal source of gelatin in the form of powder or gelatin used in the manufacture of food products and capsule shells is the PCR technique that utilizes species-specific primers. Hence, the PCR method, which utilizes species-specific primers, is a practical, suitable, specific, economic, and precise technique for detecting gelatin of bovine or porcine source, and may gain all consumers' trust, especially consumers of halal products (Shabani et al. 2015).

Proteins and DNA are the most significant molecular biomarkers used in food analysis (Table 2). DNA-based techniques are commonly considered as the most proper detectors for animal species. Numerous approaches are committed related to halal authentication with the rapid formation of modern technology in biological analysis. Henceforth, reliable and effective screening methods for certifying halal food production principles introduced the halal industry's development as a beneficial market (Lubis et al. 2016).

10 Conclusion

Halal products have become quite popular worldwide because of health, safety, and cleanliness properties. All studies on the types of slaughtering exhibit that in halal slaughtering, maximum blood loss occurs. Therefore, the best quality of meat, longer shelf life, and lower bacterial counts in the halal samples was observed. Our group's studies show that the digestion of meat proteins and their antioxidant properties in the halal sample is higher than in the non-halal sample. In comparison, the protein aggregation of the non-halal sample is more than the halal sample. Also, lipid and protein oxidation as the main causes of deterioration of meat in the halal samples are less than the non-halal samples. The detection of non-halal ingredients is a serious issue to protect the accuracy and verification of halal products. Hence, broad detection techniques for non-halal products have been developed, including protein-based (FTIR and GCMS) and DNA-based (PCR) apparatuses.

References

Abdul-Talib AN, Abd-Razak IS (2013) Cultivating export market oriented behavior in halal marketing. J Islamic Market 4(2):187–197

Addeen A, Benjakul S, Wattanachant S, Maqsood S (2014) Effect of Islamic slaughtering on chemical compositions and post-mortem quality changes of broiler chicken meat. Int Food Res J 21(3):897–907

Addeen A, Benjakul S, Prodpran T (2017) Slaughtering method affects lipid oxidation, volatile profile and overall quality of chicken patties during storage. Emirates J Food Agric 29(5):387–395

Ahmed H, Hassan Z, Manap M (2018) Physico-chemical changes and microbiological quality of refrigerated broiler chicken meat slaughtered by two different methods. Int Food Res J 25(3):913–920

Ambali AR, Bakar AN (2014) People's awareness on halal foods and products: potential issues for policymakers. Proc-Soc Behav Sci 121(19):3–25

Arasteh A, Farahi S, Habibi-Rezaei M, Moosavi-Movahedi AA (2014) Glycated albumin: an overview of the in vitro models of an in vivo potential disease marker. J Diabetes Metab Disord 13(1):49

Barzegar A, Moosavi-Movahedi AA (2011) Intracellular ROS protection efficiency and free radical-scavenging activity of curcumin. PLoS ONE 6(10): e26012

Bonne K, Verbeke W (2008) Religious values informing halal meat production and the control and delivery of halal credence quality. Agric Hum Values 25(1):35–47

Collins AR (2005) Antioxidant intervention as a route to cancer prevention. Eur J Cancer 41(13):1923–1930

Ermis E (2017) Halal status of enzymes used in food industry. Trends Food Sci Technol 64:69–73

Farouk MM, Al-Mazeedi HM, Sabow AB, Bekhit AED, Adeyemi KD, Sazili AQ, Ghani A (2014) Halal and kosher slaughter methods and meat quality: a review. Meat Sci 98(3):505–519

Fuseini A, Wotton SB, Knowles TG, Hadley PJ (2017) Halal meat fraud and safety issues in the UK: a review in the context of the European Union. Food Ethics 1 (2):127–142

Gatellier P, Santé-Lhoutellier V (2009) Digestion study of proteins from cooked meat using an enzymatic microreactor. Meat Sci 81(2):405–409

Gibson TJ, Dadios N, Gregory NG (2015) Effect of neck cut position on time to collapse in halal slaughtered cattle without stunning. Meat Sci 110:310–314

Hashim P, Mat Hashim D (2013) A review of cosmetic and personal care products: halal perspective and detection of ingredient. Pertanika J Sci Technol 21 (2):281–292

Hashim D, Man YC, Norakasha R, Shuhaimi M, Salmah Y, Syahariza Z (2010) Potential use of fourier transform infrared spectroscopy for differentiation of bovine and porcine gelatins. Food Chem 118(3):856–860

Hosseini E, Sattari R, Ariaeenejad S, Salami M, Emam-Djomeh Z, Fotouhi L, Poursasan N, Sheibani N, Ghamsari SM, Moosavi-Movahedi AA (2019) The impact of slaughtering methods on physicochemical characterization of sheep myoglobin. J Iran Chem Soc 16(2):315–324

Ibrahim SM, Abdelgadir MA, Sulieman AME (2014) Impact of halal and non-halal slaughtering on the microbiological characteristics of broiler chicken meat and sausages. Food Public Health 4(5):223–228

Karahalil E (2020) Principles of halal-compliant fermentations: microbial alternatives for the halal food industry. Trends Food Sci Technol 98:1–9

Korsak N, Taminiau B, Hupperts C, Delhalle L, Nezer C, Delcenserie V, Daube G (2017) Assessment of bacterial superficial contamination in classical or ritually slaughtered cattle using metagenetics and microbiological analysis. Int J Food Microbiol 247:79–86

Latif IA, Mohamed Z, Sharifuddin J, Abdullah AM, Ismail MM (2014) A comparative analysis of global halal certification requirements. J Food Prod Market 20(sup1):85–101

Lubis HN, Mohd-Naim NF, Alizul NN, Ahmed MU (2016) From market to food plate: current trusted technology and innovations in halal food analysis. Trends Food Sci Technol 58:55–68

Mathew VN (2014) Acceptance on halal food among non-Muslim consumers. Proc-Soc Behav Sci 121:262–271

Mead G (2004) Microbiological quality of poultry meat: a review. Braz J Poultry Sci 6(3):135–142

Murugaiah C, Noor ZM, Mastakim M, Bilung LM, Selamat J, Radu S (2009) Meat species identification and halal authentication analysis using mitochondrial DNA. Meat Sci 83(1):57–61

Nakyinsige K, Sazili AQ, Zulkifli I, Goh YM, Bakar FA, Sabow AB (2014a) Influence of gas stunning and halal slaughter (no stunning) on rabbits welfare indicators and meat quality. Meat Sci 98(4):701–708

Nakyinsige K, Fatimah A, Aghwan Z, Zulkifli I, Goh Y, Sazili A (2014b) Bleeding efficiency and meat oxidative stability and microbiological quality of New Zealand white rabbits subjected to halal slaughter without stunning and gas stun-killing. Asian-Australas J Anim Sci 27(3):406–413

Nakyinsige K, Sazili A, Aghwan Z, Zulkifli I, Goh Y, Bakar FA, Sarah S (2015) Development of microbial spoilage and lipid and protein oxidation in rabbit meat. Meat Sci 108:125–131

Ngo D-H, Vo T-S, Ryu B, Kim S-K (2016) Angiotensin-I-converting enzyme (ACE) inhibitory peptides from pacific cod skin gelatin using ultrafiltration membranes. Process Biochem 51(10):1622–1628

Peram MR, Loveday SM, Ye A, Singh H (2013) In vitro gastric digestion of heat-induced aggregates of β-lactoglobulin. J Dairy Sci 96(1):63–74

Rakhmanova A, Khan Z, Sharif R, Lv X (2018) Meeting the requirements of halal gelatin: a mini review. MOJ Food Process Technol 6:477–482

Razali A, Amin A, Sarbon N (2015) Antioxidant activity and functional properties of fractionated cobia skin gelatin hydrolysate at different molecular weight. Int Food Res J 22(2):651–660

Riaz MN, Chaudry MM (2003) Halal food production. CRC Press

Sabow A, Sazili A, Zulkifli I, Goh Y, Ab Kadir M, Abdulla N, Nakyinsige K, Kaka U, Adeyemi K (2015) A comparison of bleeding efficiency, microbiological quality and lipid oxidation in goats subjected to conscious halal slaughter and slaughter following minimal anesthesia. Meat Sci 104:78–84

Sabow AB, Sazili AQ, Zulkifli I, Goh YM, Kadir MZAA, Adeyemi KD (2015b) Physico-chemical characteristics of *Longissimus lumborum* muscle in goats subjected to halal slaughter and anesthesia (halothane) pre-slaughter. Anim Sci J 86(12):981–991

Sabow AB, Sazili AQ, Aghwan ZA, Zulkifli I, Goh YM, Ab Kadir MZA, Nakyinsige K, Kaka U, Adeyemi KD (2016) Changes of microbial spoilage, lipid-protein oxidation and physicochemical properties during post mortem refrigerated storage of goat meat. Anim Sci J 87(6):816–826

Sabow AB, Zulkifli I, Goh YM, Ab Kadir MZA, Kaka U, Imlan JC, Abubakar AA, Adeyemi KD, Sazili AQ (2016) Bleeding efficiency, microbiological quality and oxidative stability of meat from goats subjected to slaughter without stunning in comparison with different methods of pre-slaughter electrical stunning. PloS ONE 11(4):e0152661

Salami M, Moosavi-Movahedi AA, Moosavi-Movahedi F, Ehsani MR, Yousefi R, Farhadi M, Niasari-Naslaji A, Saboury AA, Chobert J-M, Haertlé T (2011) Biological activity of camel milk casein following enzymatic digestion. J Dairy Res 78(4):471–478

Sante-Lhoutellier V, Aubry L, Gatellier P (2007) Effect of oxidation on in vitro digestibility of skeletal muscle myofibrillar proteins. J Agric Food Chem 55(13):5343–5348

Sattari R, Hosseini E, Fotouhi L, Ariaeenejad S, Khatibi A, Moosavi-Movahedi AA (2015) Meat quality of halal slaughtering and comparison with different types of killing. Sci Cultivation 5(2):35–39

Shabani H, Mehdizadeh M, Mousavi SM, Dezfouli EA, Solgi T, Khodaverdi M, Rabiei M, Rastegar H, Alebouyeh M (2015) Halal authenticity of gelatin using species-specific PCR. Food Chem 184:203–206

Shariff AHM, Mona Z (2013) Raw ingredients in cat food manufacturing: palatability, digestibility and halal issues in Malaysia. J Trop Resour Sustain Sci 1(1):1–15

Sugibayashi K, Yusuf E, Todo H, Dahlizar S, Sakdiset P, Arce F Jr, See GL (2019) Halal cosmetics: a review on ingredients, production, and testing methods. Cosmetics 6(3):37

Tabatabaee SM, Mazaheri M, Farokhi R, Moosavi-Movahedi AA (2012) Trade of halal products. Sci Cultivation 2(2):15–19

Taghavi F, Habibi-Rezaei M, Amani M, Saboury AA, Moosavi-Movahedi AA (2017) The status of glycation in protein aggregation. Int J Biol Macromol 100:67–74

von Bargen C, Dojahn Jr, Waidelich D, Humpf H-U, Brockmeyer J (2013) New sensitive high-performance liquid chromatography-tandem mass spectrometry method for the detection of horse and pork in halal beef. J Agric Food Chem 61(49):11986–11994

West AR, Oates PS (2008) Mechanisms of heme iron absorption: current questions and controversies. World J Gastroenterol 14(26):4101–4110

Xu Q, He C, Xiao C, Chen X (2016) Reactive oxygen species (ROS) responsive polymers for biomedical applications. Macromol Biosci 16(5):635–646

Xu L, Zhang H, Yue H, Wu S, Yang H, Wang Z, Qi G (2018) Gas stunning with CO_2 affected meat color, lipid peroxidation, oxidative stress, and gene expression of mitogen-activated protein kinases, glutathione S-transferases, and Cu/Zn-superoxide dismutase in the skeletal muscles of broilers. J Anim Sci Biotechnol 9(1):37

Lifestyle in the Regulation of Diabetic Disorders

Fereshteh Taghavi, Mahdie Rahban, and Ali Akbar Moosavi-Movahedi

Abstract

Achieving nutritional information and health-promoting elements is an essential concern in today's world. In this regard, understanding the concept of health, disease, aging, and lifestyle is of particular importance in choosing the right method for lifestyle and disease treatment. Lifestyle as a way arises from the nation, groups or people's habits based on their belief, specific culture, economy, policy or geographical region at a particular time, can take two approaches: health and disease. Lifestyle disease, with its important elements such as immobility, unhealthy food habits, disturbed biological clock, and wrong body posture, triggers some health issues and life-threatening due to oxidative stress and inflammation. Metabolism disorders and diabetes, in particular, are some of the results and consequences of this kind of lifestyle. Accordingly, a healthy lifestyle is actually profound wisdom and to be healthy, and empowerment in this era is based on recognizing and applying the effective elements which are involved in a healthy lifestyle. Inflammatory diseases caused by modern and technologic life emphasize the necessity of an in-depth look at the anti-inflammatory elements in a healthy lifestyle. In a healthy lifestyle, probiotics, plant-based diets and phytochemicals, whole grain, healthy fat, nature close contact, negative ions and using mobile phone carefully due to their effect on cellular inflammation, have an essential role in health achieving and its consequent events. In this chapter, we will take a closer look at the effective concepts and elements of a healthy lifestyle.

Keywords

Lifestyle disease · Healthy lifestyle · Probiotics · Plants · Whole grains · Healthy fats · Nature · Negative air ions · Inner peace · Hydration

F. Taghavi (✉)
Faculty of Biological Science, Tarbiat Modares University, Tehran, Iran
e-mail: taghavif@ut.ac.ir

M. Rahban · A. A. Moosavi-Movahedi
Institute of Biochemistry and Biophysics (IBB), University of Tehran, Tehran, Iran
e-mail: mrohban@ut.ac.ir

A. A. Moosavi-Movahedi
e-mail: moosavi@ut.ac.ir

1 Introduction

The wide range of information presented in scientific papers has made it possible to achieve important nutritional information and health providing elements. But it seems necessary to go deeper into the concept of health, disease and reasons for obtaining the proper lifestyle (Liu et al. 2017).

1.1 Health

In the Oxford Dictionary, salvation from illness and injury has been defined as health, but this term has had an evolutionary line over time. The term of 'hælth' as the whole/something complete in itself, is the origination of 'health' in its English root. Hælth' itself came from Germanic origin word as 'hal' and latter hail arise from' hal' as health in toasts and greetings which itself has come from "heel" as Duch and 'heil' as German words. Heil is related to another German word as 'heilfroh,' which combines happiness and health as wholly happy. In the religious meaning, 'Heil' and salvation are the same in meaning (Brüssow 2013).

Hippocrates and ancient Greek medicine believed that health is harmony, and disease is a certain element disharmony in the human body. Later, this attitude generalized in modern medicine as homeostasis and health, which were defined as homeostasis in physiological, biochemical, psychological, and social aspects. By this way, some researches consider disease as the state that passes through homeostasis deterioration, treatment and prevention toward homeostasis restoration. In this view, all homeostasis levels play a role in their mutual interaction in which body, life and environment satisfaction have a central position.

Researchers report that based on social and psychological approach, health maintenance depends intensely on internal regulatory functions and self-regulation in social actions. In addition, spiritual aspects form human existence as a core component, which called a will to mean. Researches refer that health risks are reduced by spirituality (the way people look for meaning in their lives via healthy lifestyles promotion, health-protective behaviors, restore the correct balance of health status, maintenance and enhancement).

In this general sense, people not only evaluate their experiences and attitudes but also respond to them. Now, if the criteria for evaluation and interpretation are based on the correct knowledge of health and its promotion, the result will be the adoption of health-promoting behavior (Piko and Brassai 2016). Health also has more definitions today based on social norms and cultural values as: (a) the absence of any impairment or disease. In this situation, an individual healthy condition can be declared by the medical profession; however, the diagnosis process itself is under evolution and may not be able to detect some disease at this time. So, an individual who is declared healthy today may be found to be ill tomorrow because of the methods advancement (Piko and Brassai 2016; Sartorius 2006); (b) Individuals ability to adapt and cope with all everyday life's demands; (c) an equilibrium and balance state by which a person keeps his steady-state with internal, physical and social environment regardless to the presence of diseases (Moosavi-Movahedi 2020).

It also means the adaption capacity of external and internal circumstances changing. It is worth mentioning that the first definition is depending on the diagnostic power of advanced methods which are existing today. Also, these health paradigms are free from individuals' feelings of their health and the judgment of surrounding people about individuals' behavior and appearance and just depend on their accordance with criteria of abnormalities (Brüssow 2013; Piko and Brassai 2016; Sartorius 2006).

WHO (1948) believe the lack of disability and illness does not necessarily mean health. In fact, health means complete well-being in physical, mental and social aspects, and health in this sense is essential for the happiness, harmonious relationships and security of all people. In other words, health is considered as self-care, pain, individual mobility, vision, sleep, energy, cognition, interpersonal activities by this organization. In this regard, a small portion of people can be fitted by WHO definition, so most of them are in an unhealthy situation. Also, there are some interpretations about health as a dynamic concept in the eyes of the beholder, a state or ability, or the best ability to self-manage and adapt (Brüssow 2013; Sartorius 2006).

There is another interesting approach to health definition: The ability to adapt and self-managing is considered as the preferred view of health. But health in physical approach can be considered as allostasis, which means physiological homeostasis maintenance through changing circumstances. In this regards, an essential criterion in the health of the mind is a sense of coherence. On the other hand, social health means the capacity of individuals to realize their potentials and commitments, the ability to manage life and participate in social activities, includes work. Health also was defined with other statements: the capacity of work and love, successful or healthy aging, satisfy needs, realize aspirations, and cope with the environment by an individual in everyday life's resource. It is also stated that pathogenesis as becoming ill and salutogenesis as becoming health (Mittelmark and Bauer 2017; Yousefi and Moosavi-Movahedi 2020).

Pathogenesis is the study of diseases and risk's origin, but in contrast, health comes from salutogenesis as the sense of coherence. So, despite pathogenesis, the term of salutogenesis is oriented scholarly attention on the health origins and assets for health. Salutogenesis refers to sb's life experiences, which form his or her sense of coherence (a global orientation); it has a nearest meaning as the strong sense of coherence, which helps to manage tension and cope with stressors successfully. This kind of coherence has a vital role in one's movement toward the pathway of Ease or Dis-ease. The harmony between the sense of coherence and orientation (Salutogenesis) and social sciences development can be led to a better understanding of the positive aspects of human experience (Mittelmark and Bauer 2017; Yousefi and Moosavi-Movahedi 2020). Another definition of health is being active on different levels includes individual, interpersonal, community, environmental, and political levels (Tang et al. 2003; Smith et al. 2006).

1.2 Diseasess

On the other hand, Oxford Dictionary defines disease as a disorder in an organism's structure and function, which does not come from physical injury and has some specific symptoms; Old French' desaise' as the lack of ease is the origination of 'dis-ease.' Illr (Norse word) with the meaning of malevolent or wicked is in contrast with the well (wohl, German word) means in a good way or good health. Also, the concept of wellness is equal to beyond physical health, with a strong relation with happiness (Brüssow 2013).

1.3 Health Promotion

Another critical concept is health promotion as the synergy process or planned combination of health policy, education, organization and regulation supports in all sectors of society. In addition, health education for all leads to people empowerment about their health control by creating health literacy enhancement, supportive environments, and robust social networks (Thacker et al. 2017). These actions lead to the health of individuals, groups, or communities (Kok and Vries 2015). Health promotion is an equilibrium and balance state by which a person keeps his steady-state with internal, physical and social environment regardless of the presence of diseases. It is clear that the kinds of health's definition determine the direction of health promotion. If health is considered as the absence of any impairment or disease, health promotion can be defined as decrement in diseases numbers of affected people. But if health is regarded as the ability to adapt and afford with all the requirements of everyday life, health promotion is the enhanced and strengthened coping capacity of individuals by the involvement of functioning. Also, if health has its equilibrium definition, health promotion as an active approach refers to the highest rating for health in the eyes of individuals and society and harmonic behavior with their values (Brüssow 2013).

In fact, promoting the health of individuals and communities is a complicated procedure in which success depends on many factors, including individuals, families, communities, health professionals, academics, managers, development partners, jobs, media and governments. So, it seems that a good definition of health can be based on these elements. In the other word, social determinants (income, access to health care, goods, services, education, work, leisure, homes, communities, etc.) and Environmental determinants (external physical, chemical, and biological factors including safe houses, clean air and water, healthy workplaces, roads and managing climate change) can be added to the meaning of health (Kok and Vries 2015; Bircher and Kuruvilla 2014).

Global health is another important concept which refers to globalization's transnational effect on health problems and its determinants as an independent issue. This concept is beyond the control of individual nations and consider as Global health and can be affected by global climate change, refugee populations' vulnerability, harmful product marketing due to transnational corporations, and the diseases transmission resulting from inter countries traveling (like Corona virus disaster in recent months). Health promotion at both the national and international levels and partnerships for priority setting has the main priority in global health. In fact, global health problems are different from international health issues because global health problems appear to be challenging for controlling by the institutions of individual countries (Huynen et al. 2005).

1.4 Aging

Aging as a gradual important event is directly related to health. The increment of population age is an inclusive phenomenon around the world and change the world's structure dramatically. It is clear that socioeconomic conditions, health and disease can be affected by aging entirely. There are not straight and developed definitions of aging by biologists. 'Age' can be defined in different ways, but changed something on a timescale is its simplest definition. Interestingly, there are different attitude on aging based on different languages as deterioration (English definition); and advancement (Japanese definition). Age also is considered as regression of physiological function with age increment; body structure and function progressive decline. With any definition of aging, in this downward trend, these events take place: body mass steadily decrement, especially in muscles and visceral organs; neurodegeneration; bone strength decrement due to active demineralization, unbalanced gait, fracture events due to slow reaction times and poor balance, decrement in memory capability, sensory system (vision, hearing, taste) and resting metabolic rate (as a marker of illness); lower resistance to stress due to progressive alteration in homeostasis pathways (hormones, inflammatory mediators, antioxidants) and malnutrition due to food intake decrement (Brüssow 2013).

Based on fries view (twentieth century), human survival curves have changed to a more rectangular form that of the average length of life, but the maximum life span has not increased. He believed that chronic diseases at older ages are the main reason for most premature deaths in this century. This requires more attention to health improvement by consideration of life quality rather than life duration; chronic diseases compared with acute diseases, morbidity instead of mortality. Based on his report, lifestyle (equilibrated diet, weight control, ordered exercise, paying attention to blood pressure (hypertension), alcohol and smoking elimination) can change the quality of life, postpone chronic illness and modify aging's psychological and physiological markers. He also mentioned that delay in illness is more significant than its cure (Fries 1980). On the other hand, death can be occurred due to a disease process (Brüssow 2013) or at the end of a normal lifespan without obvious disease when the normal span is lived (Fries 1980).

It is reported that life expectancy can be increased by nutrition and healthcare. Also, it is shown that morbidity compression occurs in some low mortality countries, and only healthy life expectancy compression can be expected than life expectancy (Brüssow 2013). Interestingly, behavioral, mental and musculoskeletal disorders, diabetes and endocrine diseases, major depressive and anxiety disorders, anemia, chronic obstructive pulmonary disease, migraine are the main and important disorders in a global estimate of life burden accompanied with disease or disability over the years. So, it seems lifestyle has greater importance than what is intended before (Brüssow 2013).

2 Normal Cell Signaling as the Normal Cellular Language

The integration of a complex array of bio-signals, which are sensed, responded and adapted by living cells in regards to their environmental modifications leading to birth, health and death (Perbal 2003). Despite of the high independence of prokaryotic and unicellular eukaryotic cells in their function, meeting the needs in multicellular plants and animals requires the regulation of each cell's behavior separately and together (Cooper and Hausman 2018). Harmonious development of tissues, organs and bodies and their transcendent functions (thought, behavior and movement) depends on the cells proper received and sent signals during their whole existence. Cellular needs for proper function, its precise coordination of signals reception and release have led them to form micro societies in order to survive (Perbal 2003). Cellular networking communication can occur by single cell response to the other cells via secreted signaling molecules and producing cell–cell communication in multicellular networking in the highest level of maturity. In this way, the comprehensiveness of the whole message is understood by the cellular network (Cooper and Hausman 2018). In this regards, the secretion or expression of a variety of signaling molecules at one cell surface and its binding to the receptors expressed by other cells plays an important role. The integrity and purposefulness of these signaling in many single cells produce complicates cells set as human beings. It worth mentioning that a series of vital intracellular reactions and complex regulatory mechanisms are triggered by the binding of most signaling molecules to their receptors. All of these native biological signaling and the consequent process made a smart, complex homeostatic language system that controls all aspects of cell behavior (survival, metabolism, proliferation, movement, and differentiation). The elements of this language system are healthy signaling molecules and their receptors, normal functions of cell surface receptors, intracellular signal transduction pathways, cytoskeleton, development, and differentiation signaling and programmed cell death regulation. Many agents can interfere with this language system, breakdown it, and disrupt vital cell functions. Regards to mentioned points, the required coordination for multicellular organisms' functionality is provided by cell signaling and its precise function as an essential and ubiquitous process for living systems to make vital decisions about cell growth and division, differentiation, development, migration and apoptosis (Perbal 2003; Cooper and Hausman 2018; Radhakrishnan et al. 2010). It is clear that any malfunction of these networks causes pathological conditions (Cooper and Hausman 2018).

3 New Abnormal Language by Cellular Signaling Modification

Two crucial related processes can affect cellular signaling, change the chemical and systemic language of cellular communication toward cell destruction: (a) oxidative stress; (b) inflammation. Life has been the result of free radical interactions. Reactive oxygen species are usually produced in human normal cellular metabolism, their limited quantity involved in cellular chemical language and have an important role in biological processes (reply to alteration of intra and extracellular environmental conditions (Jabs 1999), evolution, aging, mutations, death, random changes inducing, regulation processes like cell homeostasis maintenance, gene expression, stimulation of signaling pathways and receptors activation (Upham and Trosko 2009).

Oxidative stress is an excessive cellular generation of reactive oxygen species (ROS) that cannot be neutralized by the antioxidant system. This imbalance protective mechanism leads to an increase in the chances of mutagenesis and biomacromolecular (Taghavi and Moosavi-Movahedi 2019; Taghavi et al. 2013, 2016, 2017; Najjar et al. 2017) and consequent cellular irreversible damage (Wang et al. 2004; Ďuračková 2010; Hussain et al. 2016). Interestingly, limited quantities of ROS are involved in cellular signaling (Thannickal and Fanburg 2000).

Inflammation as an essential protecting response of the host to injury or infection is produced due to the interaction between many different types of cells. Redness, heat, swelling, pain, and function disorder are prevalent symptoms of inflammatory responses. However, with activation of inflammatory mediators (such as reactive protein C (CRP), TNF-α, IL-6), persistent and developed chronic inflammation, tissue damage, and disease are created (Xu et al. 2018; Hosseini et al. 2018).

Indeed, inflammation as the biological reply of the immune system to harmful stimuli (toxic compounds, pathogens and damaged cells) (Medzhitov 2010) take places as acute or chronic events in different human main organs (such as heart, pancreas, liver, kidney, lung, brain, intestinal tract and reproductive system) and lead to tissue damage and disease. In normal condition, inflammation act as a vital defense mechanism for health providing (Nathan and Ding 2010) via injurious stimuli remove, restoration of tissue homeostasis, and the healing process is initiating. But chronic uncontrolled acute inflammation leads to inflammatory diseases (Zhou et al. 2016). Excessive chronic inflammation is a crucial common important event in all diseases, especially cardiovascular diseases, Alzheimer's and other neurological diseases, certain cancer, the pathogenesis of metabolic diseases (obesity and type 2 diabetes). The mechanism of this involvement is related to atherosclerosis facilitation, insulin resistance development, endoplasmic reticular stress, gut microbiota alteration (Xu et al. 2018; Hosseini et al. 2018).

4 Lifestyle

At a glance, lifestyle is also considered as a day to day individuals' behaviors, activities functions, job, fun and diet. In other words, lifestyle is defined as normal and conventional accepted daily activities by people that can affect life quality, human health, its promotion and diseases inhibition. So, its quality, maintenance and control have a significant impact on human health (Tol et al. 2013).

This concept has a close relationship with health based on the WHO view, and there is a deep relationship between individual quality of life and individual health. It is well marked that unhealthy lifestyle (malnutrition, unhealthy diet, stress, smoking, alcohol consumption, and drug abuse) lead to diseases formation such as metabolic diseases, cardiovascular diseases, overweight hypertension, physical and mental problem, violence, disability and even death. Regards to confronting of our lives with significant new challenges such as misuse and overuse of the technology or unknown diseases (Corona virus and things we have to wait for in the future), serious attention to diet and body mass index (BMI), exercise, sleep, taking medication, study, recreation, application of modern technologies and determining life style quality are essential (Farhud 2015). In this regards, the health-promoting lifestyle (HPL) is an excellent promoter for high-quality achievement and induces self-improvement, self-persuasion and improves satisfaction, health, and welfare. Nutrition, stress management, physical activity, spiritual growth, health responsibility, interpersonal relations are the fundamental factors for health-promoting lifestyle (HPL). It is worth mentioning that health promotion and public health are two critical elements for communities' development. Nowadays, diseases prevention by a healthy lifestyle is more important than treatment and acts as the main factor in health promotion (Tol et al. 2013).

Oxidative stress, higher production of ROS, and protein oxidations are related events that have been reported in chronic (Xu et al. 2018) and autoimmune diseases, exposure to toxic chemicals, allergens, radiation, obesity, alcohol consumption, a high-calorie diet and tobacco use. This abnormal process leads to numerous disorders in homeostasis and cellular signaling (Cecarini et al. 2007).

Excessive ROS, oxidized protein, glycated products, and lipid peroxidation (Sottero et al.

2018) act as inflammatory stimuli, produce more inflammatory signals molecules (Salzano et al. 2014), initiate synthesis, and secretion of pro inflammatory cytokines and promote inflammatory process (Kim et al. 2009; Forrester et al. 2018). In the brain, these stimulatory molecules provide neuroinflammation and consequent cell death via alteration in communication between neurons (synaptic and non-synaptic connections) (Popa-Wagner et al. 2013; Rahman and MacNee 2000). Inflammation as an intrinsic defense mechanism against pathogens accompanied by many pathogenic diseases (microbial and viral infections, autoimmune diseases) and significantly unhealthy lifestyles (Liu et al. 2017; Hosseini et al. 2018; Rahman and MacNee 2000; Berlett and Stadtman 1997). Glutathione is an example for a demonstration of the deep relationship between OS and inflammation. GSH as a vital protective antioxidant (intra- and extracellular) acts against oxidative or nitrosative stresses and involve in pro-inflammatory processes. It is also involved in other important events such as immune redox modulation, extracellular matrix remodeling, mitochondrial respiration and apoptosis (Cecarini et al. 2007).

It is necessary to point out that redox equilibrium has pivotal roles in normal cellular functions, and its abnormality provides pathological conditions. ROS has complicated interactions with various signaling molecules (receptors, ions, proteins) and signaling pathways that can activate or deactivate them. It significantly means that ROS can change the language of cellular communication and dictate a pathological program to cells (Hussain et al. 2016; Finkel 2011).

4.1 Lifestyle Diseases

There are some patterns as lifestyle diseases which lead to the formation of the unhealthy condition and diseases formation. These lifestyles originate from daily habits of people and improper relationship between people and their environment, which develop gradually and is hard to cure. All lifestyle diseases start with a lack of movement, inappropriate food habits, disturbed biological clock, and wrong body posture (Sharma and Majumdar 2009). This kind of lifestyle makes some health issues, life-threatening consequences, and chronic non-communicable diseases (NCDs) due to eliminate daily individual activities and make a sedentary routine situation. It is worth mentioning that 70% of all global deaths are related to NCDs with chronic nature and no transfer capability made by a combination of genetical, physiological, environmental and behavioral factors (Reddy 2017). In this group, cardiovascular diseases (heart attacks and stroke), cancer, respiratory diseases and diabetes with a mortality rate of 17.5 million, 8.2 million, 4 million and 1.5 million respectively are the highest causes of death and called lifestyle diseases for its heavy linkage to human lifestyle choices (Al-Mawali 2015; Aryal et al. 2015).

NCDs lifestyle includes modified behavioral (excessive alcohol use, inappropriate food habits, tobacco consumption, immobility, improper body posture, biological clock disturbance and work related stress), non-modifiable factors (Uncontrollable or changeable situations by intervention like Sex, age, ethnicity and changes in genomes) and metabolic risk factors (increased blood pressure, hyperglycemia, hyperlipidemia, obesity or, and increased levels of fat in the blood) (Sharma and Majumdar 2009; Reddy 2017; Melo et al. 2019).

4.2 Diabetes

Diabetes as a collection of serious, long- term multiple metabolic diseases has a variety of attributable causes with a significant impact on individuals, families, and societies, even worldwide lives and well-being (Reddy 2017; Atlas 2017; Gudjinu and Sarfo 2017). Researches revealed that many factors like stress, aging, population growth, physical inactivity, increasing prevalence of obesity, urbanization have a crucial role in diabetes prevalence. Recent findings (2017) revealed that about 475 million people consider as diabetic patients (Reddy 2017; James

2018). It is estimated that worldwide diabetes prevalence will be improved, and the number of diabetic patients reaches up to 629 million by 2045 (Ardeshirlarijani et al. 2019; Tecilazich 2020).

Diabetes as a lifestyle disease (Mathers and Loncar 2006) is a metabolic disorder in the way of using food for energy or physical growth by the body. In this disease, heart, blood vessels, eyes, kidneys and nerves encounter severe damage due to blood glucose elevated levels over time (Diagnosis and Classification of Diabetes Mellitus 2009). It is worth mentioning that metabolic syndrome produces a cluster of metabolic derangements that lead to obesity, glucose intolerance, dyslipidemia and hypertension (Zhang et al. 2013). Diabetes can be classified into four groups: Diabetes Type 1 (T1DM or formally as Mellitus), diabetes Type 2 (T2DM or formally as non-insulin dependent diabetes mellitus), diabetes Type 3 (a possible form of Alzheimer's disease with oxidative stress, cognitive impairment, disordered glucose metabolism, mitochondrial dysfunction, insulin resistance and brain dysfunction); Gestational, Pre-Diabetes (impaired glucose tolerance); latent autoimmune diabetes of adults (LADA); maturity onset diabetes of the young (MODY); and Neonatal diabetes(in the first six months of life with not sufficient insulin) (Reddy 2017; Gudjinu and Sarfo 2017; Diagnosis and Classification of Diabetes Mellitus 2009). Among the kind of diabetes, diabetes mellitus (T2DM) as a global health problem with life quality decrement and health expenditure increment has the highest prevalence in the world. Its main modifiable risk factors usually include unhealthy diets; immobility; obesity or overweight; hypertension; dyslipidemia; psychological stress; high consumption of alcohol and sugar; low consumption of fiber, TV watching, sleep disordered and breathing burden (Bellou et al. 2018; Gillett et al. 2012; Joseph et al. 2017). As mentioned before, the world is experiencing a dramatic rise in the number of diabetic patients, especially in low-and middle-income countries, with 1.6 million annual deaths. T2DM is generally chronic in nature and comes from insulin resistance and dysfunctionality of β-cells result from the combination of genetic and environmental factors. In this regards, environmental changes have an essential role in this epidemic disorder (Bellou et al. 2018). Researches showed that insulin resistance is the hub of diabetes and other metabolic disorders. Increasing fat non physiological deposition in visceral, muscle and intra hepatic fat tissues; decomposition of intracellular glucose transporter-4 results in insulin resistance due to obesity and physical inactivity. Overproduction of free fatty acids, cytokines, and oxidative stress by excess adipose tissue, intervene with natural signaling, and send toxic messages. This interference disturbs the regulation of glucose uptake in the liver and muscles by alteration in glucose transport and insulin's ability (Galaviz et al. 2018).

Diabetes is a premature illness and mortality risk factor, especially for cardiovascular disease (CVD) formation, and also consequent nephropathy, retinopathy, and neuropathy. Its prevalence is similar between men and women and lower in the rural population than urban. Asymptomatic diabetes and undetected symptoms for long periods of time cause nearly fifty percent of undiagnosed global diabetes. Based on researches, lifestyle interventions via healthy diet improvement, weight loss and physical activity mitigate genes effects and diminish diabetes risk significantly. Also, physically active lifestyles can offset genetic predisposition to diabetes. Interestingly, the importance of physical activity on diabetes risks reduction is related to: (a) directly effect on insulin resistance by liver and muscles free fatty acid oxidation and lipotoxicity reduction; (b) indirectly impact on visceral fat reduction; (c) increment of adiponectin levels (as insulin sensitivity promoter hormone) in serum which is decreased in obesity; (d) physiological stressor for triggering glucose transport alteration and energy supply; (e) Improve uptake of glucose by active muscles and insulin sensitivity; (f) Up-regulating of insulin signaling routes, consequent beta-cell function and apoptosis prevention (Galaviz et al. 2018).

4.3 Unhealthy Lifestyle

Diabetes can be managed by benefits of pharmacological treatments, but these efforts are often costly, induce side effects, and may not be as effective as lifestyle interventions (Galaviz et al. 2018; Kolb and Martin 2017; Reis et al. 2011). It is crucial to know that some changes in environment and lifestyle directly or indirectly translate to diseases formation and development specially diabetes (Kolb and Martin 2017). Unhealthy elements such as time spent seating (sedentary behavior), sleeping disturbances (duration, loss, apnea), psychosocial stress, oxidative agents (Taghavi et al. 2013, 2016), smoking, abnormal glucose metabolism, food, noise, fine dust, shift working, socioeconomic status are the critical risk factors of diabetic conditions. Lifestyle can target the involved components of diabetes development (Kolb and Martin 2017).

The involvement of unhealthy lifestyle with diabetes and its effect on health occur through: (a) directly by targeting β-cell function; (b) indirectly by producing metabolic stress via blood high amounts of nutrients or their metabolites; targeting distant action sites like vasculature (via adhesion molecules and immune mediators), liver (fetuin A, glucose, immune mediators, lipids), immune system (immune intermediates), brain (signals and neuroendocrine cells' hormones), intestine (incretins), muscle (myokines), or microbiota (lipopolysaccharides and fatty acids(short-chains), fat tissue (adipokines). It worth mentioning that all of these disorders have a close relationship with each other and lead to produce insulin resistance and inflammatory state. Other disadvantages of unhealthy lifestyles risk factors on human health are increased white blood cells or serum levels of C-reactive protein increment, increased inflammatory reactions even due to one night of insomnia, acute pro-inflammatory immune mediators up-regulation by refined sugars/starch and saturated fat persistent and chronic systemic inflammation in visceral fat mass, increased systemic inflammation by altering the microbiota composition, consequent intestinal leakage and releasing lipopolysaccharides into the bloodstream. It is worth mentioning that higher concentrations of circulating pro-inflammatory and inflammatory mediators can be made by sedentary lifestyle and depression. Interestingly, this inflammatory response can be prevented by physical activity. There is an interrelationship between inflammation and depression because increased inflammatory responses can cause symptoms of depression. So, it seems that inflammation is a vital crosslink and synergistic element between directly and indirectly unhealthy lifestyle risk factors. It interacts with the whole body and promotes β-cell damage via the networks of metabolic, immune endocrine and neurological systems. Base on researches, the β-cell function can be affected by alteration in environmental conditions via consequent stimulating of the sympathetic nervous system, catecholamines secretion, activated the complex set of the hypothalamus, pituitary and adrenal glands and cortisol hormone increment. Food addiction is another unhealthy lifestyle which translates to a risk of diabete. So, it seems that every agent with an anti-inflammatory effect can be considered as diabetes-protective factors (Kolb and Martin 2017).

4.4 Effective Elements in a Healthy Lifestyle

In this era, people have been encountered some lifestyles, which include decreased consumption of whole-grain (WG) cereals, vegetable, fruit and high consumption of animal products, refined cereals, sugars and fats. Ease of this modern lifestyle (as westernization diet), new methods of eating (away-from-home foods, increased portion sizes and unhealthy snacking) and put aside the traditional dietary patterns, stopped the promotion and maintenance of good health and produced serious health risks. Interestingly, inflammation is a cross-linkage between all unhealthy lifestyles (Kechagia et al. 2013). Regards to the importance of inflammatory related diseases and their gradual effect on human health, especially diabetes and its complications, high attention to the prevention of these kinds of diseases by anti-inflammatory strategies are very crucial (Fedorak 2008). It is reported that an anti-inflammatory diet and eliminate inflammatory foods will improve diabetic and pre-diabetic inflammatory biomarkers (Zwickey et al. 2019). An excellent anti-inflammatory lifestyle is based on two important considerations: (a) Selection of anti-inflammatory foods and behaviors; (b) Avoid from food with pro inflammatory properties (Ricker and Haas 2017). One of the most critical subjects which seem to have a powerful impact on the prevention of inflammation or disease treatment, especially diabetes, is nutrition and diet with appropriate quality (Kechagia et al. 2013).

4.4.1 Probiotics

Probiotic as live microorganisms have the initial meaning of "for life." This kind of food in adequate amounts is part of the food and involves microbial balance improvement in the host animal and provide health benefits for them (Kechagia et al. 2013). A wide range of food products contain extensive and growing probiotic strains such as: (a) dairy products: cheese, butter, powdered milk and yogurt, ice cream, fermented milk which they are expanding still; (b) non-dairy products like nutrition bars, cereals, soy-based products, and variety of juices. There are some essential factors in the effectiveness and evaluation of probiotic compounds such as safety, microorganism compatibility, and viability during the industrial process (Kechagia et al. 2013).

High volume of researches has presented supportive evidence about the prevention and treatment effects of probiotic in certain human diseases. Different mechanisms are involved in probiotic health benefits such as the production of anti-inflammatory short chain fatty acid and bacteriocin, decrement of gut's pH, immune modulation and stimulation of mucosal barrier function by nutrient competition, inducing phagocytosis, IgA secretion and stimulation of innate immune response by modifying of T-cell, Th1 and Th2 responses (Kechagia et al. 2013).

It is reported that probiotic plant fibers are an essential member of probiotic foods with interesting benefits such as diverse and healthy microbiota growth promotion with less endotoxin leakage, inflammatory avoidance of liver Kupffer and endothelial cells with simultaneous maintenance of hepatocytes activity, increased short-chain fatty acids production by presented bacteria in the gut, promotion of β-cells growth and function by direct binding of these kinds of fatty acids to β-cells free fatty acid receptor 2 (Kolb and Martin 2017).

Noteworthy, probiotic bacteria are involved in the prevention of gastrointestinal inflammation, positive effects on mucosal immune system dysfunction and epithelial cell function, improve metabolism by restoring a healthful balance and normal inhabitation of microflora bacteria, prevention of pathogen-induced membrane damage and pathogens adhesion, maintaining tight junction correct organization and cytoskeleton proteins, modulation of T regulatory cells and consequent prevention or amelioration of inflammatory reactions and allergic disease, producing anti-inflammatory dominant profile by modulating epithelial cytokine secretion, improved mucus production, act as ligands for the receptors of the innate immune system, recovery of the systemic and innate immune system, involvement in pro-inflammatory pathways and homeostasis of the mucosal immune response (Blum and Schiffrin 2003; Mengheri 2008; Fedorak 2008; Plaza-Díaz et al. 2017).

Probiotics also can affect diabetes. Trillions of microorganisms, especially bacterial species in the human gut, are responsible for a mass of biological metabolisms and functions. They also involved in type 2 diabetes (T2D) via different bacterial metabolites and their role in glucose homeostasis. Certain gut bacterial species, which are increased by high-fat diets, trigger the progression of insulin resistance by lipopolysaccharides high levels generation. Gut microbiota can positively modulate insulin resistance and glucose biomarkers (Gudjinu and Sarfo 2017). It is shown that probiotic in mice are involved in gluconeogenesis inhibition in type 2 diabetes and tumorigenesis. They also have potential benefits on blood glucose, insulin, and C-reactive protein (CRP) (as inflammation biomarkers) (Fedorak 2008; Yao et al. 2017).

Probiotics are involved in glucose homeostasis improvement. In T2DM, the alterations in the gut microbiome, such as gram-negative bacteria overgrowth, which leads to inflammatory pathways, were reported. Also, fragmented lipopolysaccharides (LPS) of this kind of bacteria lead to gut barrier leakage and chronic systemic inflammation. Researches clearly showed that probiotic can prevent and manage diabetes via improvement of glucose homeostasis and modulating gut microbiota; for example, glucose metabolism is influenced by gut microbiota via modulation of glucagon-like peptide-1 (GLP-1) (as enteroendocrine peptides produced by L-cell in the gut). This process leads to insulin secretion increment (Rittiphairoj et al. 2019; Rad et al. 2017).

Interestingly, probiotic also can act as an antioxidant, modulate oxidative stress, and especially has an important influence on glucose control, insulin sensitivity and glucose markers (Ardeshirlarijani et al. 2019).

4.4.2 Plant-Based Diets and Phytochemicals

Plant-based diets and their phytochemicals contents such as turmeric spice (curcumin), Kokum fruit(garcinol), cashews (anacardic acid), grape (polyphenol, resveratrol), peanut, green tea (epigallocatechin-3-gallate) and fermented soybeans (spermidine) or wheat germs, have calorie restriction activities such as exercise. They have the major anti diabetes-protective components which are involved in cell defense, anti-inflammatory genes activation via the Nrf2 signaling pathway, improvement of an anti-inflammatory effect, and cellular resistance to oxidative stress (Kolb and Martin 2017).

Natural plant's polyphenols, as the plant kingdom's largest group of chemical substances, are bioactive organic compounds with different chemical structures and beneficial roles in the human body. The primary source of plant polyphenols are vegetables, fruits, seeds and nuts, leaves, roots, herbs and whole grain products. Nutrients, minerals, vitamins are also found in plant-derived products. A well-balanced diet should have polyphenols and vitamins because of their potent anti-inflammatory and antioxidant properties and critical metabolic roles in human cells. Polyphenols reduce cardiovascular, cancer, and neurodegenerative diseases via its antioxidant activities and ROS reduction effects. Also, herbal polyphenols have other health-promoting effects such as anti-allergy, anti-atherogenic, anti-inflammatory, anti-mutagenic and anti-thrombotic effects. They also affect white blood cells proliferation and activity and modulate the human immune system and immunological defense (Gorzynik-Debicka et al. 2018).

Fruit and vegetables because of their high cellulose-a type of insoluble fiber cause glucose absorption delay from the small intestine and blood glucose control. They also provide necessary regulatory factors for growth to maintain normal health and act as a good container of various immune-protective agents such as vitamins, folate, minerals, flavonoids (antioxidants), flavanols, and flavanones, anthocyanins, carotenoids, saponins, polyphenols, isothiocyanates (sulfur-containing compounds), and several types of dietary fibers (Holt et al. 2009). Interestingly, their polyphenolic antioxidants and folate have an inverse relation with inflammation and oxidative stress. The fruits and vegetable colors are relating to its flavonoids (anthocyanidins, flavanols (or catechins), flavanones, flavones, flavonols, and isoflavones) which are located in the skins and peels and protect them from ultraviolet light, pathogens and other stress conditions. Flavonoids consumption can involve in the reduction of obesity prevalence, high blood cholesterol, high blood pressure, and has an inverse relationship with inflammation and oxidative stress markers. TNF-α and IL-6 concentrations in both pre- and postmenopausal women are decreased by grape flavonoids; also, there is an inverse association between IL-6 and tea flavonoids and quercetin and even between total flavonoids, individual flavonoids, kaempferol and quercetin with oxidative stress (Asif 2014).

Several kinds of research referred to the reducing effect of fruit and vegetable consumption on systemic inflammation, interventions effect on immune cell populations, increasing effect on natural killer cell (NK cell) cytotoxicity and lymphocyte proliferation, decreasing effect on pro-inflammatory biomarkers such as CRP and TNF-α, reducing of CVD and other chronic diseases risks such as diabetes mellitus (Hosseini et al. 2018).

4.4.3 Whole Grains

It is reported that a higher intake of whole-grain foods is involved in the inhibition and prevention of diabetes and widely in chronic non-communicable diseases (post- blood lipid profile, intestinal microbiota, prandial insulinemic response, metabolic syndrome, decreased risk of cardiovascular disease (CVD) and cancer (Marventano et al. 2017). It is recommended that whole-grain intake should be an integral part of the diet as part of total carbohydrate intake. Whole-grain (such as dark bread, brown rice, cooked cereal, wheat germ, cereals, and popcorn bran) and refined-grain foods (such as white rice, white bread, pancakes, English cakes, waffles, sweet rolls, biscuits, and pizza) have an inverse effect on diabetes formation.

Whole-grain as the intact grain is defined by the germ, bran and endosperm with all variability of its macronutrient-micronutrient compositions (vitamins and minerals), kernel and bioactive contents. It is considered as dietary fiber rich source, antioxidants and resistant starch. Interestingly, there is an inverse relationship between whole-grain or dietary fiber intake and diabetes mellitus (Della Pepa et al. 2018). Wholegrain influenced on inhibition of diabetes type 2 via its nutrients (magnesium and vitamin E), affecting postprandial glucose and insulin response (Fung et al. 2002).

The health mechanism of whole-grain is related to gut health providing by high fiber contents, anti-inflammatory compounds, antioxidants, hormone, anti-carcinogenic (phenolic compounds), metabolic effects (minerals and vitamins, improve glycemic control, insulin sensitivity and insulin homeostasis. While rapid increment of blood glucose concentrations, increases the need for insulin secretion from pancreatic β cells and increase the risk of insulin resistance were produced by refined grain meal. Also, whole-grain produce digestion slow rate, fiber fermentation, and resistant starch by microbiota and fatty acids (short-chain) (SCFA) in the large intestine. Glucose homeostasis and insulin sensitivity improvement by glucose oxidation increment in the liver via SCFAs, reduction of fatty acid release, and insulin clearance increment are other benefits of whole grains consumption. Some whole grains cereals polyphenolic antioxidants such as alkylresorcinols, anthocyanins, ferulic acid and lignans, can protect pancreatic beta cells with the high sensibility to oxidative damage. Interestingly the synergistic effect of WG components is responsible for glycemic control improvement (Marventano et al. 2017). There is a close adverse relationship between whole grain consumption and inflammation. It is reported that bioactive compounds (vitamins B, E, selenium, zinc, fiber) of whole grains can decrease the concentrations of circulating inflammatory markers (Xu et al. 2018; Ley et al. 2014).

Wholegrain fiber promotes these processes: Elevates fiber fermentation by short chain fatty acids production, nutrient absorption delay (glucose, FFA) at the intestinal level, the consequent reduction in insulin demand and fat oxidation stimulation, reduction in fat storage, adjusts gut microbiota compositions, consequent ameliorates liver insulin sensitivity and attenuates subclinical inflammation. The antioxidant and anti-inflammatory properties of whole-grain bioactive compounds (phytosterols, phenolic compounds, carotenoid and betaine) alleviate the development and progression of T2DM. In this regards, insulin sensitivity improvement, oxidative stress inhibition, and diminish inflammatory cytokines, and subclinical inflammation are fully involved in T2DM decrement (Xu et al. 2018; Della Pepa et al. 2018).

4.4.4 Healthy Fats

Dietary fatty acids include saturated (SFA), trans, mono (MUFA) and polyunsaturated (PUFA) fatty acids (omega 3, 6 and 9), and also conjugated linoleic acid (CLA). Some fatty acids are involved in inflammation and human's disease. The inflammation mechanisms are related to eicosanoid metabolism, activation of gene expression, the effect on the membrane and cytosolic signaling; gene regulation by binding to transcription factors; producing different inflammatory response based on the type of fatty acid (pro-inflammatory effect by SFA, trans fat, eicosanoids and anti-inflammatory effect in particular by the long-chain fatty acids and PUFA. Triglycerides and SFA are involved in postprandial inflammatory reactions, which can be strengthening in obese subjects. Chronic low-grade inflammation can be produced by the persistent increment in pro-inflammatory chemokines and cytokines (TNFα, IL-1β, and IL-6) systemic levels (Jabs 1999) which are involved in many lifestyle diseases. Based on researches, the diet has a healthy pattern if they include an increased amount of PUFA instead of SFA, and provide TNFα, IL-6 decreased levels, and chronic low-grade inflammation. Mediterranean diet because of its protective factors (fruits, whole grains, fiber, vegetables, fish, carotenoids, vitamin C, vitamin E, PUFA, and especially n-3 PUFA) can decline low-grade inflammation in healthy and in particular obese individuals. Nuts, tea, coffee, cocoa, flavonoids, milk peptides, vitamin D, and probiotic have no positive effect on inflammation, but lipids, SFAs, and trans fatty acids oxidation can intensify inflammatory mechanisms (Telle-Hansen et al. 2017; Ruiz-Núñez et al. 2016).

The diets' fatty acid composition, particularly their enrichment of saturated fatty acids (SFAs), affects individual obesity and overall toxicity than polyunsaturated fatty acids (PUFAs). High SFA diets lead to SFAs increment in the individual's circulation, increasing in adipose tissue inflammatory processes, insulin sensitivity decrement, and intrahepatic triglyceride increment. Also, glucose homeostasis deregulation and insulin resistance as a core of diabetes mellitus and metabolism disorder is occurred due to increased circulating of FFAs and pro-inflammatory factors. Cholesterol and SFAs high intake and PUFAs low intake lead to the development of neurodegenerative disease and increased risk of impaired cognitive function (Melo et al. 2019).

Saturated, monounsaturated, and polyunsaturated fatty acids reveal different influences in coronary heart disease. Monounsaturated fatty acids are not needed to be in the diet, and no adequate intake is recommended. The liver is the synthesis location of cis-monounsaturated fatty acids (MUFA) and saturated fats in response to carbohydrate consumption (Liu et al. 2017).

Trans fats are involved in endothelial dysfunction and LDL-C, triglycerides and inflammation increment. It is recommended to limit the intake of oils, which are partially hydrogenated and industrial trans fats. It is worth mentioning that in human health, essential fatty acids (such as Cis-polyunsaturated fatty acids) are of great importance (Liu et al. 2017).

The heterogeneity of food sources and the biological effects of varied saturated fatty acids cause their impact to become complex in heart disease. There are powerful affirmative correlations between higher intake of saturated or trans-fat and the rate of chronic heart diseases. Interestingly, the substitution of unsaturated fats instead of saturated fats has been reported to reduce mortality from CHD, neurological diseases, and cancer. Also, it is reported that total saturated fat is more harmful than total carbohydrate and refined starch in cardiovascular disease) (Liu et al. 2017). High-fat diets (trans, unsaturated and saturated fatty acids) and a sedentary lifestyle produce higher levels of plasma FFAs, insulin resistance and chronic low-grade inflammation which result in metabolic imbalance, AD and T2DM risk factors. Its reason related to their role in dysregulated brain insulin signaling and neuroinflammation events. It is worth mentioning that healthy lifestyles, especially the Mediterranean diet with reiterated consumption of ω-3 (n-3 PUFA) rich oils, fish, vegetables and fruits can prevent metabolic disorders and neurodegenerative diseases (Melo et al. 2019; Telle-Hansen et al. 2017).

Based on the World Health Organization, it is determined that 20 to 35% of total calories should belong to total fat intake. 20% of total calories cover the essential needs of the human body include essential fatty acids, fat-soluble vitamins, and adequate consumption of whole energy. In addition, fatty acids have differences in behavior in terms of burning/energy supply and adipose tissue accumulation. Certain Long-chain saturated fats have a lower oxidation rate and tend to be accumulated and produce obesity. But medium-chain saturated fatty acids (C_6–C_{12}), alpha-linolenic acid, oleic acid, and linoleic acid with particularly high oxidation rates tend to be burned and use for energy supplying. Oleic acid is the major MUFA in Western diets (Liu et al. 2017).

It is worth mentioning that high refined carbohydrates diet leads to muscle long-chain SFAs storage, intramyocellular lipid accumulation and muscle insulin resistance than MUFA. Fatty acids also have different inflammatory behaviors. The cellular content of two pro-inflammatory molecules (diacylglycerol (DAG) and ceramide) can be increased by long-chain SFAs like palmitate and produce inflammation and insulin resistance compared with unsaturated fats. Triacylglycerol (TAG), with less inflammatory effect, can be increased by oleate (Liu et al. 2017). Excess stored TAG in multiple tissues is highly associated with insulin resistance. In other words, accumulations of specific lipids can cause interference with insulin signaling and insulin resistance (Bircher and Kuruvilla 2014).

Insulin resistance is a common crosslink between obesity and metabolic syndrome (James 2018). Long-chain SFAs with lower affinity to DGAT2 (DAG convertor enzyme to TAG) can be stored as DAG compared with TAG and also can produce ceramide compared with unsaturated fatty acids. TAG and ceramide are two important inflammatory factors. Insulin signaling and cell involvement of different fats are also varied and it is clear that the standard American diet with long-chain SFAs and refined carbohydrates leads to inflammation, insulin resistance and obesity. Instead, take a Mediterranean diet has a positive effect on insulin sensitivity, metabolic syndrome (improvement), total cholesterol, and systolic blood pressure (Boskou et al. 2006).

Olive oil as an important element of the Mediterranean diet is the combination of triacylglycerols, mono- and diacylglycerol, secondarily free fatty acids, hydrocarbons, sterols, aliphatic alcohols, tocopherols, pigments, phenolic, volatile compounds, palmitic, palmitoleic, stearic, oleic, linoleic, linolenic, myristic, heptadecanoic, eicosanoic acids which construct unique character (Boskou et al. 2006; Gouvinhas et al. 2017).

Olive oil can inhibit palmitate cell death by beta-oxidation and TAG synthesis increment and, finally, inhibiting the incorporation of palmitate-DAG or palmitate-ceramid. It worth mentioning that a high level of palmitate induces skeletal muscles inflammation and insulin resistance via diacylglycerol-mediated activation of protein kinase C and activation of toll-like receptors. However, oleic acid has even been found to prevent mitochondrial dysfunction, insulin resistance, and inflammation in neuronal cells and skeletal muscle induced by palmitate.

Oleate also had an anti-insulin resistance protective effect, which is induced by palmitate, improves endothelial dysfunction in response to pro-inflammatory signals and finally, reduces proliferation and apoptosis in vascular smooth muscle cells that may contribute to an ameliorated atherosclerotic process and plaque stability. Olive oil, avocados, macadamia nuts or hazelnuts, peanuts, almonds are considering as MUFA rich diet are effective in improving insulin resistance, fat and weight loss compare with cream or butter as rich long-chain SFAs diet (Liu et al. 2017). Olive oil has a chemo preventive activity, which is depending on its supreme phenolic compositions (phenolic alcohols, secoiridoid derivatives and oleuropein). There is a correlation between anticancer properties of olive oil and their antioxidant activity of phenolic constituents because of scavenging free radicals and reactive species (Gorzynik-Debicka et al. 2018).

4.4.5 Nature Close Contact

Nature (a powerful, inexpensive public health intervention) has an important effect on human healing, and greener surroundings are the healthy selection for moving to or staying in by people. Such a way being in nature (mountains, seas, covered streets with trees, forested, agricultural lands, gardens, and parks) and closely contact with it (as a major health determinant) bring a long-term health outcome for the human being. As the same way, the lack of a green surrounding brings the severe risk of health (attention deficit/hyperactivity disorder, depression and anxiety disorder, diabetes mellitus, obesity, various infectious diseases, cancer, delay in healing from surgery, birth outcomes, cardiovascular disease, respiratory disease, musculoskeletal complaints, migraines) and mortality especially accompany with economic concerns in today's world. Natures promote health in some special ways via multiple possible mechanisms includes air quality, physical activity, stress, and social integration. There are several chemical and biological effective factors with health benefits effect in the natural environment as below:

(a) Phytoncides as antimicrobial volatile organic compounds which are produced by many plants alter autonomic activity, decrease blood pressure; boost immune functioning; (b) High concentrations of negative air ions near moving water in forests and mountainous areas which influence on depression reduction and have a positive effect on health; (c) Mycobacterium vaccae as a microorganism which boosts immune functioning;

(d) Environmental biodiversity affects the living microorganisms in gut, skin and immune functionality; (e) Sounds and sights of nature with high physiological impacts on parasympathetic activity reduces sympathetic nervous activity, improves immune system's behavior with long-term health consequences and promote healing from surgery.

In built environments, trees and landscaping may promote health not only by contributing positive factors like phytoncides but also by reducing negative factors. Vegetation is an efficient system for air pollutants filtering, urban heat island dampening, and violence reduction. Also, it is proven after a forest walk not urban the levels of health-protective factors are increased such as didehydroepiandrosterone (DHEA) with cardioprotective, anti-obesity, and anti-diabetic properties, adiponectin as atherosclerosis protective agent, the immune system's anticancer/Natural Killer cells (with high protective roles in cancer), inflammatory cytokines (involve in depression, diabetes and cardiovascular disease), elevated blood glucose reduction and significant effect on lowering blood pressure (Ideno et al. 2017; Frumkin et al. 2017). Other benefits of closely contact with nature are deep relaxation or stress reduction, sleep improvement, boosts immune function, compensation with adverse effects of stress on energy metabolism, insulin secretion, inflammatory pathways (Cohen et al. 2006), attention restoration, enhanced vitality, lower levels of inflammatory cytokines as the effect of awe[1]; infection resistance (Bhasin et al. 2013) and lower risk of mortality (Kuo 2015; Jiang et al. 2018).

4.4.6 Negative Ions

Among natures active ingredients, negative air ions (NAIs) are an interesting item. Atoms or electrically charged molecules or in the atmosphere are called air ions because they receive enough energy to expel an electron. The molecules or atoms gain an electron called NAIs and those who lose an electron name positive air ions (PAIs). Negative ions are produced by this way: (a) The water's shearing forces (via Lenard effect refer to creating a negative charge in air molecules around water droplets, because of the formation of tiny droplet sprays due to the collision of these droplets with each other or with a wet solid); (b) Plant-based energy sources (NAIs generation ability of plants during their normal growth conditions change them to NAI natural resources); (c) Sunlight radiant or cosmic rays (absorption of radiant electron resulting from light radiation with a specified wavelength on metallic surfaces by air molecule or air molecules direct ionization); (d) Natural and artificial corona discharge (thunder and lightning due to corona discharge and NAI formation via high electric fields difference potential between leaf points and trees' branches and their

---

[1] A mixture of great respect with surprise or fear.

surroundings); (e) atmosphere radiant or cosmic rays (air ionization due to radioactive elements decay (our planet uranium, radium, actinium, and thorium) and emission of α, β, and/or γ rays). NAIs can reduce particulate matter (PM) concentration in high-efficiency (Jiang et al. 2018).

It is important to know that generated NAIs will be decayed gradually because of their instability; So that, they can raise their lifetime by combination with water molecules and ionic cluster formation (Lenard effect's negative oxygen ions $O_2-(H_2O)n$ with a half-life of 60 s compared with corona discharge's NAIs with remaining time exclusively several seconds) (Duhaini 2016). NAIs lifetime also can be affected by some factors such as NAI concentration, electric fields' intensity and aerosols (Jiang et al. 2018).

The composition of negative-ion (NAIs)clusters usually are multiple negatively charged molecules with a combination of several water molecules (up to 20 or 30) in different forms of $O-(H_2O)_n$, $CO_3-(H_2O)_n$ and $O_3-(H2O)_n$. Also, there are further ions such as NO_2^-, OH^-, HCO_3^- and their water cluster forms in NAIs atmosphere (Jiang et al. 2018).

Researchers showed that NAIs have several biological effects. Based on some works of literature, their positive impact on the health of human and animals are basically referred to the cardiovascular system (normalizing blood rheology and arterial pressure, improving aerobic metabolism (Iwama 2004), decreasing blood pressure and erythrocyte deformability) (Iwama et al. 2002; Wiszniewski et al. 2014), respiratory system, mental health and mood disorders. They also have been affected by supporting tissue oxygenation, relaxing stress conditions, and reinforce resistance to unfavorable factors.

NIAs also caused a reduction of depression severity, psychological stress, anxiety, and improvement of enhanced well-being. In contrast, positive air ions exposure is followed by heightened anxiety and unpleasantness, feelings of irritability, while some cases of unchanged mood have been reported in connection with air ionization (Perez et al. 2013).

NAIs exposure also influences microorganism's growth; for example, NAIs high concentration can inactivate the growth of bacteria and prevent tuberculosis (TB) infection and its disease. These ionic species also revealed the inhibition effect on fungi and virus growth. Furthermore, plants can be affected by NAIs via their fresh, dry weight, mean stem length, and integral elongation, macroelements, and microelements, oxygen consumption increment (Cohen et al. 2006).

4.4.7 Use Mobile Phone Carefully

In the recent era, the usage of electrical and electromagnetical devices, their applications for information distribution or communication technologies are extra spread. These technologies are manufactured based on non-ionizing radiation (NIR) emitting as "electromagnetic fields" (EMF). The usage of them has been increased every moment, and different parts of the electromagnetic (EM) spectrum from low-frequency fields to high-frequency EMF encompassing are employed in recent technologies (Duhaini 2016).

Indeed, the use of new telecommunication, electricity, appliances, medical equipment technologies (biomedical, diagnostic and therapeutic applications) in human life is currently unavoidable, and their related electromagnetic field (EMF) produces a serious threat to human health and life. Some researches refer to the increased rate of cancer, brain tumors, leukemia, and other health problems due to EMF exposure. It worth mentioning that EMF biological hazards depend on the type of fields as electric or magnetic or both of them (Duhaini 2016).

The power of penetration, exposure duration, and biological properties of irradiated tissues usually determine the characteristics of radiation absorption in different tissues (Scarfi et al. 2019).

Electromagnetic fields have a wide harmful effect on different organs and tissue. Hematologic and cardiovascular systems, blood-brain barrier permeability in the nervous system, brain chemistry and histology (diminished concentrations of epinephrine, norepinephrine, 5-hydroxytryptamine, dopamine); axons' structure; purkinje cells (decrement); and hypothalamic region structural changes can be affected by RF radiation. RF radiation at non-thermal power densities also provides bradycardia, alter Ca^{2+} binding to neuron's surface in isolated brain hemispheres and the cell culture of neuroblastoma. In the visual system, high-intensity RF radiation causes cataract development in which thermal mechanism has an important role. Continuous wave and pulsed microwave fields also have the same effect. Flickering illumination or phosphenes, evoked potential (VEP) are reported as a visual phenomenon due to extremely low-frequency fields (ELF) exposure. Researchers reported that endocrine alterations and plasma corticosterone increments have caused due to the thermogenic effect of RF radiation. RF heating changes homeostasis maintenance by alteration in the complex interactions of the adrenal, pituitary, thyroid and hypothalamic system. RF power densities alter components of the immune system, produce tissue heating, and increase steroid hormones release into the circulation. High levels of RF exposures in mice increased neutrophils, decreased lymphocytes probability due to heat stress, and adrenal steroids released into the blood. The proliferative capacity of bone-marrow cells and its cellular composition can be affected by thermogenic levels of continuous waves or pulsed microwaves. Also, it is reported that microwave radiation may have a potential carcinogenic effect on whole animals.

Cell phones are one of the most critical EMF applications (Shojaeifard et al. 2018; Council 1993). The worldwide users of mobile phones have reached about 5 billion, and this device as a low-powered radio device can transfer and obtain radiofrequency radiation at the range of 900–2000 MHz. People generally keep it in close contact with their bodies (Meo and Al Rubeaan 2013).

Non-Ionizing Radiation (NIR) includes radiant energy with low- energy photons (12.4 eV) and long wavelengths more than 100 nm on the electromagnetic field (EMF) spectrum between 1 Hz and 3×10^{15} Hz. This range contains a microwave, very high and low-frequency radio waves. One application of EMF is telecommunication, and in this regard, cell phones and its advanced devices have earned extensive usage in all societies around the world. They have caused many problems related to disturbing people's health or community security (Scarfi et al. 2019; Mousavy et al. 2009; Sefidbakht et al. 2013, 2014).

Based on research, electromagnetic fields emitted by mobile phones disturb blood-brain barriers, neurotransmitter release, cellular function, memory, learning, sleep patterns, cellular redox homeostasis, hormones level (progesterone or thyroid hormones) and endocrine system (Mousavy et al. 2009; Krewski et al. 2001). Mobile phone consumption also leads to burning sensations, heating around the ear (due to radiofrequency exposure and electrical power dissipation), headaches, fatigue, sleep disturbances, tension, impaired vision and hearing, detrimental effects on the hematopoietic, cardiovascular and central nervous system, testis and utero-placental functions, cancer, possible effects on cellular DNA. It seems the thermal and non-thermal effects are responsible for mobile phones electromagnetic waves inconvenience. Interestingly, mobile phones can induce some serious disorders such as hyperglycemia (elevated oxidative stress and glucose disturbed homeostasis) with the ultimate faith of diabetes mellitus formation (Krewski et al. 2001). Researches revealed that mobile phones exposure in different time periods lead to remarkable increase in the serum levels of glucose and insulin, insulin structure alteration, early and severe β-cell dysfunction and β-cell loss via apoptosis, decrement in pancreatic islets release, high levels of HbA1c, genetic regulation and exacerbate oxidative stress (Krewski et al. 2001; Yakymenko and Sidorik 2010; Mortazavi et al. 2016; Meo et al. 2015). According to research, increasing the use of mobile phones in the last decade and the sudden increase in the prevalence of diabetes can be a point to consider (Krewski et al. 2001).

4.4.8 Spirituality and Inner Peace

Even the smallest cell in the human body is fully aware of his thoughts, feelings, and beliefs. The diversity of one's attitudes toward him/herself dictates the biochemistry of his body, and recent researches confirm the biological principles of beliefs. The human belief system is actually formed by refining all of his learned experiences through his personality (Moosavi-Movahedi 1999).

Among these, beliefs, spirituality, and culture have a significant impact on people's empowerment to live better and fight with the disease.

Spirituality means the way people seek to express meanings, goals, experience, and connection with the moment, themselves, others, nature, and special occasions. There is a close relationship between spirituality and coping with reducing anxiety and depression, willingness to live, chronic medical disease, and improving quality of life (Jafari et al. 2014).

Spiritual calm or in better word, peace of mind as the power of hope and positive thinking is related to an essential part of human existence, which leads to the fulfillment of life's goals, meaningful personal existence, understanding of the value of life, and its better consideration. Nowadays, the effect of spiritual calm and inner peace on the strengthening of human personal values, his worldview, and health are interesting topics in the research field and are considered as an important clinical target. Spiritual calm and inner peace have a powerful effect on: (a) coping and help to deal with pressures of life, pain, illness, produce life satisfying and happier conditions, positive outlook and a better quality of life especially in the condition of advanced disease; (b) recovery which leads to worry less, live in the present moment, and better health outcome, especially in surgery and disease and (c) mortality reduction and live longer by regular spiritual practices, stress control improvement, provide better coping mechanisms, overwhelming on elevated interleukin (IL)-6 (9) as the associated factor with disease incidence.

The research about the influence of the spiritual practice on human health (the 1960s) showed transcendental meditation leads to the decrement of metabolism, heart and respiratory rate, and also slower brain waves. This practice also showed its beneficial effect on insomnia, chronic pain, anxiety, depression, hostility, premenstrual syndrome, infertility, cancer or HIV. He considered these responses as "relaxation response and concluded stress could promote any diseases. He also found that stimulation of relaxation response can be an effective therapy. Spirituality is a health contributing effect and is presented in all beliefs, cultures, societies and influences on health, illness and people interact with each other (Puchalski 2001).

Indeed, spiritual domains of every person's life are a notable subject in the concept of quality of life (QOL) and received more attention today. In fact, QOL as a broad combination concept, is built of spiritual domains, cognitive, emotional, physical, and social of an individual's life (Jafari et al. 2014). Researches revealed one's spirituality as spiritual well-being has influenced the prevalence of chronic diseases (Alvarez et al. 2016) and may have an important role in diabetes mellitus and provide better tolerance for illness (Koenig 2012). Based on researches, spiritual calm, a strong sense of transcendence or spirituality, have a close relationship with glycemic control improvement, lower disease morbidity, and mortality because it produces higher self-care, greater self-efficacy, and disease management in a better way. There is a significant inverse relationship between depression and spirituality, which can act as treatment and protection indicators for depression associated with illness (such as substances abuse, diabetes, hypertension, cardiovascular disease, cancer and mood disorders) (Lynch et al. 2012). It is clear that blood higher sugar level, insulin resistance, and diabetes formation can be produced due to elevated physical and mental stress (Pouwer et al. 2010). Several studies indicated that diabetic patients had reduced quality of life compared with the general population in the same age group, and their quality of life decreases with disease progression and complications. Diabetes as a devastating multifaceted disease affects emotional, physical, social, and functional well-being. It can confuse the patient with questions about their goal, themselves and their life meaning. It is believed that suffering without meaning destroys humans and meaning as the sense of life, purpose, reason, and productivity helps to cope with the disease, having an optimistic view about life, reframing their lives against their disease (Jafari et al. 2014).

Interestingly, there is a positive relationship between spiritual well-being, glycemic control, self-management and coping with diabetes. Based on research, lower HbA1c, and better adjustment to disease can be provided by higher spiritual well-being (Alvarez et al. 2016).

4.4.9 Hydration

Water as an essential compound for life is involved in all human biological functions such as a solvent for biochemical reactions, thermoregulation and internal body temperature, pH, blood pressure, vascular volume maintenance, providing transport medium for intra and extra nutrients movements (oxygen, glucose, sodium, potassium), waste removal from the body and finally optimal health (Liska et al. 2019; Armstrong 2018). Water also is essential for cellular homeostasis, and its amount decreases from childhood to old age in the body. Health and well-being are entirely depending on the water status of the human body (Popkin et al. 2010).

Three sources are involved in providing our water need: (a) beverages (water, soft drinks, juices, and dairy products); (b) mainly vegetables and fruits, solid food; and (c) macronutrients metabolism (Puga et al. 2019). There are some crucial concepts in body's water situation: (a) Water balance equal to water gain compared with water loss; (b) hydration is the process of maintaining water balance; (c) Euhydration" is body water normal content with narrow fluctuation; (d) hypohydration means water deficit(due to absence of thirst sensation or chronic consumption of certain drugs or polypharmacy) (Puga et al. 2019); (e) hyperhydration defines body water excess; (f) Dehydration point at the losing process of body water balance; (g) Rehydration describes water regaining process by body and (h) Overhydration regardless of electrolyte replacement is another events which result in excessive water intake (Liska et al. 2019; Riebl and Davy 2013). Dietary intake, age, physical activity level, and environmental conditions have an important influence on water balance (Riebl and Davy 2013). Water intake refers to all type of water soft or hard, spring or well, carbonated or distilled water which can be get directly (beverage) and indirectly (to a very small extent also from oxidation of macronutrients (metabolic water) and from food (which are different with fruit and vegetable diet)). In European countries (especially Greece) and South Korea, a higher intake of water comes from fresh fruits and vegetables, but in the United States, water intake occurred through food (Popkin et al. 2010).

Maintenance of human constant water and mineral balance is very crucial. It can be controlled by different sites in the body, such as integrative processing centers in the brain and neural pathways. These processing centers are sensitive to blood pressure, dieresis and natriuresis regulation by using neurohormones. Drinking as corrective actions can take place by interactive function between administrative organs (like kidney, salivary glands and sweat glands) and certain nerves. Most of the components of fluid balance and responding to the body's water status can be controlled by precise homeostatic mechanisms which are sensitive to deficits (ionic concentration increment of the extracellular compartments which causing cells to shrink) or excesses of water (body fluids lower ionic concentration and much water entrance in intracellular compartments). The Regulation of fluid intake and prevention of body dehydration is a critical issue to maintain the normal functioning of the human organs. Regulatory or physiological thirsty come from water deficiency. In this regard, the kidneys have an important role in fluid balance regulating and are more efficient in the presence of a large source of water. Water economizing of kidneys and more concentrated urine production results in higher energy expenditure and more wear on their tissues. The presence of enough water helps to protect this important organ. In healthy people who live in temperate climates, thirst plays little daily role in water intake controlling. Fluids are not only provided by drinking to tranquilize thirst but also by daily foods (milk, soup) and soft drinks (tea, coffee), which are used in hot weather for cooling or in cold weather for body warming. However, rehydration by soft drink replaces the water losses before the occurrence of water deficiency in the body, but their extra calories can be harmful to human bodies. Thermoregulation is also controlled by body hydration status. Sweat production as a significant cooling mechanism in physical activity and hot weather conditions acts based on the temperature and humidity of the environment, the amount of activity, and the type of clothing worn. If the loss of sweat is not compensated by fluid intake, the state of hypo-hydration occurs with a simultaneous increase in body core temperature. Lack of hydration via sweating leads to the loss of electrolytes, decline in plasma volume and can cause an increase in plasma osmolality. During this time, the plasma output is not sufficient to compensate for heat increment. As mentioned before, euhydrated state is an ideal hydrated state with cellular sufficient water provision for overcoming water loss, and upsetting this balance will determine the dehydration as the abstinence of fluids over the time. Proximity of the body to each of these two concepts will determine the individual health state. Dehydration provide some serious problems as chronic diseases, cognitive performance(disruptions in mood and concentration, cognitive functioning, alertness and short-term memory, increased negative emotions, deterioration in attention and memory); delirium(dementia in the elderly and very ill persons), gastrointestinal function, headache(due to hypohydration), skin and physical performance(fatigue increment, thermoregulatory capability alteration, motivation reduction), unfavorable body composition and increased especially oxidative stress and related inflammation (Liska et al. 2019; Popkin et al. 2010).

In recent decades, the consumption of fruit juices and sugar-sweetened beverages has become a major unfavorable habit and provide a source of caloric fluid for the human body. Researches showed the close relationship between risk of diabetes mellitus (T2D) and certain caloric beverages (sugar-sweetened beverages and fruit juices). Regards to properties of water and its role in providing hydrated condition, substituting of caloric beverage with plain water provide a healthy life style (Pan et al. 2012).

It is worth mentioning that, alterations in hydration status can be formed by pharmaceutical excipients via gastrointestinal passing time decreasing or intestinal permeability increment. Hypohydration can be triggered by drugs due to increased water excretion through diarrhea, sweat or urine; appetite or thirst sensation decrement; or alteration in central thermoregulation. It is very important to note that water depletion lead to oxidative attack to (Puga et al. 2019) biomacromolecules and their damages (protein, DNA and phospholipids).

Dehydration also leads to fluidization and perturbation of cell membranes by ROS attack. Intermediate ranges of water loss produce membrane lipids extensive peroxidation and de-esterification. Cell death is the consequent events of these oxidative attacks (França et al. 2007). It is shown that fluid replacement can compensate the destructive effects of dehydration. So, stabilization of physiological conditions and minimization of stresses in the neuromuscular, cardiovascular and thermoregulatory systems need dehydration by fluids replacement (Noakes 2007).

5 Conclusion

Natural cellular signaling is the communication language of the human intelligent cellular network that pursues homeostasis, interactions, defense, proliferation, metabolism, and all normal cellular events in all organs which provide ultimately life. All of this process can be occurred by the presence of defined amounts of normal signaling molecules and reactive radical and non-radical species. Oxidative stress and the presence of excess radical and non-radical reactive species is a process that changes the communication language of cells, removes the cellular signaling from the normal to abnormal state and dictates inflammatory commands to them. The result of these changes are development of disharmony in human body, triggering of metabolic disorders especially diabetes (as the origin of many other diseases) and neurodegenerative diseases. Meanwhile, lifestyle has a significant impact on maintaining health or disease occurrence. Excessive presence of inflammatory elements in modern human life (bad food habits, physical inactivity, modern technologies and their electromagnetic waves, disturbed biological clock and wrong body posture) and creating an inflammatory process are common to all unhealthy lifestyles. In the other hand, eliminating of oxidative stress and inflammation is the common elements in all healthy lifestyles which prevent all diseases specially diabetes. Man's return to nature, his serious and new look at natural gifts, his reasonable and defined enjoyment of all natural gifts and determinants such as trees, plants and their amazing diversity, sounds and lights, high concentrations of negative air, fruits and vegetables, beneficial microorganisms, healthy foods, avoiding from the unsecured electromagnetic waves of modern technologies, inner peace and body hydration and their entrance in human lifestyle create healthy lifestyle. So, this kind of lifestyle makes a clear vision for maintaining human health and his empowerment, especially in old age.

References

Al-Mawali A (2015) Non-communicable diseases: shining a light on cardiovascular disease Oman's Biggest Killer. Oman Med J 30(4):227–228

Alvarez JS, Goldraich LA, Nunes AH, Zandavalli MCB, Zandavalli RB, Belli KC, Rocha NSd, Fleck MPdA, Clausell N (2016) Association between spirituality and adherence to management in outpatients with heart failure. Arq Bras Cardiol 106(6):491–501

Ardeshirlarijani E, Tabatabaei-Malazy O, Mohseni S, Qorbani M, Larijani B, Jalili RB (2019) Effect of probiotics supplementation on glucose and oxidative stress in type 2 diabetes diabetes mellitus: a meta-analysis of randomized trials. DARU J Pharm Sci 27 (2):827–837

Armstrong LE, Johnson EC (2018) Water intake, water balance, and the elusive daily water requirement. Nutrients 10(12):1928

Aryal KK, Mehata S, Neupane S, Vaidya A, Dhimal M, Dhakal P, Rana S, Bhusal CL, Lohani GR, Paulin FH (2015) The burden and determinants of non communicable diseases risk factors in Nepal: findings from a nationwide steps survey. PLoS ONE 10(8): e0134834

Asif M (2014) The prevention and control the type-2 diabetes by changing lifestyle and dietary pattern. J Educ Health Promot 3

Atlas ID (2017) Brussels, Belgium: International diabetes federation; 2013. Int Diabetes Fed (IDF):147

Bellou V, Belbasis L, Tzoulaki I, Evangelou E (2018) Risk factors for type 2 diabetes diabetes mellitus: an exposure-wide umbrella review of meta-analyses. PLoS ONE 13(3):e0194127

Berlett BS, Stadtman ER (1997) Protein oxidation in aging, disease, and oxidative stress. J Biol Chem 272 (33):20313–20316

Bhasin MK, Dusek JA, Chang B-H, Joseph MG, Denninger JW, Fricchione GL, Benson H, Libermann TA (2013) Relaxation response induces temporal transcriptome changes in energy metabolism, insulin secretion and inflammatory pathways. PLoS ONE 8 (5):e62817

Bircher J, Kuruvilla S (2014) Defining health by addressing individual, social, and environmental determinants: new opportunities for health care and public health. J Public Health Policy 35(3):363–386

Blum S, Schiffrin EJ (2003) Intestinal microflora and homeostasis of the mucosal immune response: implications for probiotic bacteria? Curr Issues Intestinal Microbiol 4(2):53–60

Boskou D, Blekas G, Tsimidou M (2006) Olive oil composition. In: Olive oil. Elsevier, pp 41–72

Brüssow H (2013) What Is Health? Microb Biotechnol 6 (4):341–348

Cecarini V, Gee J, Fioretti E, Amici M, Angeletti M, Eleuteri AM, Keller JN (2007) Protein oxidation and cellular homeostasis: emphasis on metabolism. Biochim Biophys Acta (BBA)-Mol Cell Res 1773(2):93–104

Cohen S, Alper CM, Doyle WJ, Treanor JJ, Turner RB (2006) Positive emotional style predicts resistance to illness after experimental exposure to rhinovirus or influenza a virus. Psychosom Med 68(6):809–815

Cooper GM, Hausman RE (2018) The cell: a molecular approach. Oxford University Press

Council NR (1993) Assessment of the possible health effects of ground wave emergency network. National Academies Press

Della Pepa G, Vetrani C, Vitale M, Riccardi G (2018) Wholegrain intake and risk of type 2 diabetes: evidence from epidemiological and intervention studies. Nutrients 10(9):1288

Diagnosis and Classification of Diabetes Mellitus (2009). Diabetes care 32 (Supplement 1):S62–67

Duhaini I (2016) The effects of electromagnetic fields on human health. Physica Med 32:213

Ďuračková Z (2010) Some current insights into oxidative stress. Physiol Res 59(4)

Farhud DD (2015) Impact of lifestyle on health. Iran J Publ Health 44(11):1442

Fedorak RN (2008) Understanding why probiotic therapies can be effective in treating Ibd. J Clin Gastroenterol 42:S111–S115

Finkel T (2011) Signal transduction by reactive oxygen species. J Cell Biol 194(1):7–15

Forrester SJ, Kikuchi DS, Hernandes MS, Xu Q, Griendling KK (2018) Reactive oxygen species in metabolic and inflammatory signaling. Circ Res 122(6):877–902

França M, Panek A, Eleutherio E (2007) Oxidative stress and its effects during dehydration. Comp Biochem Physiol a: Mol Integr Physiol 146(4):621–631

Fries JF (1980) Aging, natural death, and the compression of morbidity. N Engl J Med 303(3):130–135

Frumkin H, Bratman GN, Breslow SJ, Cochran B, Kahn PH Jr, Lawler JJ, Levin PS, Tandon PS, Varanasi U, Wolf KL (2017) Nature contact and human health: a research Agenda. Environ Health Perspect 125(7):075001

Fung TT, Hu FB, Pereira MA, Liu S, Stampfer MJ, Colditz GA, Willett WC (2002) Whole-grain intake and the risk of type 2 diabetes: a prospective study in men. Am J Clin Nutr 76(3):535–540

Galaviz KI, Narayan KV, Lobelo F, Weber MB (2018) Lifestyle and the prevention of type 2 diabetes: a status report. Am J Lifestyle Med 12(1):4–20

Gillett M, Royle P, Snaith A, Scotland G, Poobalan A, Imamura M, Black C, Boroujerdi M, Jick S, Wyness L (2012) Non-pharmacological interventions to reduce the risk of diabetes diabetes in people with impaired glucose regulation: a systematic review and economic evaluation. Health Technol Assess 16(3):1–236

Gorzynik-Debicka M, Przychodzen P, Cappello F, Kuban-Jankowska A, Marino Gammazza A, Knap N, Wozniak M, Gorska-Ponikowska M (2018) Potential health benefits of olive oil and plant polyphenols. Int J Mol Sci 19(3):686

Gouvinhas I, Machado N, Sobreira C, Domínguez-Perles R, Gomes S, Rosa E, Barros AI (2017) Critical review on the significance of olive phytochemicals in plant physiology and human health. Molecules 22(11):1986

Gudjinu HY, Sarfo B (2017) Risk factors for type 2 diabetes diabetes mellitus among out-patients in Ho, the volta regional capital of Ghana: a case-control study. BMC Res Notes 10(1):324

Holt EM, Steffen LM, Moran A, Basu S, Steinberger J, Ross JA, Hong C-P, Sinaiko AR (2009) Fruit and vegetable consumption and its relation to markers of inflammation and oxidative stress in adolescents. J Am Diet Assoc 109(3):414–421

Hosseini B, Berthon BS, Saedisomeolia A, Starkey MR, Collison A, Wark PA, Wood LG (2018) Effects of fruit and vegetable consumption on inflammatory biomarkers and immune cell populations: a systematic literature review and meta-analysis. Am J Clin Nutr 108(1):136–155

Hussain T, Tan B, Yin Y, Blachier F, Tossou MC, Rahu N (2016) Oxidative stress and inflammation: what polyphenols can do for us? Oxidative Med Cell Longevity 2016:7432797

Huynen MM, Martens P, Hilderink HB (2005) The health impacts of globalisation: a conceptual framework. Globalization Health 1(1):14–26

Ideno Y, Hayashi K, Abe Y, Ueda K, Iso H, Noda M, Lee J-S, Suzuki S (2017) Blood pressure-lowering effect of Shinrin-Yoku (Forest Bathing): a systematic review and meta-analysis. BMC Complement Altern Med 17(1):409

Iwama H (2004) Negative air ions created by water shearing improve erythrocyte deformability and aerobic metabolism. Indoor Air 14(4):293–297

Iwama H, Ohmizo H, Furuta S, Ohmori S, Watanabe K, Kaneko T, Tsutsumi K (2002) Inspired superoxide anions attenuate blood lactate concentrations in postoperative patients. Crit Care Med 30(6):1246–1249

Jabs T (1999) Reactive oxygen intermediates as mediators of programmed cell death in plants and animals. Biochem Pharmacol 57(3):231–245

Jafari N, Farajzadegan Z, Loghmani A, Majlesi M, Jafari N (2014) Spiritual well-being and quality of life of Iranian adults with type 2 diabetes. Evid-Based Complement Altern Med 2014

James SL (2018) Global, regional, and national incidence, prevalence, and years lived with disability for 354 diseases and injuries for 195 countries and territories, 1990–2017: A Systematic Analysis for the global burden of disease study 2017. The Lancet 392(10159):1789–1858

Jiang S-Y, Ma A, Ramachandran S (2018) Negative air ions and their effects on human health and air quality improvement. Int J Mol Sci 19(10):2966

Joseph JJ, Echouffo-Tcheugui JB, Talegawkar SA, Effoe VS, Okhomina V, Carnethon MR, Hsueh WA, Golden SH (2017) Modifiable lifestyle risk factors and incident diabetes in African Americans. Am J Prev Med 53(5):e165–e174

Kechagia M, Basoulis D, Konstantopoulou S, Dimitriadi D, Gyftopoulou K, Skarmoutsou N, Fakiri E (2013) Health benefits of probiotics: a review. ISRN Nutritions 2013; 2013:481651.481651

Kim YS, Young MR, Bobe G, Colburn NH, Milner JA (2009) Bioactive food components, inflammatory targets, and cancer prevention. Cancer Prev Res 2(3):200–208

Koenig HG (2012) Religion, spirituality, and health: the research and clinical implications. ISRN Psychiatry 2012

Kok G, de Vries NK (2015) Health education and health promotion

Kolb H, Martin S (2017) Environmental/Lifestyle factors in the pathogenesis and prevention of Type 2 diabetes. BMC Med 15(1):131

Krewski D, Byus CV, Glickman BW, Lotz WG, Mandeville R, McBride ML, Prato FS, Weaver DF (2001) Potential health risks of radiofrequency fields from wireless telecommunication devices. J Toxicol Environ Health Part B 4(1):1–143

Kuo M (2015) How might contact with nature promote human health? Promising mechanisms and a possible central pathway. Front Psychol 6:1093

Ley SH, Hamdy O, Mohan V, Hu FB (2014) Prevention and management of type 2 diabetes: dietary components and nutritional strategies. The Lancet 383 (9933):1999–2007

Liska D, Mah E, Brisbois T, Barrios PL, Baker LB, Spriet LL (2019) Narrative review of hydration and selected health outcomes in the general population. Nutrients 11(1):70

Liu AG, Ford NA, Hu FB, Zelman KM, Mozaffarian D, Kris-Etherton PM (2017) A healthy approach to dietary fats: Understanding the science and taking action to reduce consumer confusion. Nutr J 16(1):53

Lynch CP, Hernandez-Tejada MA, Strom JL, Egede LE (2012) Association between spirituality and depression in adults with type 2 diabetes . The Diabetes Educ 38(3):427–435

Marventano S, Vetrani C, Vitale M, Godos J, Riccardi G, Grosso G (2017) Whole grain intake and glycaemic control in healthy subjects: a systematic review and meta-analysis of randomized controlled trials. Nutrients 9(7):769

Mathers CD, Loncar D (2006) Projections of global mortality and burden of disease from 2002 to 2030. PLOS Med 3(11):e442

Medzhitov R (2010) Inflammation 2010: new adventures of an old flame. Cell 140(6):771–776

Melo HM, Santos LE, Ferreira ST (2019) Diet-derived fatty acids, brain inflammation, and mental health. Front Neurosci 13:265

Mengheri E (2008) Health, probiotics, and inflammation. J Clin Gastroenterol 42(3):S177–S178

Meo SA, Al Rubeaan K (2013) Effects of exposure to electromagnetic field radiation (Emfr) generated by activated mobile phones on fasting blood glucose. Int J Occup Med Environ Health 26(2):235–241

Meo SA, Alsubaie Y, Almubarak Z, Almutawa H, AlQasem Y, Hasanato RM (2015) Association of exposure to radio-frequency electromagnetic field radiation (Rf-Emfr) generated by mobile phone base stations with glycated hemoglobin (Hba1c) and risk of type 2 diabetes mellitus. Int J Environ Res Public Health 12(11):14519–14528

Mittelmark MB, Bauer GF (2017) The meanings of salutogenesis. The handbook of salutogenesis. Springer, Cham, pp 7–13

Moosavi-Movahedi A (1999) Mysteries of spiritual scientific knowledge. Hamdard Islamicus 22(1):9–15

Moosavi-Movahedi AA (2020) Human health: Balance with creation and human inner nature. Sci Cultivation 10(1):2–10

Mortazavi S, Owji S, Shojaei-Fard M, Ghader-Panah M, Mortazavi S, Tavakoli-Golpayegani A, Haghani M, Taeb S, Shokrpour N, Koohi O (2016) Gsm 900 Mhz microwave radiation-induced alterations of insulin level and histopathological changes of liver and pancreas in rat. J Biomed Phys Eng 6(4):235

Mousavy SJ, Riazi GH, Kamarei M, Aliakbarian H, Sattarahmady N, Sharifizadeh A, Safarian S, Ahmad F, Moosavi-Movahedi AA (2009) Effects of mobile phone radiofrequency on the structure and function of the normal human hemoglobin. Int J Biol Macromol 44(3):278–285

Najjar FM, Taghavi F, Ghadari R, Sheibani N, Moosavi-Movahedi AA (2017) Destructive effect of non-enzymatic glycation on catalase and remediation via curcumin. Arch Biochem Biophys 630:81–90

Nathan C, Ding A (2010) Nonresolving inflammation. Cell 140(6):871–882

Noakes TD (2007) Does dehydration impair exercise performance? Med Sci Sports Exerc 39(8):1209–1217

Pan A, Malik VS, Schulze MB, Manson JE, Willett WC, Hu FB (2012) Plain-water intake and risk of type 2 diabetes in young and middle-aged women. Am J Clin Nutr 95(6):1454–1460

Perbal B (2003) Communication Is the key. Cell Commun Signaling 1(1):1–4

Perez V, Alexander DD, Bailey WH (2013) Air ions and mood outcomes: a review and meta-analysis. BMC Psychiatry 13(1):29

Piko BF, Brassai L (2016) A reason to eat healthy: The role of meaning in life in maintaining homeostasis in modern society. Health Psychol Open 3(1):2055102916634360

Plaza-Díaz J, Ruiz-Ojeda FJ, Vilchez-Padial LM, Gil A (2017) Evidence of the anti-inflammatory effects of probiotics and synbiotics in intestinal chronic diseases. Nutrients 9(6):555

Popa-Wagner A, Mitran S, Sivanesan S, Chang E, Buga A-M (2013) Ros and brain diseases: the good, the bad, and the ugly. Oxidative Med Cell Longevity 2013

Popkin BM, D'Anci KE, Rosenberg IH (2010) Water, hydration, and health. Nutr Rev 68(8):439–458

Pouwer F, Kupper N, Adriaanse MC (2010) Does emotional stress cause type 2 diabetes mellitus? a review from the European depression in diabetes (Edid) research consortium. Discov Med 9(45):112–118

Puchalski CM (2001) The role of spirituality in health care. In: Baylor University medical center proceedings, vol 4. Taylor & Francis, pp 352–357

Puga AM, Lopez-Oliva S, Trives C, Partearroyo T, Varela-Moreiras G (2019) Effects of drugs and excipients on hydration status. Nutrients 11(3):669

Radhakrishnan K, Halász Á, Vlachos D, Edwards JS (2010) Quantitative understanding of cell signaling: the importance of membrane organization. Curr Opin Biotechnol 21(5):677–682

Rad HA, Abbasalizadeh S, Vazifekhah S, Abbasalizadeh F, Hassanalilou T, Bastani P, Ejtahed H-S, Soroush A-R, Javadi M, M Mortazavian A (2017) The future of diabetes management by healthy probiotic microorganisms. Curr Diab Rev 13(6):582–589

Rahman I, MacNee W (2000) Oxidative stress and regulation of glutathione in lung inflammation. Eur Respir J 16(3):534–554

Reddy PH (2017) Can diabetes be controlled by lifestyle activities? Current Res Diabetes Obes J 1(4)

Reis JP, Loria CM, Sorlie PD, Park Y, Hollenbeck A, Schatzkin A (2011) Lifestyle factors and risk for new-onset diabetes: a population-based cohort study. Ann Intern Med 155(5):292–299

Ricker MA, Haas WC (2017) Anti-inflammatory diet in clinical practice: a review. Nutr Clin Pract 32(3):318–325

Riebl SK, Davy BM (2013) The hydration equation: update on water balance and cognitive performance. Acsm's Health Fitness J 17(6):21

Rittiphairoj T, Pongpirul K, Mueller NT, Li T (2019) Probiotics for glycemic control in patients with type 2 diabetes mellitus: protocol for a systematic review. Syst Rev 8(1):1–6

Ruiz-Núñez B, Dijck-Brouwer DJ, Muskiet FA (2016) The relation of saturated fatty acids with low-grade inflammation and cardiovascular disease. J Nutr Biochem 36:1–20

Salzano S, Checconi P, Hanschmann E-M, Lillig CH, Bowler LD, Chan P, Vaudry D, Mengozzi M, Coppo L, Sacre S (2014) Linkage of inflammation and oxidative stress via release of glutathionylated peroxiredoxin-2, which acts as a danger signal. Proc Natl Acad Sci 111(33):12157–12162

Sartorius N (2006) The meanings of health and its promotion. Croatian Med J 47(4):662

Scarfi MR, Mattsson M-O, Simkó M, Zeni O (2019) Electric, magnetic, and electromagnetic fields in biology and medicine: from mechanisms to biomedical applications. Multidisciplinary Digital Publishing Institute

Sefidbakht Y, Hosseinkhani S, Mortazavi M, Tavakkolnia I, Khellat MR, Shakiba-Herfeh M, Saviz M, Faraji-Dana R, Saboury AA, Sheibani N (2013) Effects of 940 Mhz Emf on luciferase solution: structure, function, and dielectric studies. Bioelectromagnetics 34(6):489–498

Sefidbakht Y, Moosavi-Movahedi AA, Hosseinkhani S, Khodagholi F, Torkzadeh-Mahani M, Foolad F, Faraji-Dana R (2014) Effects of 940 Mhz Emf on bioluminescence and oxidative response of stable luciferase producing hek cells. Photochem Photobiol Sci 13(7):1082–1092

Sharma M, Majumdar P (2009) Occupational lifestyle diseases: an emerging issue. Indian J Occup Environ Med 13(3):109–112

Shojaeifard M, Jarideh S, Owjfard M, Nematollahii S, Talaei-Khozani T, Malekzadeh M (2018) Electromagnetic fields of mobile phone jammer exposure on blood factors in rats. J Biomed Phys Eng 8(4):403

Smith BJ, Tang KC, Nutbeam D (2006) Who health promotion glossary: new terms. Health Promot Int 21(4):340–345

Sottero B, Rossin D, Poli G, Biasi F (2018) Lipid oxidation products in the pathogenesis of inflammation-related gut diseases. Curr Med Chem 25(11):1311–1326

Taghavi F, Moosavi-Movahedi A, Bohlooli M, Alijanvand HH, Salami M, Maghami P, Saboury A, Farhadi M, Yousefi R, Habibi-Rezaei M (2013) Potassium sorbate as an age activator for human serum albumin in the presence and absence of glucose. Int J Biol Macromol 62:146–154

Taghavi F, Habibi-Rezaei M, Bohlooli M, Farhadi M, Goodarzi M, Movaghati S, Maghami P, Taghibiglou C, Amanlou M, Haertlé T (2016) Anti-amyloidogenic effects of ellagic acid on human serum albumin fibril formation induced by potassium sorbate and glucose. J Mol Recognit 29(12):611–618

Taghavi F, Habibi-Rezaei M, Amani M, Saboury AA, Moosavi-Movahedi AA (2017) The status of glycation in protein aggregation. Int J Biol Macromol 100:67–74

Taghavi F, Moosavi-Movahedi AA (2019) Free radicals, diabetes, and its complexities. In: Plant and human health, vol 2. Springer, Berlin, pp 1–41

Tang KC, Ehsani JP, McQueen DV (2003) Evidence based health promotion: recollections, reflections, and reconsiderations. J Epidemiol Community Health 57(11):841–843

Tecilazich F (2020) Microvascular disease in diabetes diabetes . Wiley, India

Telle-Hansen VH, Christensen JJ, Ulven SM, Holven KB (2017) Does dietary fat affect inflammatory markers in overweight and obese individuals?—a review of randomized controlled trials from 2010 to 2016. Genes Nutr 12(1):26

Thacker SB, Sencer DJ, Jaffe HW (2017) Centers for disease control. In: Quah SR (ed) International Encyclopedia of public health, 2nd edn. Academic Press, Oxford, pp 448–454

Thannickal V, Fanburg B (2000) Reactive Oxygen species in cell signaling. Am J Physiol Lung Cell Mol Physiol 279:L1005–1028

Tol A, Tavassoli E, Shariferad GR, Shojaeezadeh D (2013) Health-promoting lifestyle and quality of life among undergraduate students at school of health, Isfahan University of medical sciences. J Educ Health Promot 2(11)

Upham BL, Trosko JE (2009) Oxidative-dependent integration of signal transduction with intercellular gap junctional communication in the control of gene expression. Antioxid Redox Signal 11(2):297–307

Wang C, Levis GBS, Lee EB, Levis WR, Lee DW, Kim BS, Park SY, Park E (2004) Platycodin D and D3 isolated from the root of platycodon grandiflorum modulate the production of nitric oxide and secretion of Tnf-A in Activated Raw 264.7 Cells. Int Immunopharmacol 4(8):1039–1049.

Wiszniewski A, Suchanowski A, Wielgomas B (2014) Effects of air-ions on human circulatory indicators. Pol J Environ Stud 23(2)

Xu Y, Wan Q, Feng J, Du L, Li K, Zhou Y (2018) Whole grain diet reduces systemic inflammation: a meta-analysis of 9 randomized trials. Medicine 97(43): e12995

Yakymenko I, Sidorik E (2010) Risks of carcinogenesis from electromagnetic radiation of mobile telephony devices

Yao K, Zeng L, He Q, Wang W, Lei J, Zou X (2017) Effect of probiotics on glucose and lipid metabolism in type 2 diabetes mellitus: a meta-analysis of 12 randomized controlled trials. Med Sci Monit Int Med J Exp Clin Res 23:3044

Yousefi R, Moosavi-Movahedi AA (2020) Achilles' heel of the killer virus: The highly important molecular targets for hitting Sars-Cov-2 that causes covid-19. J Iran Chem Soc 17:1257–1258

Zhang C, Klett EL, Coleman RA (2013) Lipid signals and insulin resistance. Clinical Lipidol 8(6):659–667

Zhou Y, Hong Y, Huang H (2016) Triptolide attenuates inflammatory response in membranous glomerulonephritis rat via downregulation of Nf-Kb signaling pathway. Kidney Blood Press Res 41(6):901–910

Zwickey H, Horgan A, Hanes D, Schiffke H, Moore A, Wahbeh H, Jordan J, Ojeda L, McMurry M, Elmer P (2019) Effect of the anti-inflammatory diet in people with diabetes and pre-diabetes: a randomized controlled feeding study. J Restorative Med 8(1): e20190107

Healthier Lifestyle by Considering Psychoemotional Dimension of Wellness

Monireh-Sadat Mousavi and Gholamhossein Riazi

Abstract

In today's fast-paced society imposing considerable stress on daily human life, psychoemotional-related lifestyle diseases are rapidly growing. Therefore, a large part of research attention has recently been devoted to the mental dimension of lifestyle. This chapter aims to highlight the role of psychoemotional issues in quality of life and to point out some techniques for creating psychophysiological coherence. To achieve this, the chapter is divided into five parts. The first part introduces Emotional Intelligence (EI) as an essential component in the superiority of one's day-to-day life that plays a crucial role in making a fine-tuned lifestyle. In this section, two main classifications of a healthy diet, including a healthy (1) food diet and (2) mental diet, are also well described. The second and third parts respectively deal with how the brain and heart are effectively associated with emotional energy regulation. The fourth part introduces the basic concept of heart rate variability (HRV) as a reliable indicator of psychoemotional state. The fifth part pertains to heart-brain connection, psychophysiological coherence, and positive emotion-focused techniques for reaching the health tipping point. In this context, the field of "Psymentology," as a potent Iranian Complementary and Alternative Medicine (CAM), is introduced for generating psychophysiological coherence state based on building healthy worldviews and developing mindfulness. Finally, we conclude the chapter by emphasizing mind training and emotion regulation through caring sensory organs that seem to have a significant effect on the prevention of psychoemotional-related lifestyle diseases and the creation of a longer, healthier life.

Keywords

Emotional intelligence (EI) · Heart rate variability (HRV) · Heart-Brain connection · Emotion-focused techniques · Psychophysiological coherence

1 Introduction

In these days' world, people generally pay more attention to the physical dimension of their life, while the non-physical or emotional dimension plays a key role in their multidimensional life quality Pocnet et al. 2017; Isasi et al. 2013). So, in order to achieve significant gains in human health, more research attention must be directed towards emotional factors.

M.-S. Mousavi · G. Riazi (✉)
Laboratory of Neuro-Organic Chemistry, Institute of Biochemistry and Biophysics (IBB), University of Tehran, Tehran, Iran
e-mail: ghriazi@ut.ac.ir

M.-S. Mousavi
e-mail: mousavi.m@ut.ac.ir

Etymologically, emotion is made up of energy and motion, to represent the movement of energy. Emotion (energy in motion) is generated originally from the electrical pulses in our body. The amount of energy in motion for each person creates his emotional state. Each emotion has a particular vibratory pattern as its own fingerprint or signature Zhao et al. 2016). Hypo and hyper movement of energy throughout the body could cause negative emotions such as depression and anxiety, respectively Chambers et al. 2009). Therefore, a healthy emotional lifestyle could create a normal energy flow to positively affect the health of our body at all levels, from organs to subcellular organelles or even subatomic particles.

According to Albert Einstein, everything in the world is made of energy and everything in life is vibration Einstein 2019). A molecule is made of atoms. An atom is made of three basic parts: electrons, protons, and neutrons. The last two are made of quarks, which are the fast-moving points of energy. Electrons and quarks are fundamental particles which fully made of energy. Therefore, all matter in the universe is basically the energy in different states of vibration.

In this context, one of the major phenomenon for healthy lifestyle that has emerged today is calibrating the body's energetic vibration through emotion regulation.

The chapter deals with the role of psychoemotional issues in the overall vibration of the human body and introduces some techniques of creating vibrational coherency which can greatly boost health and well-being. In this regard, the pivotal role of the brain and heart organs due to their specific energetic characteristics has been explained.

2 The Role of Psychoemotional Factors in Health

For a long time, the concept of intelligence quotient (IQ) had been known as an indicator of a healthy personal, and professional life. However, over the last few years, the concept of emotional quotient (EQ), as the main success criteria, has arisen and developed to describe the significance of the contribution of Emotional Intelligence (EI) throughout the human life cycle. In fact, new observations strongly indicate that the EI plays a key role in making a fine-tuned lifestyle Brackett et al. 2011; Ciarrochi et al. 2006; Grewal and Salovey 2005). However, according to global statistics, antidepressants having lots of side-effects on EI are one of the most widely used drugs in the world. This is partially related to the fact that the expectation of humankind has gone far beyond their lives, causing more psychological stress than ever before. Therefore, nowadays, the psychoemotional root of lifestyle diseases, which was a relatively neglected area in lifestyle assessment, needs more attention. Considering the powerful link between body and mind, new research has recently focused on the association between diseases and psychoemotional factors Turner and Kelly 2000). Many further research studies have recently discovered that psychoemotional distress and mental illness can fuel diverse physical diseases such as immune system disorders Koh 2018), multiple sclerosis (MS) Karageorgou et al. 2018; Meknatkhah et al. 2018), diabetes Martinez et al. 2018; McCoy and Theeke 2019), hypertension Handler et al. 2019), cognitive performance, oxidative stress Mousavi et al. 2018), and cardiovascular disease (Albus et al. 2019; Mousavi et al. 2019).

In this context, developing mentally healthy worldviews would be highly beneficial (Taheri and Rahimi 2014). Besides, according to the results of recent studies, even in the physical dimension of life, the quality of daily food consumption is vital not only because of the amount of vitamins, proteins, carbohydrates (sugar) and fats but also because of their overall vibrational frequency which affects our mood and emotions. Therefore, learning, knowing, applying and developing the lifestyle covering the consumption of high-quality foods along with the use of powerful relaxation skills, which would well support the psychoemotional state, seems to be a useful element of a healthy life.

2.1 Healthy Food Diet

A brief review of food traditions and dietary restrictions in diverse religions indicate that vegetarianism is highly recommended while consumption of meat is less suggested. Not only considering the non-violence principle, but it is also in complete accordance with the new medical evidence, showing less malignant diseases such as cancer among vegetarians and those who eat less meat. In addition, it has been recently reported that livestock plays a significant role in global greenhouse gas emissions, causing climate change and global warming. So, breeding less livestock and eating less meat is the finest thing we can do for our living planet.

Another point about the consumption of high-quality foods is using proper cooking times and temperatures for food safety and nutrient protection. During the long cooking process at high temperature, the nutrients will be affected by different processes such as denaturation, degradation, and decomposition, making the food as waste material. Consequently, the more we intake fresh herbs, nuts, and other healthy plant foods, the more we fuel our body's electrical currents by natural frequencies, which raise our energy vibration.

2.2 Healthy Mental Diet

The new world skills and lifestyle, focusing on our inner world, provides an opportunity to improve the quality of life regarding both physical and psychoemotional well-being. Our inner world refers to emotions we hold in our minds resulted from our feelings, beliefs, and thoughts. The best way to promote our psychoemotional health is the perfect vibrational diet (Gerbarg et al. 2014). In contrast to the general idea, diet does not refer to just the food we eat through the mouth, but more specifically, it relates to all the vibrations we receive from our surrounding environment through all the senses. It strongly seems that the latter, known as the mental diet holds the secret of a longer and healthier life.

Experts recommend some ways to get rid of the hustle and bustle of today's busy life, to protect ourselves from the destructive effects of the harmful frequencies of urban daily life routine, and to provide opportunities to raise our vibration level. Since sensing the vibration of each specific energy resulted in feeling its exact emotion, "Intentional Emotion Regulation" through all the human senses is the leading comprehensive approach in this area (Tugade and Fredrickson 2007). As yet, human beings have five known sense organs; eyes to see, ears to hear, nose for the smell, tongue for the taste, and skin to the touch. Each sensory organ receives individual information from the surrounding environment and sends them to the brain to be processed. Consequently, these five sense organs provide five different input pathways which controlling them is the basis of a mental health diet using special sound, sights, aroma, taste, and touch for healing (Jawer 2009).

Today, some diverse methods are used throughout the world to help to achieve emotional and mental well-being. Meditation is one of the most popular and accepted methods with nobody's movements practicing mindfulness. This mental focus could be in silence on a particular object within the body, such as breath control. Spending time in silence for a few minutes every day can help to clear mental clutter and emotional disturbances. Likewise, nature sounds can be the object of mental focus in mindfulness practice. For example, sounds of forest, birds, waterfall, rain, wind, ocean, and other nature sounds are inner relaxation melodies using by many psychotherapists. For better results in meditation, being accompanied by positive inner thought and feeling is a crucial principle. According to research results, emotions of gratitude and appreciation have the highest and most productive vibrations. In this regard, "gratitude meditation" is one of the most famous proficient methods for emotional purging. This practice is a powerful happiness intervention and psychic nutrition, which harmonize different rhythm of the human body, such as breathing, blood pressure, etc.

2.3 Making Lifestyle Changes

Each of these healthy lifestyle practices needs to persist for a certain period of time (generally more than three weeks) to have a lasting effect. Experts believe in 21/90 rule, which says, "it takes 21 days to create a habit and 90 days to make it a lifestyle change". This rule work as a double-edged sword capable of making both good and bad habits. So, we need to watch out for each of our repeated activities that can eventually lead to a habit and then a lifestyle change.

In this regard, there is a famous quote which says: "Watch your thoughts, for they become words. Watch your words, for they become actions. Watch your actions for they become habits. Watch your habits, for they become your character. Watch your character, for it becomes your destiny" (Donaldson 2017). The real source of this quote is unknown, and it is attributed to several people and scholars such as Ralph Waldo Emerson, Lao Tzu, Frank Outlaw, Gautama Buddha, Bishop Beckwith, Margaret Thatcher, Mahatma Gandhi, and Ali Ibn Abi Talib, without explicit reference. This well-known quote, regardless of its real origin, well describes the critical effect of repeated mental whispers on a healthy lifestyle and destiny.

3 The Role of Brain in Psychoemotional Health

The brain is a complex network of many neural circuits consisting of billions of nerve cells (called neurons) and specific connections (called synapses). The normal adult human brain is about 2% of the total body weight; however, it consumes approximately 25% of the total energy consumption. As the primary energy consumer in the human body, it generates myriad electrical impulses across its sophisticated neural web to let neurons interconnect and share information for a moment-to-moment synchronization of thoughts, emotions, and behaviors (Varela et al. 2001; Ward 2003). Synchronized electrical pulses from communication between neurons within our brains produce neural vibrations or brainwaves, including Delta, Theta, Alpha, Beta and Gamma, grouped based on their frequencies measured in Hertz[1] (Fig. 1). The brainwaves with diverse oscillatory patterns look like different musical notes in a symphony orchestra, which cohere with each other in a synchronized harmony (Moser et al. 2008).

The relative level of each vibrational frequency contributes significantly to creating an overall coordinated pattern. As out of balanced musical notes make a non-synchronized orchestra, out of sync brainwaves results in corresponding problems in the psychoemotional or neuro-physical health. In fact, out of sync brainwaves, based on their frequencies, which are inhibitory or stimulatory, cause under-arousal or over-arousal in different brain areas resulting in different negative psychoemotional states. For example, attention deficit is connected to under-arousal; however, anger, hyper-vigilance, and anxiety disorders are related to over-arousal. Some certain psychoemotional health disorders like attention-deficit/hyperactivity disorder (ADHD) is associated with a combination of under-arousal and over-arousal (Goozen et al. 2000; Lang et al. 2007).

Our brainwave profile is in close association with our emotional lifestyle, making our regular experience of the world around us. By now, the brainwave patterns related to different emotional and neurological conditions have been mostly identified (Murugappan et al. 2010; Ismail et al. 2016; Robinson 2008). In this context, what is certain is that the most prevailing brainwave during the experience of positive emotions in daily life is the Alpha wave, considered as an indicator of psychoemotional state.

Each environmental signal such as sound, sights, aroma, taste, and touch, received by the sensory organs, affect our brainwave profile. Experimental studies have demonstrated that exposure to natural vibrational signals like nature's sound and light make coherent brain waves and promote our brain's energy efficiency.

---
[1]It was *first observed* by Hans Berger in 1924 using electroencephalography (EEG).

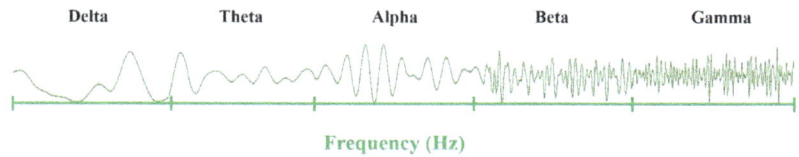

Fig. 1 Brainwaves grouped based on their frequencies

Therefore, living closer to nature would be one of the best ways to influence positively our psychoemotional health. Moreover, traditional eastern skills such as meditation train our brainwaves leading to balance for dealing with stressful life events. Therefore, all emotion-based lifestyle techniques such as meditation (Travis 2001; Boellinghaus et al. 2014) and living close to nature (Smith 2016) seem to boost our health by fine-tuning our brainwave function.

Moreover, from the perspective of the brain's chemicals, the neurotransmitters have been proved to be the primary inner source of brain electrical signals resulting in brainwave variability. Since each of neurotransmitters is mostly located in the special part of the brain, their passing from one neuron to another thorough firing of the action potential in synapses leads to arising a specific emotion. Therefore, each or a couple of neurotransmitters has been associated with one unique sensation or emotion (Aday et al. 2017).

Meanwhile, in healthy lifestyle research, some attention turned toward the heart because from the energetic-based viewpoint, the heart is the most potent energetic organ in the human body.

4 The Role of Heart in Psychoemotional Health

The heart tissue is a pump that circulates the blood flow throughout our bodies for delivering oxygen, nutrients, and hormones to our every single cell. Contrary to popular belief, the heart's pumping function is its primary, not the central role. Since the sixth century BC, the ancient philosopher's viewpoints about heart, promote the heart's role beyond the pumping machine. Reviewing the history of studies on the heart's role in the human body-mind system represents some major philosophers, including Avicenna, Alcmaeon, Plato, Aristotle, Galen, as pioneers of research on this issue.

In the sixth century BC, Alcmaeon was the first to identify the brain as the seat of human intelligence (Celesia 2012). After more than a century and a half, while Plato accepted Alcmaeon's view of the brain's role as the tissue of intellect, he identified the heart as the location of human emotions. At that time, Plato described emotion and intellect as two horses pulling the human being in opposite directions (Konstan 2006). This image seems to have been borrowed by Alcmaeon. Shortly after Plato, Aristotle developed Plato's philosophical analysis of emotions, providing a further comprehensive understanding of the emotional system. He, besides describing the heart as the source of emotion, introduced it as a sensory organ and the seat of intelligence too (Gregoric 2007; Crivellato and Ribatti 2007). After Aristotle, Galen like him, was firmly committed to regarding the heart as the seat of perception, emotion, and intelligence (Hankinson 1991; Tieleman 2002).

Afterward, during the 10th to sixteenth centuries, the philosopher-physician comprehension of heart's significance was greatly impressed by Aristotle and Galen's perspectives. For instance, Avicenna (Ibn Sina, in Persian) and Andreas Laguna, two great physicians of the tenth and sixteenth centuries respectively, agreeing with those attitudes, integrated all opinions of Aristotle and Galen and incorporated them into medical diagnosis and treatment (Holzman 2015). Although Avicenna lived at the end of the 10th, and the commencement of the eleventh century (980–1037), his book named "The Canon of Medicine," was considered as the main medical source book all over the world until the seventeenth century. Avicenna's Canon of Medicine is divided into five volumes. In the second volume, he well describes the association among psychoemotional issues, heart, blood, brain, and various diseases. According to his perspective, the heart, blood, and brain contribute to mental and emotional health, but the heart plays a more radical role. He proposed heart-based lifestyle modification, including more happiness, aromatherapy, and music therapy as the primary way of emotion regulation for advanced human well-being (Yousofpour et al. 2015; Mosaddegh et al. 2013).

In the early twentieth century, by the discovery of the brain nervous system structure, containing one hundred billion nerve cells or neurons, all attention was shifted for a while from the heart to the brain as the seat of intelligence Carlos and Borrell (2007). For this critical discovery, the 1906 Nobel Prize in Physiology or Medicine is awarded jointly to Ramón y Cajal and Golgi. But interestingly, modern scientific finding, being in line with Aristotle's theories of emotion and intelligence, has drawn attention again to the heart as the seat of sensation and intellect. In fact, it has been recently demonstrated that the heart has some vital characteristics that enable it to play key roles in body-mind connection beyond its known general role in blood circulation (McCraty et al. 2001). Its four significant characteristics are mentioned below:

1. Heart generates a powerful electromagnetic field that surrounds the body and can be detected several feet away (the heart's electrical waves and its magnetic field are approximately 60 and 5000 times stronger than those produced by the brain, respectively).
2. Heart generates mechanical vibrations (sounds and pressure).
3. Heart has an intrinsic nervous system with intrinsic neurotransmitters the same as the brain, so-called "small brain of the heart."
4. Heart synthesis some essential hormones for our physical and mental well-being.

These features of the heart affect the brain and whole body and communicate with every single cell. Interestingly, all these ways share a property in common, which is the vibrational frequency.

Therefore, it seems that the main function of the heart is related to its vibrational frequencies, controlled by specialized electrical signal generator cells called the pacemaker. The direct effect of the heart's fine-tuned rhythmic pattern on electromagnetic pulse, blood pressure, neural and hormonal patterns finally shape our psychoemotional state.

According to experts, heart transplantation leads to significant effects on recipients' psychoemotional issues, wisdom, cognitive performance, personality, identity and bodily integrity Pearsall et al. 2000). It appears that these major heart's effects were related to the heart's brain and cardiac conduction system, which control its electrical frequency by regulating the heartbeats. Although the electrical frequency of the human body is segregated into two major categories of physiologic (harmonic) and pathologic (nonharmonic), each category has a spectrum resulting in the person to personal differences. Consequently, psychophysiological states of transplanted heart recipients change under the influence of the new vibrational frequencies.

Likewise, a large number of worldwide known idioms, phrases and traditional sayings about the heart, such as "listen to your heart," "believe from the bottom of your heart," "allow your heart to guide you," and "go where your heart leads you," somehow conveys the dominant role of heart's intelligence in psychophysiological well-being.

Given all of the things mentioned above, the heart seems to be somehow the sixth sense organ. Accordingly, the cardiac afferent information sent to the brain, besides exerting homeostatic effects on cardiovascular regulation, have separate significant effects on central emotional processing in the brain. It has been established that the accurate monitoring of the heart's rhythmic patterns by the brain cortex is one of the fundamental functions of our body's emotional system.

5 Heart Rate Variability (HRV): The Symphony of the Human Body

Although it was once believed that rhythmic heartbeat at rest was uniformly regular like clockwork, we now know that a healthy resting heart rhythm has non-negligible variation (Shaffer et al. 2014). This variability result from the communication pathways interacting between the heart and brain. Interestingly, through the two-way heart-brain communication, afferent pathways by which information from the heart travels to the brain has much more traffic than the opposite side (LeDoux 1998). HRV genesis is either in time or frequency of the heart's electrical activity (Bilchick and Berger 2006).

Regarding the time-domain of HRV, the beat-to-beat minor fluctuations in heart rate named heart rate variability (HRV), which are unnoticed when calculating the mean heart rate (Fig. 2). Consider a car that has traveled 60 km in an hour. The car probably has traveled the distance by different speeds, not necessarily every kilometer in a single minute by the speed of 60 km/h, and so is our heart. If our mean heart rate is 60 beats per minute, it doesn't mean that all of the beats were at the same speed. In fact, there are fluctuations in the time and frequency of heartbeats that contain valuable information about what is happening inside the human body.

Regarding the frequency-domain of HRV, the fast Fourier transform (FFT) technique is used to compute the heart's frequency spectra, including three main frequency ranges: VLF (reflecting sympathetic activity), HF (reflecting parasympathetic activity), and LF (representing a mixture of sympathetic-parasympathetic activity) (Fig. 3). In healthy individuals, the heart's electrical waves with diverse vibratory patterns create an integrated entity and synchronized harmony, as the symphony orchestra of the human body.

Different physiological mechanisms have extensive roles in the synergistic action of the two branches of the Autonomic Nervous System (ANS) resulting in HRV. Therefore, a normal healthy HRV is an indicator of a well-balanced autonomic activity (McCraty and Shaffer 2015). Likewise, ANS activity in different tissues has been established to be also associated with psychoemotional states. Hence, HRV, as a reliable indicator of autonomic activity, can reflect the emotional states as well (Appelhans and Luecken 2006).

In this regard, the results of our animal experiments conducted in the Laboratory of Neuro-Organic Chemistry at the Institute of

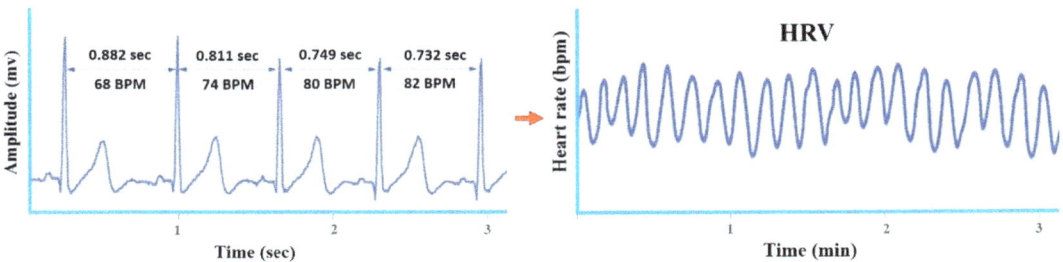

Fig. 2 The time-domain of HRV

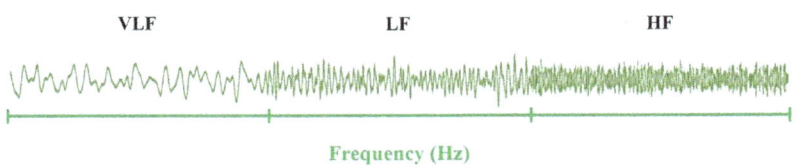

Fig. 3 The frequency-domain of HRV

Fig. 4 HRV patterns during normal psychophysiological state and two types of tension (physical or emotional) in groups of laboratory rats

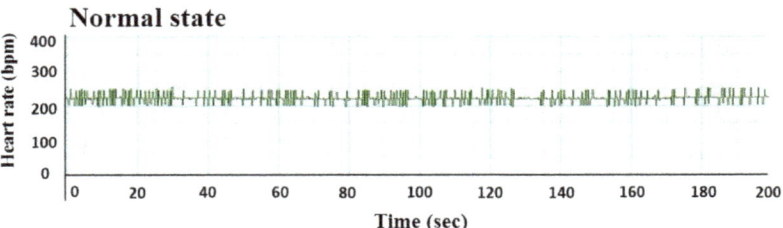
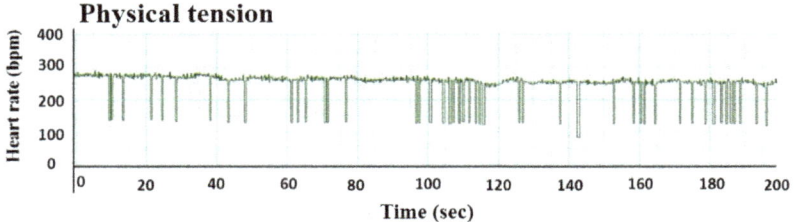
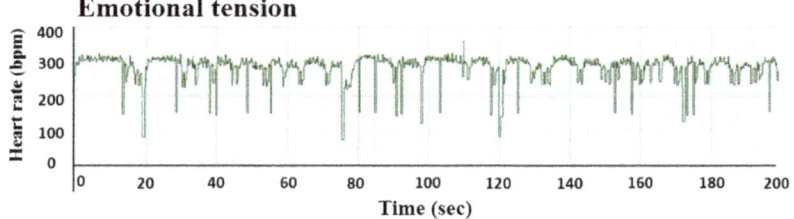

Biochemistry and Biophysics (IBB), University of Tehran, Tehran, Iran, displayed three different patterns of HRV waveforms in our three groups of rats (Fig. 4). Control rats yielded coherent sine mode HRV, while the rats of both tension groups presented non-coherent and irregular modes. Interestingly, HRV waveforms in psychologically stressed rats compared to physically stressed ones demonstrated more erratic shapes (unpublished data).

According to the HRV distribution graph plotted by 60,000 points (60,000 recorded heart rates) for each rat, there is an extremely sharp peak around the heart rate of 211 bpm in control rats, expressing the normal distribution pattern. However, the HRV distribution curve shifted to higher heart rate values in both stress groups. Overlapping of three diagrams illustrate three distinct zones of the HRV distribution curve representing three diverse modes of heart function (Fig. 5).

Therefore, our HRV pattern, the same as the brainwave profile, is in close relationship with our daily life emotional experience. So far, HRV patterns during several psychoemotional states have been reported (McCraty and Childre 2002). In this context, what is certain is that positive emotional experiences create ordered sine-like wave patterns, while negative ones make disordered HRV shapes. Researches show that the stronger the positive emotional experiences, the sharper the peak around 0.1 Hz region in the power spectral density (PSD) analysis of HRV. In this respect, the notable difference in PSD between of the appreciation as a super positive emotional state and the relaxation state reflects the fact that their mechanisms of action are totally different. During relaxation, the heart rate is necessarily reduced, but when experiencing deep positive emotions, the heart rhythm pattern has changed to a smooth, coherent wave without heart rate lowering. This coherent state is the result of increased heart-brain synchronization making a sharp peak around 0.1 Hz in PSD of HRV (Massaro and Pecchia 2019).

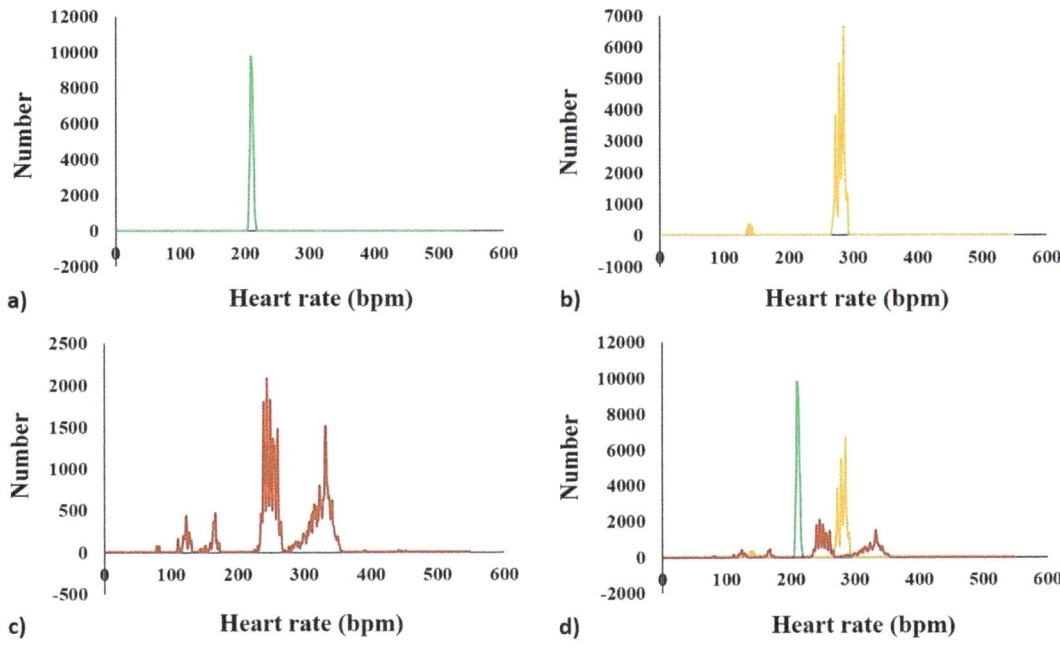

Fig. 5 HRV distribution graphs signify three distinct modes of heart function in the three groups of laboratory rats; **a** control, **b** physical stress, and **c** psychoemotional stress. Last image **d** displays overlapping of three diagrams

6 Heart-Brain Connection and Coherence: The Optimized Psychoemotional State

Coherence is a state of alignment and harmony between the heart, brain and mind. Incoherence mode, the energy accumulates and is not wasted, giving you clear and coordinated yield as well as more energy. In this state, the body's various physiological oscillatory subsystems such as respiration, heart rate variability, and blood pressure rhythm fluctuate at the same frequency (Tiller et al. 1996). The steady sinusoidal waveform of these rhythms leads to a physiological wave clarity and a greater sense of mental peace which lets the body's subsystems to comprehend the message of heart as the main orchestra conductor of the body's symphony. Therefore, in the two-way heart-brain dialogue, psychophysiological coherence is one of the most important mechanisms to clearly convey the moment-to-moment message to every single cell throughout the body. In this state, the body's natural health processes would be well facilitated (McCraty and Atkinson 2006).

So far, a number of the institute has been created through the world, research to develop ways of increasing the efficiency of the physiological and emotional system. The HeartMath Institute (HMI) in California is one of the most successful and well-known institutes worldwide, which has mostly focused on the heart-brain connection in order to achieve optimal human functioning (McCraty 2017; Edwards 2015). HMI has developed certain powerful relaxation and deep calm techniques known as "Freeze-Frame" (Childre 1998), "Cut-Thru" (Childre and Rozman 2002) and "Heart Lock-In" Childre et al. (1999) to induce psychophysiological coherence. The increased heart-brain synchronization in this state creates physiological, mental, emotional and social systems entrainment producing optimal well-being, which manifests itself in the form of life satisfaction (McCraty et al. 2009).

Based on the perspective of the National Institute of Health (NIH) in the U.S.A, collaborating very closely with World Health

Organization (WHO), any technique of health care and maintenance beyond conventional medicine falls into the category of Complementary and Alternative Medicine (CAM). So far, five distinct classifications have been introduced for CAM; 1—Energy Therapies, 2—Mind–Body Intervention, 3—Alternative Medical Systems, 4—Biologically-based Therapies, 5—Manipulative and Body-based practices (Koithan 2009; Keene et al. 2019; Bardia et al. 2006). Each of these classifications has its own sub-categories, and sub-sub-categories and so on. For instance, the field of Psymentology (Psyche + Mental + Logy) is an Iranian CAM that falls into the sub-category of Mental Treatment in the category of Mind–Body Intervention (Taheri and Bayyazi 2013; Taheri and Biriya 2013). The basis of lifestyle techniques in Psymentology, as a potent Iranian healthcare field, is building healthy worldviews and developing mindfulness for generating psychophysiological coherence state. In this outlook, our worldviews, depending on whether they are constructive or destructive, can make a healthy or unhealthy lifestyle, respectively.

7 Conclusion

Taken together, this chapter has attempted to show the importance of considering emotion in the quality of a healthy lifestyle. Interestingly, in various philosophical and religious texts, it has been repeatedly stated that positive emotions like generosity, kindness, and love make you the most satisfied with your life. According to numerous traditions, mind training and emotion regulation have been strongly recommended for optimal living. Therefore, positive emotions generated through each of sensory organs seem to have a significant effect on the prevention of psychoemotional-related lifestyle diseases.

For those interested in learning more about heart-brain coherence for advanced lifestyle, the references provided at the end of the chapter serve as a great reliable source to direct them for further information.

We conclude this chapter with a quote from Dr. Childre, the founder of HMI and one of the pioneers of developing EI:

> What you put out comes back. The more you sincerely appreciate life from the heart, the more the magnetic energy of appreciation attracts fulfilling life experiences to you, both personally and professionally. Learning how to appreciate more consistently offers many benefits and applications. Appreciation is an easy heart frequency to activate, and it can help shift your perspectives quickly. Learning how to appreciate both pleasant and even seemingly unpleasant experiences is key to increased fulfillment.

References

Aday J, Rizer W, Carlson JM (2017) Neural mechanisms of emotions and affect. In: Emotions and affect in human factors and human-computer interaction. Elsevier, pp 27–87

Albus C, Waller C, Fritzsche K, Gunold H, Haass M, Hamann B, Kindermann I, Köllner V, Leithäuser B, Marx N (2019) Significance of psychosocial factors in cardiology: update 2018. Clin Res Cardiol 12(5):1–22

Appelhans BM, Luecken LJ (2006) Heart rate variability as an index of regulated emotional responding. Rev Gen Psychol 10(3):229–240

Bardia AB, Debra L, Prokop LJB, Brent A, Moynihan TJ (2006) Efficacy of complementary and alternative medicine therapies in relieving cancer pain: a systematic review. J Clin Oncol 24(34):5457–5464

Bilchick KC, Berger RD (2006) Heart rate variability. J Cardiovasc Electrophysiol 17(6):691–694

Boellinghaus I, Jones FW, Hutton J (2014) The role of mindfulness and loving-kindness meditation in cultivating self-compassion and other-focused concern in health care professionals. Mindfulness 5(2):129–138

Brackett MA, Rivers SE, Salovey P (2011) Emotional intelligence: implications for personal, social, academic, and workplace success. Soc Pers Psychol Compass 5(1):88–103

Celesia GG (2012) Alcmaeon of Croton's observations on health, brain, mind, and soul. J Hist Neurosci 21 (4):409–426

Chambers R, Gullone E, Allen NB (2009) Mindful emotion regulation: an integrative review. Clin Psychol Rev 29(6):560–572

Childre DL (1998) Freeze-frame: one minute stress management: a scientifically proven technique for clear decision making and improved health. HeartMath

Childre D, Rozman D (2002) Overcoming emotional chaos: eliminate anxiety, lift depression, and create security in your life. HeartMath

Childre DL, Martin H, Beech D (1999) The heartmath solution: proven techniques for developing emotional intelligence. Piatkus

Ciarrochi JE, Forgas J, Mayer JD (2006) Emotional intelligence in everyday life. Psychology Press/Erlbaum (UK) Taylor & Francis

Crivellato E, Ribatti D (2007) Soul, mind, brain: greek philosophy and the birth of neuroscience. Brain Res Bull 71(4):327–336

De Carlos JA, Borrell J (2007) A historical reflection of the contributions of cajal and golgi to the foundations of neuroscience. Brain Res Rev 55(1):8–16

Donaldson W (2017) In Praise of the "Ologies": a discussion of and framework for using soft skills to sense and influence emergent behaviors in sociotechnical systems. Syst Eng 20(5):467–478

Edwards SD (2015) Heartmath: a positive psychology paradigm for promoting psychophysiological and global coherence. J Psychol Afr 25(4):367–374

Einstein A (2019) The albert einstein collection volume two: essays in science, letters to Solovine, and letters on wave mechanics. Open Road Media

Gerbarg PL, Gootjes L, Brown RP (2014) Mind-body practices and the neuro-psychology of wellbeing. In: Religion and spirituality across cultures. Springer, pp 227–246

Gregoric P (2007) Aristotle on the common sense. Oxford University Press

Grewal D, Salovey P (2005) Feeling smart: the science of emotional intelligence: a new idea in psychology has matured and shows promise of explaining how attending to emotions can help us in everyday life. Am Sci 93(4):330–339

Handler SS, Hallis BJ, Tillman KA, Krolikowski M, Kuhn EM, Kirkpatrick EC, Brosig CL (2019) Assessment of quality of life in pediatric patients with pulmonary hypertension. Pulm Circ 9(3):2045894018822985

Hankinson RJ (1991) Galen's Anatomy of the soul. Phronesis 36(2):197–233

Holzman RS (2015) The history of sedation. In: Pediatric sedation outside of the operating room. Springer, pp 3–15

Isasi CR, Ostrovsky NW, Wills TA (2013) The association of emotion regulation with lifestyle behaviors in inner-city adolescents. Eat Behav 14(4):518–521

Ismail WW, Hanif M, Mohamed S, Hamzah N, Rizman ZI (2016) Human emotion detection via brain waves study by using electroencephalogram (Eeg). Int J Advan Sci, Eng Inform Technol 6(6):1005–1011

Jawer MA (2009) The spiritual anatomy of emotion: how feelings link the brain, the body, and the sixth sense. Simon and Schuster, pp 653–656

Karageorgou A, Kokaridas D, Theodorakis Y, Mousiolis S, Patsiaouras A, Goudas M (2018) Comparative study of individuals with and without multiple sclerosis: overall profile of quality of life, exercise, health behaviors. Int J Sports Sci Phys Educ 3:55–61

Keene MR, Heslop IM, Sabesan SS, Glass BD (2019) Complementary and alternative medicine use in cancer: a systematic review. Complement Ther Clin Pract 35:33–47

Koh KB (2018) Stress, emotion, and immunity. In: Stress and somatic symptoms. Springer, pp 43–54

Koithan M (2009) Introducing complementary and alternative therapies. J Nurse Pract 5(1):18–20

Konstan D (2006) The concept of" emotion" from Plato to Cicero. Méthexis 19:139–151

LeDoux J (1998) The emotional brain: the mysterious underpinnings of emotional life. Simon and Schuster

Martinez K, Frazer SF, Dempster M, Hamill A, Fleming H, McCorry NK (2018) Psychological factors associated with diabetes self-management among adolescents with type 1 diabetes: a systematic review. J Health Psychol 23(13):1749–1765

Massaro S, Pecchia L (2019) Heart Rate Variability (Hrv) analysis: a methodology for organizational neuroscience. Organ Res Methods 22(1):354–393

McCoy MA, Theeke LA (2019) Systematic review of quantitative studies of the relationships among psychosocial factors and coping in adult men and women with type 2 diabetes mellitus. Int J Nurs Sci 6:468–477

McCraty R (2017) New frontiers in heart rate variability and social coherence research: techniques, technologies, and implications for improving group dynamics and outcomes. Frontiers Public Health 5:267

McCraty R, Atkinson M (2006) Psychophysiological coherence. Harwood Academic Publishers, Emotional Sovereignty Amsterdam forthcoming

McCraty R, Childre D (2002) The appreciative heart: the psychophysiology of appreciation. The psychology of positive emotions and optimal functioning. pp 1–21

McCraty R, Shaffer F (2015) Heart rate variability: new perspectives on physiological mechanisms, assessment of self-regulatory capacity, and health risk. Global Adv Health Med 4(1):46–61

McCraty R, Atkinson M, Tomasino D (2001) Science of the heart: exploring the role of the heart in human performance. HeartMath Research Center, Institute of HeartMath, Publication, Boulder Creek, CA

McCraty R, Atkinson M, Tomasino D, Bradley RT (2009) The coherent heart heart-brain interactions, psychophysiological coherence, and the emergence of system-wide order. Integr Rev: Transdisciplinary Transcult J New Thought, Res, Praxis 5(2)

Meknatkhah S, Sharif Dashti P, Mousavi MS, Zeynali A, Ahmadian S, Karima S, Saboury AA, Riazi GH (2018) Psychological stress effects on myelin degradation in the cuprizone-induced model of demyelination. Neuropathology 39(1):14–21

Mosaddegh M, Shariatpanahi N, Minaee MB, Ahmadian-Attari MM (2013) Avicenna's view on heart and emotions interaction. Int J Cardiol 162(3):256–257

Moser M, Fruhwirth M, Kenner T (2008) The Symphony of Life. IEEE Eng Med Biol Mag 27(1):29

Mousavi M-S, Riazi G, Imani A, Meknatkhah S, Fakhraei N, Pooyan S, Tofigh N (2018) Comparative evaluation of adolescent repeated psychological or physical stress effects on adult cognitive performance,

Oxidative stress, and heart rate in female rats. Stress pp 1–10

Mousavi M-S, Imani A, Meknatkhah S, Riazi G (2019) Correlation between adolescent chronic emotional stress and incidence of adult cardiovascular disease in female rats. Iran J Basic Med Sci 22(10):1179–1185

Murugappan M, Ramachandran N, Sazali Y (2010) Classification of Human Emotion from Eeg Using Discrete Wavelet Transform. Journal of Biomedical Science and Engineering 3(04):390

Pearsall P, Schwartz GE, Russek LG (2000) Changes in heart transplant recipients that parallel the personalities of their donors. Integr Med 2(2–3):65–72

Pocnet C, Dupuis M, Congard A, Jopp D (2017) Personality and its links to quality of life: mediating effects of emotion regulation and self-efficacy beliefs. Motiv Emot 41(2):196–208

Robinson DL (2008) Brain function, emotional experience and personality. Neth J Psychol 64(4):152–168

Shaffer F, McCraty R, Zerr CL (2014) A healthy heart is not a metronome: an integrative review of the heart's anatomy and heart rate variability. Frontiers in Psychology 5:1040

Smith J (2016) Nature contact, health, and the built environment. In: Sowing seeds in the city. Springer, pp 101–105

Taheri MA, Bayyazi A (2013) Definition of psymentology, an Iranian complementary and alternative medicine. Procedia-Social Behav Sci 84:1534–1549

Taheri MA, Biriya A (2013) Definition of 'Psyche', psychological or emotional body as approached by psymentology. Procedia-Social Behav Sci 84:1651–1659

Taheri MA, Rahimi G (2014) Absence of knowledge, understanding, and perception of worldly love as approached by halqeh mysticism. Procedia-Social Behav Sci 114:181–185

Tieleman T (2002) Galen on the seat of the intellect: anatomical experiment and philosophical tradition. Science and mathematics in ancient greek culture. pp 256–273

Tiller WA, McCraty R, Atkinson M (1996) Cardiac coherence: a new, noninvasive measure of autonomic nervous system order. Altern Ther Health Med 2(1):52–65

Travis F (2001) Autonomic and eeg patterns distinguish transcending from other experiences during transcendental meditation practice. Int J Psychophysiol 42(1):1–9

Tugade MM, Fredrickson BL (2007) Regulation of positive emotions: emotion regulation strategies that promote resilience. J Happiness Stud 8(3):311–333

Turner J, Kelly B (2000) Emotional dimensions of chronic disease. West J Med 172(2):124

Van Goozen SH, Matthys W, Cohen-Kettenis PT, Buitelaar JK, Van Engeland H (2000) Hypothalamic-Pituitary-Adrenal Axis and Autonomic Nervous System Activity in Disruptive Children and Matched Controls. J Am Acad Child Adolesc Psychiatry 39(11):1438–1445

Van Lang ND, Tulen JH, Kallen VL, Rosbergen B, Dieleman G, Ferdinand RF (2007) Autonomic Reactivity in Clinically Referred Children Attention-Deficit/Hyperactivity Disorder Versus Anxiety Disorder. Eur Child Adolesc Psychiatry 16(2):71–78

Varela F, Lachaux J-P, Rodriguez E, Martinerie J (2001) The brainweb: phase synchronization and large-scale integration. Nat Rev Neurosci 2(4):229–239

Ward LM (2003) Synchronous neural oscillations and cognitive processes. Trends Cogn Sci 7(12):553–559

Yousofpour M, Kamalinejad M, Esfahani MM, Shams J, Tehrani HH, Bahrami M (2015) Role of heart and its diseases in the etiology of depression according to avicenna's point of view and its comparison with views of classic medicine. Int J Prev Med 6:49–49

Zhao M, Adib F, Katabi D (2016) Emotion recognition using wireless signals. In: Proceedings of the 22nd annual international conference on mobile computing and networking. pp 95–108

Good Sleep as an Important Pillar for a Healthy Life

Faezeh Moosavi-Movahedi and Reza Yousefi

Abstract

Good quality sleep, which is important for health, is influenced by various chemical compounds such as melatonin and adenosine produced and released in the body in a 24-h cycle. The production of melatonin, which is made of tryptophan in the pineal gland, increases in the evening with the onset of darkness, which tells us that it is time to go to bed. Unlike melatonin, adenosine is produced during the day, and with the beginning of darkness, its amount in the body reaches its maximum, playing an essential role in sleep-inducing sleep. The secretion of chemical sleep stimulants, especially melatonin, is also affected by hormones such as norepinephrine and cortisol. These two hormones, which also play a role in restlessness, anxiety and stress, suppressing production of melatonin in the body and deprive a person of good quality sleep. The secretion of hormones such as prolactin and growth hormone is also dependent on sleep. Sleeping slows down the body activities and reduces body temperature, heart rate, respiration rate and energy expenditure. Sleep also plays an important role in stabilizing and improving memory, effective productivity and high concentration levels, maintaining hormonal balance, regulating temperature and heart rate, removing metabolic wastes from the brain, strengthening the immune system, healing wounds and reducing inflammation. Adequate sleep has been also reported to enhance athlete performance and lowers blood pressure, allowing the heart and blood vessels to rest.

Keywords

Melatonin · Chemical sleep stimulants · Insomnia · Blood pressure · Diabetes

F. Moosavi-Movahedi
Institute of Biochemistry and Biophysics (IBB), University of Tehran, Tehran, Iran
e-mail: fmoosavi@ut.ac.ir

R. Yousefi (✉)
Protein Chemistry Laboratory (PCL), Department of Biology, College of Sciences, Shiraz University, Shiraz, Iran
e-mail: ryousefi@shirazu.ac.ir

1 Introduction

This chapter describes in detail how two important sleep-inducing stimuli, melatonin, and adenosine, are produced in the human body in harmony with the circadian cycle. In addition, we explain how sleep can affect the secretion of important hormones or how the secretion of certain hormones affect our night's sleep. Modern science has determined the mechanism and different stages of sleep, which are discussed in detail in this chapter.

In addition to explaining the positive impacts of good sleep on the human body, we will explain the relationship between some serious illnesses and poor sleep. At the end of this chapter, the important chemical compounds that induce sleep and their important dietary sources are introduced. We will also try to acquaint the readers of this book with the important strategies that will help to have a good night's sleep.

2 The Role of Melatonin and Adenosine in the Sleep–Wake Cycle

Research shows that our bodies release a variety of chemicals in a 24-h cycle that motivates us to perform certain activities at specific times; each of these cycles is called a 'circadian rhythm' from the Latin *circa* (about) and *dies* (day) (Foster and Kreitzman 2017). Circadian rhythms are not limited to humans but are also found in plants, animals, fungi, and even in prokaryotes (Dunlap and Loros 2017). This biological clock not only helps the organisms to adjust their daily activities like sleep/wake routines but also the seasonal cycles. Most species experience seasonal changes in physiology and behavior, including reproductive cycle, pelage, migration, appetite, body weight, and fat, etc., all these are controlled by circadian rhythm, a phenomenon that adapts the body timing to the outside world (Foster and Kreitzman 2017; Cardinali and Pévet 1998).

In humans, circadian rhythms are known for our sleep–wake routine. External environmental factors, more potently the light, is translated to the cyclic release of some chemicals and hormones in the body. One of the most important chemicals involved in this process is a hormone called melatonin (N-acetyl-5-methoxytryptamine) (Cardinali and Pévet 1998; Brown 1994). This hormone induces sleep, and its amount in the body increases during the evening and with the onset of darkness, thus informing us that it is time to go to bed. The level of this hormone peaks in the middle of the night and then decreases until the morning, which allows us to wake up (Wahl et al. 2019).

To maintain a 24-h sleep schedule, our body translates information about the time of day into melatonin production. This process begins in the retina, and when the retina is exposed to light. The retinal ganglion cells (RGCs) are a kind of photoreceptor that transmits signals directly to the brain. Some of these RGCs express melanopsin (Gooley et al. 2001), a photosensitive pigment with a spectral peak around 480 nm (Bailes and Lucas 2013). This type of RGCs is called 'intrinsically photosensitive retinal ganglion cells' (ipRGCs), which are particularly sensitive to the blue light. The ipRGCs, which are count for around 1% of the total RGCs (Berson 2003), among others process, transmit signals to an area of the brain called the supra chiasmatic nucleus (SCN), the so-called circadian clock of the brain which plays a vital role in creating a sense of sleep or wakefulness (Wahl et al. 2019; Blume et al. 2019). The signals then travel from the brain to the spinal cord and then to the pineal gland. The pineal gland is a small conical organ similar to the pinecone-shaped organ in the brain where melatonin production occurs (Borjigin et al. 1999). Previous studies suggested that the removal of this gland abolishes the ability to respond to the day length changes (Cardinali and Pévet 1998). Once synthesized, melatonin a hydrophobic molecule, is not storing in the producing cells and is simply and quickly diffusing across cell layers; thus, the concentration of melatonin in the pineal is a direct reflection of both its production and its engagement in the plasma (Cardinali and Pévet 1998; Reiter 1991; Peuhkuri et al. 2012a). Also, melatonin concentration can be measured in some other body fluids such as saliva and urine. The melatonin is mostly deactivated by the liver and excreted in urine as 6-sulphatoxymelatonin (6-SMT); its urinary concentration reflects the plasma melatonin profile (Peuhkuri et al. 2012a).

How is melatonin synthesized? The precursor of melatonin in the body is the amino acid tryptophan, which is absorbed through the bloodstream into the pineal gland. The synthesis of melatonin from this amino acid occurs by a four-step biochemical pathway (Fig. 1). At the beginning of this pathway, tryptophan is converted to 5-hydroxytryptophan by the enzyme tryptophan hydroxylase, which is then converted to serotonin by a decarboxylase enzyme. In the third stage, serotonin is converted to N-acetyl serotonin by the enzyme serotonin N-acetyltransferase (SNAT) [also named as arylalkylamine *N*-acetyltransferase (AANAT)]. In the final stage, N-acetyl serotonin is converted to the hypnotic hormone melatonin by the action of hydroxyindole-O-methyl transferase (HIOMT) enzyme (Cardinali and Pévet 1998; Reiter 1991; Claustrat et al. 2005; Pandi-Perumal et al. 2006).

By starting the day at sunrise and the gradual increase of blue light, the production of melatonin in the pineal gland gradually decreases until noon when it is completely cut off. At dusk, as blue light decreases, melatonin synthesis begins to peak until midnight (2–4 a.m.). In other words, exposure to light prevents the release of melatonin, which leads to awakening, and a lack of exposure to light releases melatonin, which tells us to sleep (Wahl et al. 2019). From the biochemical point of view, the regulation of SNAT occurs in such a way that this enzyme is most active at dark, and its activity is critical in the synthesis of melatonin as a regulatory step (Cardinali and Pévet 1998). Research shows that this enzyme is phosphorylated and activated at night, and the phosphorylation process prevents its degradation. Thus, phosphorylation of this enzyme in the dark increases the production of melatonin in the brain, and in the morning, when we are exposed to sunlight, by dephosphorylation and destruction of the enzyme, the amount of melatonin decreases, which helps to wake up and start daily activities (Szewczuk et al. 2008).

As mentioned, one of the most critical chemicals in the production of melatonin is serotonin. Serotonin is one of the essential brain chemicals or neurotransmitters that is essential for regulating the sleep–wake cycle and many physical and mental disorders (Morin 1999). It has been shown that there are four strategies to elevate brain serotonin. First, self-induced changes in mood have a significant influence on the synthesis of serotonin; in other words, mood produces serotonin, and serotonin is the builder of the mood (Lambert et al. 2002). The second strategy is to be exposed to bright light; there is a direct relationship between the amount of serotonin production in the brain and the time duration exposing to the

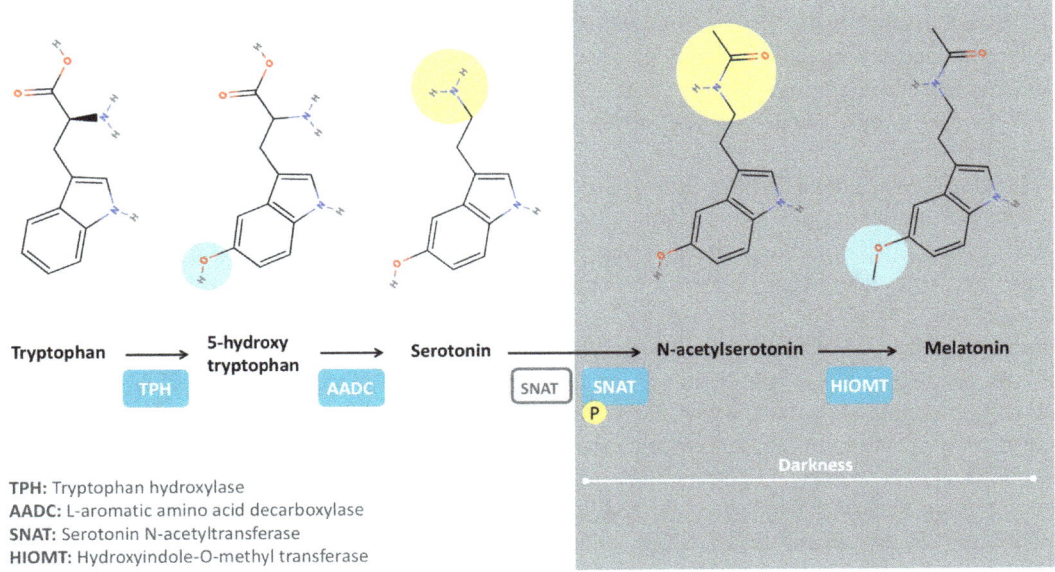

Fig. 1 Biochemical pathway of melatonin synthesis in pineal gland

sunlight and light luminosity (Lambert et al. 2002; Young 2007). The third and fourth ways to raise brain serotonin are exercise (Daniele et al. 2017) and diet. Tryptophan is a precursor to producing serotonin, and so diets rich in tryptophan can maintain healthy serotonin levels (Peuhkuri et al. 2012a; Zimmermann et al. 1993), but choosing a different lifestyle such as regular travel and irregular sleep patterns can disrupt its production (Ursin 2002). When the level of this critical compound is not normal, sleep disorders and other problems can lead to depression (Cowen and Browning 2015), aggression (Olivier 2004), insomnia (Ursin 2002), poor memory and learning (Meneses and Liy-Salmeron 2012; Meneses 2015), chronic fatigue syndrome (The et al. 2014) and poor appetite (Blundell and Halford 1998).

In addition to inducing sleep, melatonin is also involved in regulating blood pressure (Pechanova et al. 2014). If a person is in a shelter with constant light and dark conditions, he experiences a period of slightly more than 24 h, a rhythmic increase, and a decrease of body temperature and melatonin. Scientists refer to such conditions as the free-running of the circadian rhythm. Under normal conditions, light signals regularly set this period downwards, corresponding to the exact 24 h of a day on Earth (Schwartz and Roth 2009). The circadian clock has a continuous effect on the body and causes sinusoidal fluctuations in body temperature between approximately 36.2 °C and 37.2 °C (Dijk and Edgar 1999; Czeisler and Wright 1999).

In adolescents, unlike children and adults, the melatonin production time has a shift and starts later (around 10 p.m.) and in the morning continues and ends later. This phenomenon causes teenagers to sleep later and wake up in the morning harder. When teens wake up early, the enzyme acetyltransferase is still active, and they are still producing melatonin, which makes them feel drowsy in the morning. Adolescents generally need 8–10 h of sleep a night but often have a lack of sleep because of late bedtime and early school start in the morning. Therefore, adolescents usually do not get enough sleep at night, and the constant feeling of drowsiness negatively affects their ability to learn and concentrate. Research shows that raising awareness, reducing depression, and reducing the number of car-related accidents in adolescents who get enough sleep. A healthy young adult who is exposed to sunlight most of the year sleeps a few hours after sunset and experiences a minimum body temperature of 6 a.m. and wakes up shortly after sunrise (Hagenauer et al. 2009; Carskadon 2011; Kelley et al. 2015).

Exposure to artificial light at night, including TV, computers, and cell phones, lowers the amount of sleep-stimulating hormone in the brain. Artificial light, like natural light, inhibits melatonin synthesis in the pineal gland while degrading the enzyme acetylase, making the natural sleep process difficult. Exposure to even low light during the night can suppress melatonin secretion and increase body temperature and wakefulness (Kubiszewski et al. 2014; Cajochen et al. 2011; Gooley et al. 2011). Blue light, in particular, has the most significant impact, and this phenomenon has led to concerns about the use of electronic media before bedtime, which may play a significant role in sleep disorders (Benke and Benke 2013; Ja and Tapia-Ayuga 2020). Modern humans often separate themselves from their internal circadian clock due to work requirements (especially work shifts), long journeys, and the effect of indoor lighting. More sleep at the end of the week also damages the natural sleep process. If you do not get enough sleep during the week, your body will be encouraged to stay in bed for longer hours on weekend mornings to make up for your lack of sleep. It is essential to have a regular sleep schedule throughout the week and not make up for the lack of sleep at weekends, because sleeping too much on the weekends can confuse the body's biological clock and make it more challenging to wake up on weekdays (Machado et al. 1998; Kang and Chen 2009).

Melatonin is not the only chemical that determines our sleep patterns. The nucleoside compound adenosine, as a neuromodulator and a neuroprotector, plays a vital role in inducing sleep by slowing down the activity of neurons (Basheer et al. 2004) and also plays an important role as a painkiller, vasodilator, and heart rhythm regulator (Mustafa et al. 2009). Adenosine is gradually produced due to metabolic processes in the body during wakefulness so that its amount reaches its maximum at the end of the day and accumulates extracellularly in areas of the brain responsible for promoting arousal, especially the reticular activating system (Basheer et al. 2004; Lin et al. 2011). Adenosine triphosphate (ATP) depletion, along with an increase in the extracellular level of adenosine, represent a state of energy deficiency which associate with sleep. Our neurons are equipped with adenosine receptors, and when adenosine binds to these receptors, the activity of nerve cells is suppressed, causing a feeling of drowsiness. Then, when we sleep, the adenosine molecules break down, so this cycle can be resumed (Porkka-Heiskanen and Kalinchuk 2011; Huang et al. 2014; Lazarus et al. 2019).

Caffeine, which is abundant in tea and coffee, has a very similar cyclic structure with adenosine (Fig. 2). This structural similarity causes caffeine to bind the cellular adenosine receptors and counteract the effects of this nucleoside compound by serving as an antagonist, which consequently inhibits the ability of adenosine to induce sleep. The final consequence of body level elevation of caffeine is the increase of wakefulness and alertness (Fredholm et al. 1999). Caffeine also increases the level of catabolic signal cyclic AMP (cAMP) by inhibiting the enzyme phosphodiesterase. The increase of cAMP facilitates the digestion of the body's glycogen and lipid stores and raises the level of consciousness as the body stores energy releases (Burg et al. 1975; Vanderveen et al. 2001). Low levels of caffeine temporarily increase alertness, improve memory, improve mental function, fibrinolysis, and reduce fatigue. Still, high levels cause negative side effects such as insomnia, tremors, nausea, chest pain, and palpitations. Research shows that young people are particularly prone to excessive caffeine consumption and its negative side effects (Rivera-Oliver and Díaz-Ríos 2014; McLellan et al. 2016; Fredholm et al. 2017).

3 The Role of Other Hormones in the Sleep–Wake Cycle

Because sleep disorders can have detrimental effects on health and quality of life, many medications have been developed to treat these problems.

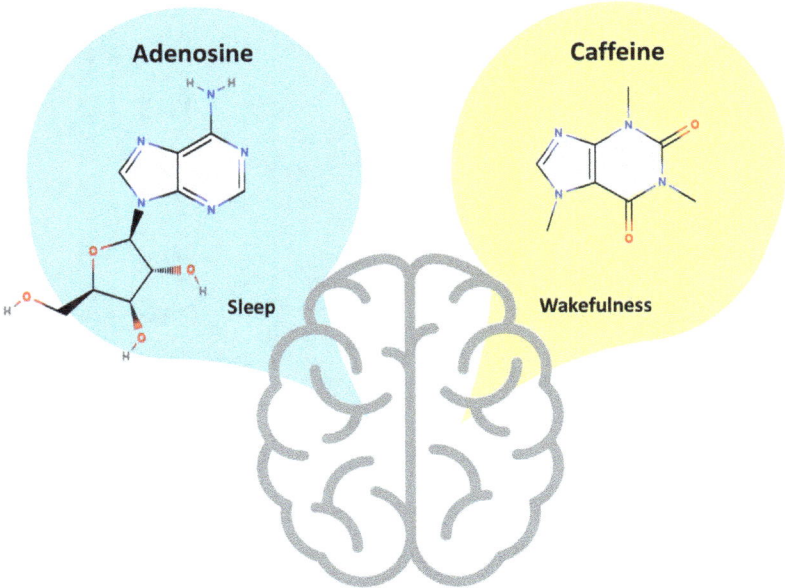

Fig. 2 Chemical structure of melatonin and adenosine as two sleep-inducer agents

3.1 Norepinephrine

Norepinephrine is one of the primary neurotransmitters involved in arousal stimulation and interferes with the function of many of these drugs (Berridge 2008; España et al. 2016). It also has an inhibitory effect on the synthesis of melatonin (a sleep-stimulating hormone) (Simonneaux and Ribelayga 2003). The secretion of norepinephrine is lowest during sleep and increases when awake, and is much higher in times of stress or danger (Marriott 1994; Mitchell and Weinshenker 2010; Liu et al. 2019). In the brain, norepinephrine stimulates arousal and alertness and enhances memory formation and recovery. This compound also relates to restlessness, depression, and anxiety (Fig. 3) (Stegeren 2008; Joëls et al. 2011).

3.2 Cortisol

Another hormone that interferes with the sleep–wake process is cortisol, which is from the glucocorticoids group and secreted by the adrenal cortex (Fink 2000) (Fig. 3). This hormone prepares the body multi-directionally for physical and mental coordination with stress. It has a central role in carbohydrate, lipid, and protein metabolism. Also, this hormone involves in the regulation of water and electrolytes balance. Cortisol regulates energy levels, blood pressure, body temperature, and appetite. It also suppresses inflammation and acts on mood and behavior (Christiansen et al. 2007; Buckingham 2009; Perogamvros et al. 2012; Stachowicz and Lebiedzińska 2016). Thus abnormal levels of this hormone, which correlate with chronic stress for

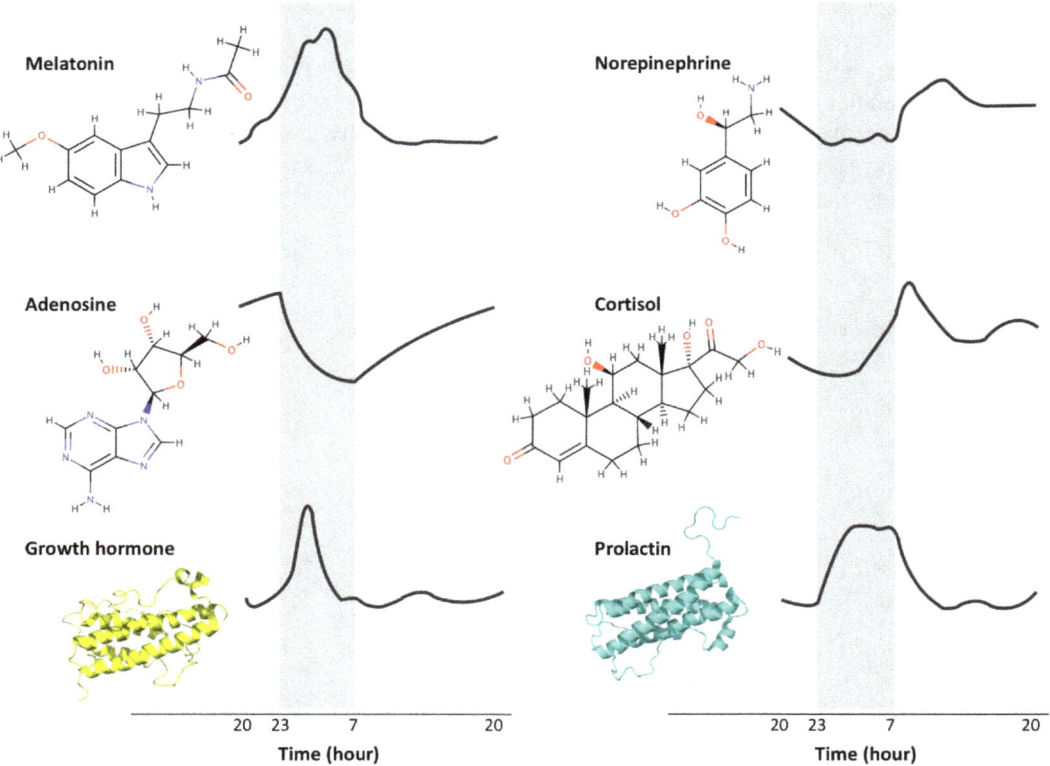

Fig. 3 Important hormones and chemicals whose production are depending on the sleep–wake cycle

a long time, are relating to various medical problems such as high blood pressure, diabetes, heart disease, digestive issues, mood disorders (depression and anxiety), and trouble sleeping (McEwen 2008).

Research shows that in addition to melatonin and norepinephrine, cortisol also plays a vital role in regulating sleep and wakefulness. Cortisol levels rise gradually about 2–3 h after the onset of sleep until the time of awaking. Also, immediately at the post-awakening time, cortisol reveals a significantly steep increase for 30–45 min, which is called cortisol awakening response (CAR) that relates to the transition from sleep to waking. After reaching the peak, the plasma cortisol concentration begins to decline with the continuation of the day, with the minimum of its plasma levels occurring around bedtime (Weitzman et al. 1974; Wilhelm et al. 2007; Dijk et al. 2012; Elder et al. 2014). This hormone plays an important role in sleep and wakefulness, and its abnormal levels, specially CAR fluctuations, have a significant effect on sleep disorders (Elder et al. 2014). An important question is whether high cortisol levels cause sleep disorders or is high cortisol the result of sleep disorders? The answer is a bit complicated, but it is probably a two-way street. High cortisol levels often present with insomnia, but it is not yet clear whether cortisol increase is the cause or result of insomnia. It is also quite possible that depending on the individual's condition; cortisol can be both cause and effect (Elder et al. 2014; Roth et al. 2007).

3.3 Prolactin

Prolactin (PRL) is a growth factor secreted by the pituitary gland that affects sleep (Fig. 3). In mammals, prolactin is associated with milk production, but it also acts as an essential regulator of the immune system, angiogenesis and osmotic balance (McEwen 2008). This hormone acts as a factor for cell growth, differentiation, and has an anti-apoptotic role in the cell cycle (Ben-Jonathan et al. 2002). In general, circadian prolactin secretion begins in the late afternoon and is subsequently enhanced by sleep, then peaks during rapid eye movement (REM) sleep, and this continues to the early morning (Roky et al. 1995; Lange et al. 2010).

3.4 Growth Hormone

The growth hormone (GH) is another important factor that has an important role in sleep (Fig. 3). The secretion of this hormone is highly sleep-dependent. The previous study also did not identify a significant difference between the level of growth hormone in day-sleepers and night-sleepers, but the hormone secretion in these two groups is associated with an acute shift that depends on sleep time (Weibel et al. 1997). Anyway, scientists estimate that the most significant secretion of human growth hormone is released during sleep, also the sleep quality affects the amount of growth hormone secretion (Kerkhofs et al. 1993). The growth hormone enters the bloodstream through the brain during sleep, and its release is part of the restorative function of sleep (Scacchi et al. 1999). This hormone is a complex protein produced by the pituitary gland in the brain (Harvey and Hull 1997) and in addition to boosting growth in childhood, it helps maintain healthy body tissue even in adulthood. The human growth hormone boosts healthy metabolism and bodily function and may even increase longevity (Frazer et al. 1982; Shalet et al. 1998).

Growth hormone production peaks at a young age and steadily decreases with age. Older adults in particular, spend less time in deep sleep, which explains the link between growth hormone deficiency and other aging-related disorders (Weibel et al. 1997; Cauter and Plat 1996). For example, lower growth hormone levels are associated with a higher risk of heart disease, obesity, and diabetes (Scacchi et al. 1999; Rosen et al. 1993; Attanasio et al. 2011; Cannavò et al. 2011). Elite athletes sometimes use growth hormone supplements (such as a recombinant form called somatropin) to improve performance (Scacchi et al. 1999). However, the association between growth hormone and adequate sleep and increased athletic performance is evident.

In fact, sleep itself is very important for athletic performance, and numerous studies have shown that increasing sleep time (up to 10 h) increases reaction time and speed in many sports. Smart coaches and world-class athletes understand the importance of regular sleep for optimal athlete performance. Sleep enables the body to produce hormones necessary for the growth and development of children and maintaining health in adults. These hormones help the body build muscle, fight disease, and repair damaged parts (Fullagar et al. 2015; Thun et al. 2015; Simpson et al. 2017).

The metabolic stage of sleep is anabolic, and anabolic hormones such as growth hormone (as mentioned above) are preferably secreted during sleep (Simpson et al. 2017). If in some organisms, the secretion of melatonin depends on sleep, in humans, its secretion is independent of sleep and depends only on the amount of light. In contrast, other hormones such as growth hormone (GH) and prolactin are so dependent on sleep that they are severely suppressed in the absence of sleep. Likewise, cortisol and thyroid-stimulating hormone (TSH) stimulants are circadian and diurnal hormones, most of which are independent of sleep (Davidson et al. 1991; Morris et al. 2012; Ikegami et al. 2019).

4 Different Stages of Sleep from the Perspective of Modern Science

Traditionally, sleep has been studied as part of psychology and medicine, but the study of sleep from a neuroscience perspective has emerged with advances in technology and the expansion of neuroscience research since the second half of the twentieth century (Bentivoglio and Grassi-Zucconi 1997). The development of improved polysomnographic techniques using fix electrodes to analyze the electrophysiological activity of the brain by electroencephalography (EEG), and also muscles by electromyogram (EMG), heart by electrocardiogram (ECG), and eye by electrooculography (EOG) as a complementary, led scientists to recognize and categorize the stages of sleep. EEG recordings do not provide accurate information about the brain different regions activity, so the rise of neuroimaging methods such as positron emission tomography (PET) and functional magnetic resonance tomography (fMRI), combined with high computing power, has led to a greater understanding of the sleep micro- and macro neural processes (Turner and Jones 2003; Dresler et al. 2014).

Sleep is a dynamic process that involves the continued activity of the brain in the production and release of hormones and proteins necessary for the body to regulate, grow and repair tissue. Rapid eye movement sleep (REM), non-rapid eye movement sleep (NREM,) and wakefulness represent the three main states of consciousness, neural activity, and physiological regulation. NREM sleep, which accounts for 70–85% of sleep time, is divided into three stages N1, N2, and N3 (previously known as stages 1–4). Each sleep cycle, which begins with the NREM stages and deepens into the REM, usually shown as N1 → N2 → N3 → N2 → REM; the cycle repeats every 90–120 min (Fig. 4). A normal night consists of six cycles, If the whole path of the cycles is considered, the ratio of deep sleep decreases from the beginning to the end of the sleep period, while REM sleep increases along the same time (Penzel et al. 2003; McNamara et al. 2010; Rama and Zachariah 2013).

4.1 The First Stage of NREM Sleep or N1

The first stage of NREM sleep or N1 is the beginning of the sleep cycle and is a transition period between wakefulness and other sleep stages or between sleeping and arousal and comprise 3–8% of total sleep time. If you wake someone up at this stage, they may claim that they have not slept at all. At this stage, the alpha wave (8–13 Hz) characterized by wakefulness decreases, and the brain produces high amplitude theta waves (4–8 Hz). In this stage, the eye movements slow down, and the muscles relax (Rama and Zachariah 2013; Alam 2013).

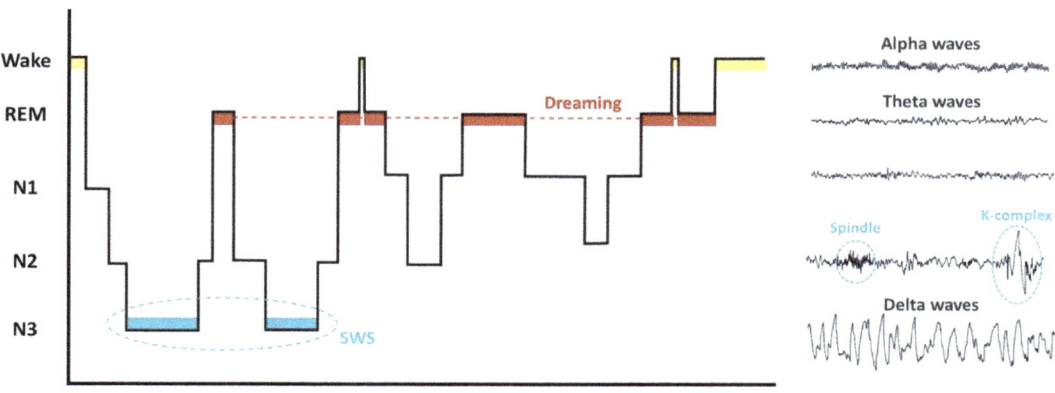

Fig. 4 Different stages of sleep

4.2 The Second Stage of NREM Sleep or N2

The second stage of NREM sleep or N2, which occupies 45–55% of sleep time, begins after 10–12 min of the N1 stage. At this stage, the brain begins to produce a series of rapid and rhythmic activities of the waves known as sleep spindles and K-complexes. Delta waves (0.5–4 Hz) first appear in the N2 stage but just in a small amount. Also, at this stage, the heart rate and respiration decrease, the muscles relax more, the eyes move become absent, and the brain activity slows down (Penzel et al. 2003; Rama and Zachariah 2013; Alam 2013).

4.3 N3 Stage of NREM Sleep or Stage 3–4

N3 stage of NREM sleep or stage 3–4, comprising 15–20% of the total sleep time, is the deepest stage of the sleep cycle. This stage is also known as the slow-wave sleep (SWS) stage. At this stage, the delta wave is predominant (20–50% in stage 3 and >50% in stage 4), the heart rate and respiration rate are minimal, and the brain activity slowly decreases, muscles relax, and blood pressure decreases. The SWS is the stage at which the body repairs itself, the immune system strengthens, and the building of muscles and bones happens. At this stage, people react less to environmental noise and activities. Also, sleepwalking occurs during deep sleep at this stage (Penzel et al. 2003; Rama and Zachariah 2013; Alam 2013).

4.4 In REM Sleep

In REM sleep, the pupils move rapidly from side to side while the eyes are closed. At this stage, which accounts for 20–25% of sleep time, the slow alpha (1–2 Hz slower than wake alpha) and theta waves are mixed. The rate of respiration and heart rate increases, blood pressure rises, and the brain becomes more active. Due to the activation of the brain, dreaming occurs mainly at this stage of sleep. REM sleep is also known as paradoxical sleep because as the brain and other body systems become more active, the arm and leg muscles become paralyzed; in other words, the body becomes sedentary. REM sleep, which is closer to waking up, increases almost with increasing sleep time and gradually in subsequent cycles (Penzel et al. 2003; Rama and Zachariah 2013; Alam 2013).

Moreover, acetylcholine, a chief neurotransmitter, plays an important role in the transition between NREM and REM sleep, and generating the brain activated states in wakefulness and REM sleep depends on cholinergic neurons. The release of acetylcholine is the highest during REM sleep and a bit lower during wakefulness, but its concentration decrease during NREM sleep and reaches the lowest during the SWS stage when theta wave is predominant (Watson et al. 2010; Yamada and Ueda 2020). Apart from its essential role in promoting REM sleep, acetylcholine is known to play an important role in learning and memory consolidation specially during SWS sleep with the lowest concentration (Gais and Born 2004; Power 2004). Overall, the stages of sleep play an important role in a number of processes, such as brain maturation, memory consolidation, learning, and brain managing and cleansing (Walker and Stickgold 2004; Rasch and Born 2013; Li et al. 2017).

5 Changing Sleep Patterns with Age and Pregnancy

It is now well established that sleep patterns change dramatically with age. Some of these changes may be social in humans (Fukuda and Ishihara 2001) but others are related to the hormonal changes (Copinschi and Caufriez 2013). These hormonal changes alter the architecture of sleep during ages, so that older people often complain of shallow and fragmented sleep during the night, unwanted daytime naps, waking up early in the morning, and feeling drowsy during the day. Researches have shown that from adulthood (16–25 years) to midlife (35–50 years), SWS duration decreases significantly, which is accompanied by an increase in the light parts of the NREM sleep (stages 1 and 2); while REM sleep and wakefulness do not change significantly. From midlife to old ages, the SWS duration does not significantly vary, but the amount of NREM and REM decreases, resulting in increased awake hours (Cauter et al. 2000; Feinberg 1974).

For example, as mentioned before, melatonin is a hormone produced by the pineal gland in response to reduced light during the night, and decreases in the early morning and before waking up. Research shows that aging is inversely related to endogenous melatonin synthesis, which it's reduction alters sleep patterns and quality, leading to changes in the sleep/wake cycle and an increase of sleep disorders (Karasek 2004). Melatonin is the opening of the sleep gate at night and sleep promoter, and its reduction is accessioned with lowered sleep efficacy and latency (Karasek 2004; Pandi-Perumal et al. 2005). Also, melatonin is an antioxidant and anti-aging agent that can slow down age-related processes. So, the reduction of this hormone is associated with the enhancement of aging disorders such as disrupted circadian rhythm, ocular degeneration, Alzheimer's and Parkinson's disease, and age-related weakening of the immune system in advanced age (Suzen 2018; Stepicheva et al. 2019). Melatonin is also a powerful cardio protectant that defends the heart against age-related cardiac pathology (Favero et al. 2017).

Growth hormone, which plays a vital role in the sleep cycle, has significant decreases with age. Between young adulthood and middle age, the secretion of this hormone rapidly decreases exponentially, but it declines at a much slower rate from the middle to the old ages. Growth hormone secretion is directly related to the SWS phase of sleep, and the age-related decrease of the hormone is in line with the reduction observed for SWS. The decline of thyroid-stimulating hormone (TSH) levels as a function of time and with ages also have an important impact on SWS sleep (Copinschi and Caufriez 2013; Cauter et al. 2000; Li et al. 2018).

Prolactin, which is secreted consistently from the beginning of sleep and its concentration enhancement, shifts the sleep to deeper stages and SWS. The nocturnal secretion of prolactin can be reduced by up to 50% in the elderly compared to young people, which is a reason for shallow and fragmented sleep (Copinschi and Caufriez 2013; Spiegel et al. 1995). Also, after the age of 50, the profile of cortisol secretion begins to change. At these ages, the evening and late evening levels of cortisol are much higher than in young people. This shortens the sleep time of these people so that the quiescent time starts later and ends sooner. This cortisol profile affects REM sleep over age. The EM reduction profile is depicted as a mirror image of increased

Table 1 The need for sleep in people of different ages

Ages		Required sleep (hours)
1	Newborn, up to three months	14 to 17
2	Infant, 4–12 months	12 to 16
3	Toddler, 1–2 years' old	11 to 14
4	Preschool, 3–5 years' old	10 to 13
5	School-age, 6–12 years	9 to 12
6	Adolescents, 13–18 years' old	8 to 10
7	Adults, 18–60 years' old	7 h or more
8	Adults, 61–64 years' old	7 to 9
9	Adults, 65 years and older	7 to 8

cortisol (Copinschi and Caufriez 2013; Cauter et al. 1996; Kern et al. 1996).

Depending on age, the need for sleep varies from person to person. For example, an older person typically needs less sleep to function correctly. Therefore, the US Centers for Disease Control and Prevention recommends the need for sleep for 24 h, depending on the age group of the people according to Table 1 (Center of disease 2017).

Some people, such as the elderly, appear to be more resistant to the effects of sleep deprivation, while young children and adults are far more vulnerable (Cauter et al. 1996). However, the amount of sleep in a person has depended on how drowsy s/he feels and how productive s/he is. For example, feeling sleepy during the day may be a sign of insufficient sleep or poor sleep. As we get older, the sleep pattern changes significantly so that the overall amount of sleep and sleep quality both decrease.

Research shows that infants do not have a fixed circadian rhythm, and the need for more sleep during the night instead of during the day occur as part of a 24-h cycle from the age of 2 or 3 months. By the age of 12 months, sleep patterns are well established, after which sleep is more fixed during the night (Cauter et al. 1996). Pregnancy also increases the need for sleep, especially in the first trimester. Pregnant women may also experience more daily drowsiness, which can continue into the first few months after delivery. These changes are thought to be due in part to the effects of increased progesterone during pregnancy. Restless legs syndrome also occurs more often during pregnancy, which can affect the quality of sleep. Therefore, to enhance sleep during pregnancy, pregnant women are advised to use a nap during the day and to sleep on the left side to improve blood flow and nutrients to the fetus (Bourjeily 2009; Izci Balserak and Lee 2017).

6 Introducing Important Sleep Disorders

We spend about a third of our lives asleep, and contrary to popular belief, the brain never not only shuts down at this time but also performs important functions. Poor sleep and insomnia have been shown to impair normal brain function greatly. Insomnia, which is defined as dissatisfaction with the quality or quantity of sleep, can be associated with difficulty initiating sleep, having trouble in maintaining the sleep, or having a problem with falling asleep again after waking in the middle of sleep time. Some predisposing factors, such as biologic, psychological, and demographic characteristics, can raise the probability of insomnia. Also, stressful life, medical condition behavioural, or cognitive changes are all can manifest themselves as insomnia. Insomnia can be short-term (maximum three weeks) or long-term (more than three to four weeks). This problem usually occurs at any age but is more common in the elderly, and it is known as an age-related disease, so that both overall sleep and sleep efficiency decrease with age (Li et al. 2018; Ohayon 2002; Patel et al. 2018). Lack of sleep has also been shown to have a detrimental effect on cognitive tasks, especially in divergent or multitasking functions, poor memory, depression, visual disturbances, decreased concentration, irritability, and increased risk of cardiovascular disease, high blood pressure, heart attacks, and strokes, obesity, emotional disorders, aggression, diabetes, and increased risk of traumatic events such as car, plane, ship, train, and nuclear power plant accidents (Colten and Altevogt 2006; Born and Wagner 2009; AlDabal 2011; Paterson et al. 2013).

6.1 Immune System

The results of scientific research show that lack of sleep has a severe negative effect on the immune system. Studies have shown that under regular sleep–wake patterns, the level of human peripheral blood mononuclear cell (PBMC) subsets consists of lymphocytes and monocytes, regulate with circadian rhythm. Also, during sleep time, the immune system produces and secretes some kind of proteins called cytokine; each has a specific role in sleep-inducing and sleep depth. Moreover, in case of infection or any stress, the immune cells release these cytokines in response to stimulation for cell signalling and inflammatory process activation. Researches have shown that sleep deprivation is directly related to the increase of these inflammatory markers, which are indicators of body stress. This happens in line with the significant increase of immune cells such as monocytes and lymphocytes, and decrease of neutrophil phagocytose ability. This means that the body experiences sleep deprivation as a stressor, which can suppress and weaken the immune system, makes it challenging to deal with infectious agents, and reduce the ability to resist infection (Lange and Mölle 1997; Taheri et al. 2004;

Besedovsky et al. 2012; Faraut et al. 2012). Infections, in turn, affect the amount and patterns of sleep. Researchers have recently shown that people who sleep less than seven hours a night on the average show almost three times more symptoms than those who sleep eight hours or more nights when exposed to cold-causing rhinoviruses. Also, those people who have better quality sleep are less likely to catch a cold (Bryant et al. 2004; Lorton et al. 2006; Imeri and Opp 2009). Research shows that poor sleep is also strongly associated with long-term inflammation of the gastrointestinal tract (Ali et al. 2013). Studies also show that depriving mice of sleep increases the growth of cancer and weakens the immune system's ability to control cancer (Chen et al. 2018) (Fig. 5).

6.2 Obesity

Short sleep duration is associated with an increased risk of weight gain and obesity in children and adults, and it is directly associated with the increased body mass index (BMI) (Watson et al. 2012). People who sleep less are more likely to be overweight than those who get enough sleep. According to the results of a scientific study, children and adults with short sleep duration were respectively 89% and 55% more likely to be obese (Cappuccio et al. (2008)). It is believed that the effect of sleep insomnia on weight gain is exerted by numerous factors such as hormones and decreased athletic motivation. Lack of sleep disrupts the daily fluctuations of appetite hormones, which weaken the regulation of the appetite system. In insomnia, higher levels of ghrelin (an appetite-stimulating hormone) and low levels of leptin (an appetite-suppressing hormone) have been seen. If you are trying to lose weight, having qualified sleep is absolutely important. People who get enough sleep also consume fewer calories than those who do not, which is important in preventing obesity (Taheri et al. 2004; Beccuti and Pannain 2011; Al Khatib et al. 2017).

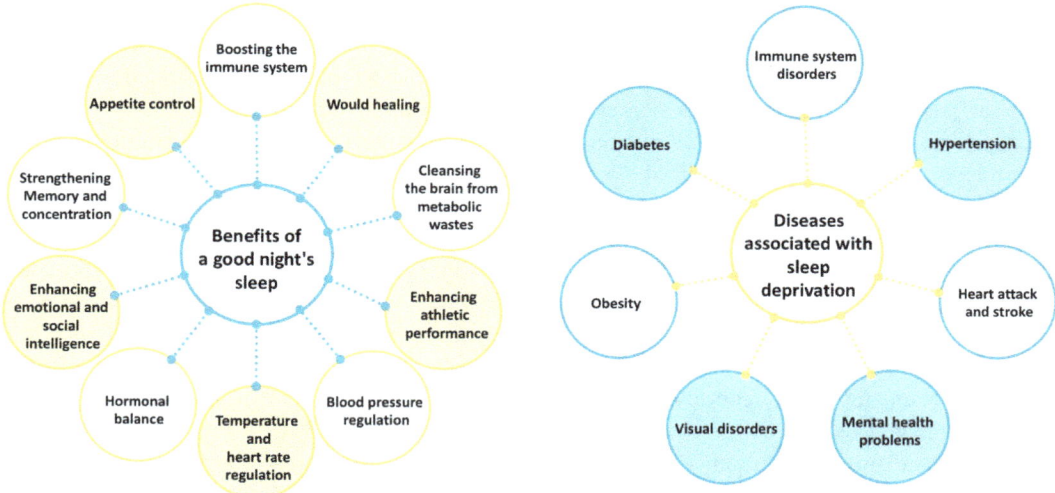

Fig. 5 Benefits of good sleep and harms of bad sleep

6.3 Cardiovascular System

Studies show that people with inadequate sleep, less than 7–8 h, have a higher risk of heart disease and stroke. Sleep deprivation and rotating night shift works can increase the risk of coronary heart disease and produces fluctuations in blood pressure, and it is one of the reasons for hypertension. Sleep time is associated with increased plasma homocysteine levels, which is associated with H-Type hypertension (Perry et al. 2007; Gangwisch 2014). Sleep deprivation is also related to elevations in heart rate and diastolic pressure (Mezick et al. 2014). Recent studies have shown that even a slight decrease in sleep is associated with an increased risk of coronary artery calcification and death from heart attacks. There is also ample evidence of an association between sleep deprivation due to airway obstruction and an increased risk of cardiovascular disease, hypertension, stroke, coronary heart disease, and irregular heartbeat (O'Donnell et al. 1994; Ahmad et al. 2007; Tobaldini et al. 2017; Liu and Chen 2019).

6.4 Diabetes

Scientific research shows that sleep duration and quality are associated with glucose metabolism and the risk of type 2 diabetes. Restricted sleep has been shown to reduce insulin sensitivity greatly, and people who sleep less than 6 h a night are at increased risk for type 2 diabetes. People who sleep less than five hours a night have recently been shown to increase their risk of developing type 2 diabetes greatly. Fortunately, studies have also shown that better sleep can improve blood sugar control and reduce the effects of type 2 diabetes (Grandner et al. 2016; Larcher et al. 2015).

6.5 Mental Health

Today, it is clear that poor sleep is associated with depression. Mental health issues such as depression are also strongly associated with poor sleep quality and sleep disorders. A recent study suggests that when you have insomnia, you are five times more likely to be depressed and more likely to have anxiety or panic disorders. Sleep duration and depression is a two-way street. However, sleep deprivation causes depression, and depression itself causes sleep deprivation. It is estimated that 90% of people with depression also complain about the quality of their sleep. Depression is associated with the decrease of SWS stage of sleep and also shortening of REM latency, but increase the total REM sleep time (Zhai et al. 2015; Riemann et al. 2020).

Insomnia also affects mood and emotions, and there have been numerous reports of increased tendency to anger, fear, or depression with sleep deprivation (Ireland and Culpin 2006; Lemola et al. 2012). Poor sleep increases even the risk of death from suicide (Porras-Segovia et al. 2019). Persistent sleep deprivation can lead to daytime sleepiness, emotional problems, mood, general health, poor job performance, and decreased perception of the quality of life. Lack of sleep at night can confuse you the next day (Paterson et al. 2013; Bonnet 1985; Scott et al. 2006). Sleep deficiency is also associated with long-term side effects on health and a higher risk of premature death. Analysis of data from three separate studies shows that sleeping five hours or less a night may increase the risk of death by up to 15 percent (Colten and Altevogt 2006). Most importantly, getting enough sleep can ultimately affect your life expectancy and well-being.

7 Important Benefits of Good Quality Sleep for Body and Health

When it comes to health, sleep is as important as regular exercise and a healthy balanced diet. Therefore, along with nutrition and exercise, good sleep is one of the pillars of health. Good and quality sleep occurs in the period of 9–10 p.m. to 5–6 a.m. and simultaneously with the circadian cycle. The brain is active during sleep, and the idea is that one of the important functions of sleep is to reorganize neural circuits or strengthen neural connections. Another potential goal of sleep is to restore the signal strength of synapses that are active when awake at the basal level. During sleep, unnecessary neural connections are weakened to facilitate the learning process better and improve memory functions. Normally, the brain forgets some of the things we learn every day, and sleep plays an important role in stabilizing and improving memory. Good sleep also dramatically increases people's productivity and concentration. What researchers have shown is that sleep is linked to several brain functions, such as better concentration, higher productivity, and improved cognition. Recent studies have also shown that children's sleep patterns can have a direct impact on their behavior and academic performance. When you are sleep deprived, you may have difficulty keeping and remembering details. The reason for this phenomenon, as mentioned above, is that sleep plays an important role in learning and memory. Without enough sleep, it is difficult to concentrate on and record new information (Born and Wagner 2009; Marshall et al. 2006; Sterpenich et al. 2009; Deak and Stickgold 2010).

Other suggested sleep functions include maintaining hormonal balance, regulating temperature, and heart rate. During sleep, metabolic wastes are cleared from the brain faster than when awake. When awake, metabolic processes produce more oxygen-rich species that damage the body's cells. During sleep, the rate of metabolism decreases, and the production of reactive oxygen species decreases significantly. Such conditions help the body significantly repairs processes. It has generally been suggested that sleep helps facilitate the synthesis of molecules that protect the brain from harmful elements produced when awake. Hormones play an important role in energy balance and metabolism, and sleep also plays a role in the timing and range of their secretions (Xie et al. 2013; Underwood 2013; Zielinski et al. 2016).

Some early theories of sleep function also predict that sleep plays a metabolic regulatory role. It has been suggested that sleep increases the number of white blood cells (the body's defense cells) and strengthens the immune system. In this regard, good sleep quality has been shown to play an important role in wound healing and reducing inflammation. Previous research has also shown that good sleep quality helps the body to better fight various infections (Besedovsky et al. 2012; Faraut et al. 2012; Krueger et al. 2011).

Research shows that people with good sleep tend to consume fewer calories. Studies also show that people with sleep deprivation have a higher appetite, which is associated with obesity and overweight. Recent studies show that sleep patterns also affect the secretion of hormones responsible for appetite control. When a person does not get enough sleep, it impairs his body's ability to regulate food intake properly, and when a person gets enough sleep, s\he feels less hungry (Taheri et al. 2004; Beccuti and Pannain 2011; Al Khatib et al. 2017).

It has also been suggested that adequate sleep can enhance a person's athletic performance. According to the National Sleep Foundation, adequate sleep for adults is between 7 and 9 h a night, but athletes may also benefit from 10 h of sleep. Accordingly, sleep is as important to athletes as calories and nutrition (Fullagar et al. 2015; Thun et al. 2015; Simpson et al. 2017).

Therefore, sleep is essential for overall heart health. Blood pressure also drops during sleep, allowing the heart and blood vessels to rest. Therefore, the shorter the sleep time, the higher the blood pressure over a 24-h cycle, and high blood pressure are associated with cardiovascular disease (Gangwisch 2014). Another important function of sleep is to influence emotions and social interactions. Sleep is also associated with emotional and social intelligence. A person who does not get enough sleep has more difficulty recognizing the feelings and expressions of others (Killgore et al. 2008).

One of the most important functions of sleep is to help cells, and tissues recover from daily wear and tear. The main restorative functions in the body, such as tissue repair, muscle growth, and protein synthesis, occur almost exclusively during sleep (Xie et al. 2013; Drummond et al. 2012). Sleep experts say there is ample evidence that when people get enough sleep, they not only feel better but also have a better chance of living a healthier and more productive life. One of the most important things the brain does during sleep is to process emotions. Your mind needs time to know and react to the right method. When sleep time is short, negative emotional reactions prevail, and fewer positive reactions are seen.

8 The Important Events Associated with Dreaming, Nightmares, and Sleepwalking

8.1 Sleep Dreaming

Some ancient civilizations saw sleep dreaming as a mediator between the terrestrial life and the gods. The Greeks and Romans believed that dreaming had a certain prophetic power. Some scientists also believe that dreaming is related to the signals that are sent to the cerebral cortex during sleep, and some of these signals are very important for memory and learning, but some are seemingly random. Your brain may try to interpret some of these signals as a coherent story and the end product of which is a dream (Wamsley and Stickgold 2011; Palagini and Rosenlicht 2011; Perogamvros et al. 2013).

Some scientists, such as Sigmund Freud, believe that dreaming is the product of repressed passions and blocked wishes, and others, such as Carl Jung, believe that dreaming has psychological significance (Boag 2017; Roesler 2020). One of the prominent theories about dreaming is known as the activation-synthesis model. This theory states that dreaming has no special meaning and that it is only the electrical pulses of the brain that bring random thoughts and images out of our memories (Boag 2017).

Since other mammals, such as cats, have sleep dreaming, evolutionary psychologists believe that dreaming serves an important purpose and interprets it as an ancient biological defense mechanism in which the brain simulates threatening events. This strengthens the neurological mechanism needed to understand threatening events. However, the results of new research also provide a compelling insight into the mechanism of dreaming and its strong relationship to memories. Research shows that dreaming often occurs in the REM sleep phase, in which the brain is more active (Franklin and Zyphur 2005).

8.2 Nightmares

Nightmares are vivid night events that can cause feelings of fear, panic, or anxiety. Usually, a person with a nightmare wakes up suddenly from REM sleep and is unable to describe its exact content, and it is difficult for him/her to go back to sleep. Nightmares can be caused by many factors, including illness, anxiety, the loss of a loved one, or negative reactions to a medication. If nightmares occur more than once a week and cause sleep deprivation and anxiety, it is necessary to treat it. As REM sleep time gradually lengthens over time, more nightmares occur in the early hours of the morning. Nightmares may frequently recur after accidents that result in injury. In general, nightmares are caused by various reasons such as stress, anxiety, irregular sleep, mental disorders, and post-traumatic stress. While nightmares are more common among children, one in two adults has nightmares on different occasions. In general, between 2 and 5% of the adult human population experience nightmares. Do your nightmares cause significant distress? Do they constantly interrupt your sleep? If so, it is important to determine what is causing the adult nightmares. You can then make changes to reduce their occurrence. Some people have nightmares after having a snack late at night, which can increase metabolism and lead to more brain activation during sleep (Nielsen et al. 2010; Sandman et al. 2013; Godin et al. 2015; Macêdo et al. 2019).

A number of medications also help regulate the frequency of nightmares in the brain. Alcohol, antidepressant medicines, and drugs are often associated with nightmares. Blood pressure medications can also sometimes cause nightmares in adults. Severe sleep deprivation can also lead to adult nightmares (Nielsen et al. 2010; Pagel and Helfter 2003; Aurora et al. 2010).

Nightmares in adults can also be caused by some sleep disorders such as sleep apnea and restless legs syndrome. People who have relatives with nightmares may also develop the disease themselves, and from this perspective, the genetic background for nightmares is also considered. In general, among people who experience nightmares, those who are anxious and depressed are more likely to experience this problem and even suffer from more psychological effects. Research shows that nightmares are also linked to suicide (Hublin et al. 1999; Schredl et al. 2006; Schredl 2009; Hasler and Germain 2009).

Because nightmares can have a significant impact on your quality of life, be sure to consult a specialist if you experience them regularly. Depending on the cause of the nightmare, there are several ways to treat or reduce the number of times facing with nightmare during the night. If the nightmare is the result of taking a certain medication, you may be able to change the dose or even the type of medication in consultation with your doctor to eliminate this unwanted side effect. In people whose nightmares are caused by conditions such as sleep apnea or restless legs syndrome, treatment for the underlying disorder may help reduce the symptoms. Even if the nightmare is not the result of illness or dependence on certain medications, there are still promising solutions to treat it.

Behavioural changes have been effective for adults with nightmares, including those caused by anxiety, depression, and post-traumatic stress disorder (PTSD) (Hasler and Germain 2009). It is also important to maintain a regular sleep schedule and regular exercise, which reduces anxiety and stress, can help treat nightmares. Yoga and meditation are also helpful in treating nightmares. People who have nightmares (sometimes as a scary dream) usually do not remember these events the next morning. Horrors of night sleep are similar to nightmares and usually occur during deep sleep. These people may pose risks to themselves and others due to the movement of the limbs. Night terrors are more common in children between the ages of 3 to 7 years old. Children with a scary dream also often talk to themselves while sleeping or sleepwalking. It has also been claimed that severe emotional stress or alcohol consumption can increase the prevalence of panic in night sleep in adults (Taylor 1993).

8.3 Sleepwalking

In the past, people believed that sleepwalking was a sign of brain disease. Now it has become clear that this phenomenon is not usually associated with serious brain and psychological problems. Sleepwalking is a behavioral disorder that occurs during sleep and leads to a series of complex behaviours that occur during sleep, the most obvious is walking. This occurring phenomenon triggered by partial arousal during SWS and usually happens in the first half of sleep. Symptoms of sleepwalking include simply sitting in the bed and looking around, walking in a room or house, and even leaving home for the relatively long distances (Malhotra and Avidan 2012; Chopra et al. 2020).

The phenomenon of sleepwalking alone does not cause any health problems, but it can indirectly lead to serious problems. Due to safety concerns, going out of the house, jumping out of windows, using lighters and kitchen knives, hitting sharp objects can cause harm to the sleepwalker. If a person wakes up in the middle of these events, they become disoriented and do not remember what happened; Some patients only remember a few images related to sleepwalking. There is also a misconception that waking up a sleepwalker may expose him or her to heart attacks, brain damage, or even death. However, waking up a sleepwalker may cause panic and be accompanied by violent attacks on the person waking up. It is recommended that you guide the sleepwalker to his/her bed without waking him/her up (Pressman 2007,2011; Zadra et al. 2013).

Sleepwalking occurs in about 5% of children and 1.5% of adults, this indicates that the disease is more common in children and 80% of adults, which involved with this disorder having a continuation of childhood behavior. It is more common between the age of 3–10 years old and is usually solved in adolescence by reduction of the amount of deep sleep and gradually improves with the onset of adolescence. Therefore, it can be concluded that the onset of sleepwalking for the first time is uncommon in adults, and, if it occurs in adulthood, there must be an external factor starting it, such as a disease or medication that was not present in childhood (Ohayon and Priest 1999; Laberge et al. 2000; Stallman and Kohler 2016). Studies show that the sleepwalking prevalence rate increase in people with sleep deprivation (Zadra et al. 2008), and also this is also true for alcoholics because alcohol increases SWS (Casez et al. 2005). It is prevalent in Parkinson's disease, migraine, and hyperthyroidism (Casez et al. 2005; Ajlouni et al. 2005; Poryazova et al. 2007).

So far, there is no specific treatment for sleepwalking, but there are many cases where the problem of sleepwalking patients has been solved by hypnosis (Hauri et al. 2007). In some cases, some sedatives or antidepressants have been shown to reduce the incidence of sleepwalkers (Kierlin and Littner 2011).

9 Medical Problems and Diseases Caused by Insomnia

Today, insomnia is one of the important complications of urban and industrial societies. The high dependence of families on social media and frequent daily visits to the public networks deprives them of the opportunity to have a good night's sleep. People who have trouble sleeping may also use roaming in these virtual networks as a way to spend time, which will greatly increase their problems (Levenson et al. 2016; Scott and Woods 2019). Sleep disturbance or drowsiness is a medical problem in human or animal sleep patterns. Currently, sleep medicine experts have identified more than 100 types of sleep disorders, most of which are characterized by excessive daytime sleepiness, difficulty sleeping or staying asleep, abnormal movements, and bizarre behaviours or feelings during sleep. In many cases, insomnia or lack of sleep has been rooted in other medical problems such as pain, infection, chronic obstructive pulmonary disease, obstructive sleep apnea, and peptic ulcer disease (Ting and

Table 2 Some important sleep disorders

Some important sleep disorders			
1	Jet lag	6	Shift work sleep disorder (SWSD)
2	Sleep apnea	7	Delayed sleep phase disorder
3	Hypopnea	8	Bruxism
4	Restless leg syndrome	9	Catathrenia
5	Narcolepsy	10	Fatal family insomnia

Malhotra 2005). Some important sleep disorders are indicated as Table 2.

Insomnia, an important medical problem, prevents a person from falling asleep continuously. In other words, difficulty sleeping, frequent awakenings during the night with inability or difficulty falling asleep again, waking up too early in the morning, and sleep that does not rejuvenate are called insomnia, which is more common in women than men. Three types of insomnia, including transient, acute, and chronic insomnia, have been identified so far (Ellis et al. 2012; Roller and Gowan 2014). Research shows that about one-third of Iranians also suffer from insomnia as the most common sleep disorder (Yazdi et al. 2012; Mousavi et al. 2012).

One of the major problems is sleep deprivation, which is known as jet lag. This condition occurs when the body's circadian rhythm changes due to long journeys (from east to west or vice versa), and consequently, the person's sleep regulation is disturbed due to the difference between the origin time and the flight destination. The most important reason for jet lag is the disruption of the body's biological clock, and during long journeys, the secretion of the hormone melatonin, which is responsible for the human biological clock, decreases, disrupting sleep and wakefulness. In aircraft, air pressure, diet, preflight stress, lack of mobility, and movement are other causes of jet lag. The consequences of jet lag during air travel to the east are much more severe than journey to the west. The reason for this phenomenon is that when traveling east, the length of the day decreases, and in general, the body's biological clock adapts to a long day better than a shortened day. Jet leg causes symptoms such as reduced concentration, neurological problems as well as issues in the stomach, and may take several days for the passenger to fully adapt to his new time zone (Samel et al. 1995; Srinivasan et al. 2010; Szaulińska et al. 2017).

Another significant sleep disorder is known as sleep apnea, which is an important sleep disorder that causes you to stop or reduce breathing for a short time during sleep. Sleep apnea can last for several seconds or even minutes with each stop of breathing, and usually, many stops occur overnight. Each of these pauses is called an apnea, which is usually accompanied by a snoring sound and sometimes accompanied by a sound and a feeling of suffocation. In such cases, the person wakes up suddenly and suffocated. Although many people with apnea do not notice shortness of breath or stop breathing overnight, these periods usually significantly reduce the quality of their sleep. As a result, despite prolonged sleep, a person with sleep apnea may feel too tired during the day, which can lead to irreversible driving accidents. Sleep apnea can lead to stroke, heart attack, type 2 diabetes, high blood pressure, obesity, poor memory, and depression if left untreated. The body temperature of people with sleep apnea rises after waking up, and sometimes their mood will change. People with sleep apnea often have depression (Lee and Douglass 2010; Carter et al. 2019; Rajagopalan 2011; Zhang et al. 2014; LaGrotte et al. 2016). In hypopnea syndrome, the patient also has slow and shallow breathing, which reduces oxygen delivery efficiently. This complication, which occurs due to a slight obstruction of the airways, is more severe than apnea.

Another important factor that leads to sleep disorders is Restless Leg Syndrome. In this case, the sufferer experiences an unpleasant sensation in the legs and describes it as a tingling, burning, pain, and stretching sensation or movement of insects on her/his skin. To reduce these sensations, S/he has to shake or pull her/his foot. In this condition, patients involuntarily have periodic leg movements for up to 60 s during sleep, which disrupts sleep. Research shows that restless legs syndrome, which is also associated with iron deficiency, is the cause of about one-third of insomnia disorders in people over 60 years of age. Another type of sleep disorder is known as narcolepsy. These patients show a sudden and irresistible urge to sleep. These patients develop muscle cramps or sleep paralysis. Adolescent boys with long sleep apnea have been found to feel hungry after waking up. This sleeping sickness is characterized by five signs of drowsiness, excessive pollution during the day, cataplexy (sleep paralysis/hypnosis), and hallucinations (hypnopompic) (Singh et al. 2016; Kim et al. 2017a; Sundaresan et al. 2019).

Shift work sleep disorder (SWSD) is a type of circadian rhythm sleep disorder that is associated with insomnia and excessive drowsiness. This complication is seen in people whose working hour overlap with the normal sleep period. It is estimated that about 20% of the population working in such shifts are employed, and it is estimated that 10–40% of night-shift workers suffer from this disorder (Burke et al. 2012).

Another important condition is delayed sleep phase syndrome (DSPS). In this case, the patient's sleep is delayed for up to two hours or more, and delayed sleep causes him not to wake up at the desired time (Rosenthal et al. 1990). For example, people with Alzheimer's and Parkinson's have had sleep disorders (Rothman and Mattson 2012). Also, sleep disorders are often associated with deteriorating cognitive function, emotional state, and quality of life. Some sleep disorders are serious enough to interfere with normal physical, mental, social, and emotional functioning. Polysomnography and actigraphy are tests that are usually ordered for some sleep disorders.

Bruxism, a sleep disorder, can damage the teeth, gums, and supporting bones. Although gnashing of teeth can be caused by stress or anxiety, it is more likely to occur during sleep and is caused by crooked teeth, missing teeth, and extra teeth. Another important sleep disorder is known as Catathrenia. A sound in sleep that, unlike snoring, occurs during exhalation is called sleep moaning. In this complication, the person usually takes a very deep breath, holds his breath for a moment, and then releases it with a long, steady, and usually high-risk groan (Castrillon et al. 2016; Melo et al. 2019). There is still no consensus among scientists as to the physical or neurological cause of sleep deprivation. Fatal family insomnia is also an infrequent genetic disorder that causes complete sleep deprivation and rapid death due to lack of sleep (Castrillon et al. 2016; Melo et al. 2019). There is no cure for the disease, during which the person progresses to insomnia, which in turn leads to hallucinations, confusion, disturbances in the level of consciousness (similar to what is seen in dementia), and eventually death.

10 Important Strategies to Cope with Insomnia Problems and to Improve Sleep Quality

A good night's sleep is essential for people's health, which occurs in harmony with the circadian rhythm cycle and the secretion of sleep-inducing hormone (melatonin). Therefore, people must have a regular sleep plan that is implemented in the same way on weekends. As mentioned earlier, good sleep occurs between 9 and 10 p.m. to 5 to 6 a.m. Decreased melatonin synthesis in older adults is associated with sleep disorders and a wide range of medical conditions. Therefore, many sleep hygiene practices may help the body regulate melatonin synthesis properly (see Table 3).

The important points that need to be followed in order to have a good night's sleep are summarized in Table 3. To have a good and quality sleep, try to spend more time outside the house with physical activity and go to bed at a particular time every night. You need to have a light dinner at the beginning of the night and drink

Table 3 Important tips that help to have a good sleep

	Important tips that help to have a good sleep		
1	Having a regular sleep schedule	7	Avoiding stressful situations before going to bed
2	Spending more time outdoors	8	Avoid smoking
3	Do not napping during the day	9	Avoid using artificial light emitting devices before going to bed
4	Eating a light dinner and drinking less fluids before bed	10	Having a quiet, dark and cool bedroom
5	Avoid drinking strong tea and coffee	11	Wearing comfortable pajamas
6	Using natural foods containing sleep-inducing substances	12	Having a regular exercise program

fewer fluids before going to bed. It is necessary to keep your bedroom quiet, dark, and cool and wear comfortable clothes while sleeping. It is important to avoid foods and beverages containing alcohol, caffeine, smoking and heavy and high-fat meals before going to bed. Also, avoid napping during the day, which reduces drowsiness (Stepanski and Wyatt 2003; Atkinson and Davenne 2007; Kay et al. 2012; Dhand and Sohal 2007; Cao et al. 2016).

Regular exercise reduces the level of anxiety and stress and helps to improve the sleep process and avoid nightmares. Yoga and meditation have also proven to be important in improving sleep quality. Do strenuous exercise during the day and relaxing exercises such as yoga before bed. Poor sleep is also associated with obesity and overweight, so it is important to gain weight by exercising and eating a healthy diet (Dolezal et al. 2017).

Try to avoid stress before bed, for example, stressful discussions that change the level of some hormones and drastically reduce the quality of sleep. Also, avoid watching TV, browsing the internet, etc. near bedtime, and never do these activities in the bed. The use of artificial light, including light emitted by televisions, telephones, and computers, inhibits melatonin synthesis and significantly delays sleep. If you cannot sleep after 20 min of effort, go to another room to reduce your connection with the inability to sleep and study in a comfortable chair until you feel sleepy. Go to sleep when you feel tired and have at least 7 h of good quality sleep (Aulsebrook et al. 2018; Christensen 2020).

Many chemicals, amino acids, enzymes, nutrients and hormones work together to enhance good sleep and regulate the sleep cycle. Some of these compounds include tryptophan, melatonin, gamma-aminobutyric acid (GABA), calcium, potassium, magnesium, pyridoxine, ornithine, serotonin, histamine, acetylcholine, folate, antioxidants, vitamin D, B vitamins, apigenin, lactocin, zinc, and copper (Fig. 6). Although many foods contain small amounts of these sleep-enhancing compounds, only a few contain high levels of them, which are potentially known to be effective sleep-inducing foods (Binks et al. 2020; St-Onge et al. 2016; Peuhkuri et al. 2012b).

Taking into account traditional knowledge and the results come out from the new scientific research, as well as dietary profiles, here are the best foods and drinks that help you sleep well. One of the most important sleep-inducing foods is almonds, which contain large amounts of melatonin. This food contains significant amounts of magnesium and calcium, which may help relax muscles and strengthen sleep (Ghafarzadeh et al. 2019). Warm milk is a common home remedy for insomnia and contains four sleep-boosting compounds such as tryptophan, calcium, vitamin D, and melatonin. The results of some studies also show the relationship between kiwi consumption and sleep. Kiwi contains many sleep-enhancing compounds such as melatonin,

Fig. 6 Foods rich in sleep-inducing compounds

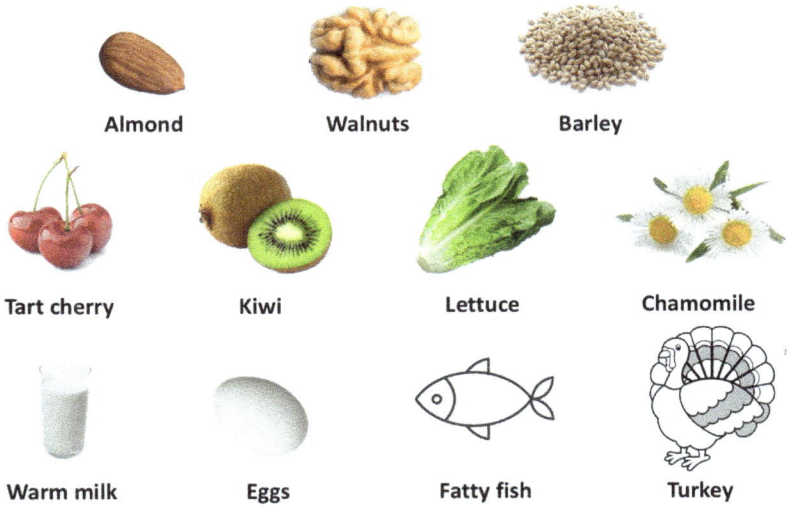

anthocyanin, flavonoids, carotenoids, potassium, magnesium, folate, and calcium (St-Onge et al. 2016). Chamomile is also a traditional herb for treating insomnia. Researchers have shown that a flavonoid compound called apigenin is responsible for the sleep-inducing properties of chamomile. This compound appears to activate GABA receptors to stimulate sleep (Marder 2012; Adib-Hajbaghery and Mousavi 2017; Salehi et al. 2019). Walnuts also contain important compounds that strengthen and regulate sleep. Fatty fish may also help improve sleep because they are a great source of vitamin D and omega-3 fatty acids. Research shows that these two nutrients help regulate serotonin, and that serotonin is mainly responsible for creating a consistent sleep–wake cycle (St-Onge et al. 2016; Zeng et al. 2014).

Turkey, tart cherry, and eggs are also high in melatonin and help to induce sleep. Barley sprout powder is also rich in several sleep-boosting compounds, including GABA, calcium, tryptophan, zinc, potassium and magnesium. The results of scientific research show that barley grass powder may induce sleep. Lettuce may also help treat insomnia and induce good sleep. Researchers have suggested that lettuce has a mild sedative-hypnotic effect, possibly due to a compound called lactocin (Fig. 7). (St-Onge et al. 2016; Zeng et al. 2014; Kim et al. 2017b; Doherty et al. 2019).

Many foods contain nutrients, chemicals, and other compounds that help control the body's sleep cycle. Preliminary studies show that different types of nuts, fruits, and seafood may improve sleep. Hence, people have been using other foods and beverages for decades to treat insomnia and improve sleep. To get the potential benefits of some hypnotic foods, it has been suggested to be eaten a few hours before bedtime to avoid the potential risk of indigestion and gastric acid reflux.

11 Conclusion

Good sleep along with proper and healthy nutrition and continuous exercise are the three sides of a triangle that ensures the health and well performance of individuals in community. Having a good sleep is affected by both environmental (external) and body endogenous factors. Light pollution in the modern industrial societies, and physical and mental illnesses may severely affect sleep quality. It is essential that citizens are properly educated about sleep hygiene and the

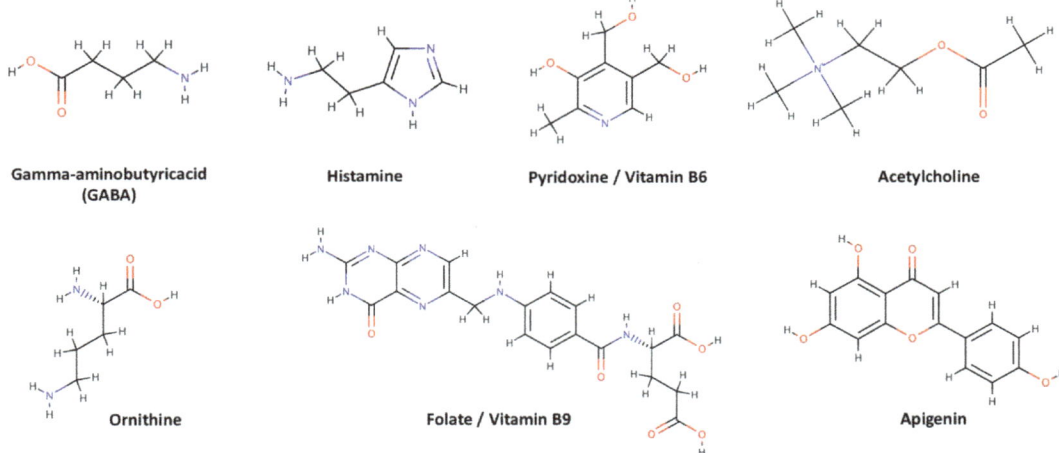

Fig. 7 The chemical structure of some sleep-inducing compounds

right ways to experience perfect sleep. Therefore, proper sleep significantly improves the health and functioning of individuals in communities and removes the high costs of treatment of poor-sleep related medical conditions from governments.

References

Ajlouni KM, Ahmad AT, Al-Zahiri MM, Ammari FL, Jarrah NS, Abujbara MA, Ajlouni HK, Daradkeh TK (2005) Sleepwalking associated with hyperthyroidism. Endocrine Practice 11(1):5–10

Ahmad J, Riley R, Sieunarine K (2007) Pca-induced respiratory depression simulating stroke following endoluminal repair of abdominal aortic aneurysm: a case report. J Med Case Rep 1(45):1–3

Atkinson G, Davenne D (2007) Relationships between sleep, physical activity and human health. Physiol Behav 90(2–3):229–235

Aurora RN, Zak RS, Auerbach SH, Casey KR, Chowdhuri S, Karippot A, Maganti RK, Ramar K, Kristo DA (2010) Best practice guide for the treatment of nightmare disorder in adults. J Clin Sleep Med 6 (4):389–401

AlDabal L (2011) Metabolic, endocrine, and immune consequences of sleep deprivation. Open Respir Med J 5(1):31–43

Attanasio AF, Jung H, Mo D, Chanson P, Bouillon R, Ho KKY, Lamberts SWJ, Clemmons DR (2011) Prevalence and incidence of diabetes mellitus in adult patients on growth hormone replacement for growth hormone deficiency: a surveillance database analysis. J Clin Endocrinol Metab 96(7):2255–2261

Alam N (2013) NREM sleep: anatomy and physiology. In. Elsevier, pp 453–459

Ali T, Choe J, Awab A, Wagener TL, Orr WC (2013) Sleep, immunity and inflammation in gastrointestinal disorders. World J Gastroenterol 19:9231–9239

Adib-Hajbaghery M, Mousavi SN (2017) The effects of chamomile extract on sleep quality among elderly people: a clinical trial. Complement Ther Med 35:109–114

Al Khatib H, Harding S, Darzi J, Pot G (2017) The effects of partial sleep deprivation on energy balance: a systematic review and meta-analysis. Eur J Clin Nutr 71(5):614–624

Aulsebrook AE, Jones TM, Mulder RA, Lesku JA (2018) Impacts of artificial light at night on sleep: a review and prospectus. J Exp Zool Part a: Ecol Int Physiol 329(8–9):409–418

Burg AW, Werner E (1975) Effect of orally-administered caffeine and theophylline on tissue concentrations of 3', 5'cyclic-AMP and phospho-diesterase. Fed Proc 34(3):332–332

Bonnet MH (1985) Effect of sleep disruption on sleep, performance, and mood. Sleep 8(1):11–19

Brown GM (1994) Light, melatonin and the sleep-wake cycle. J Psychiatry Neurosci 19(5):345–345

Bentivoglio M, Grassi-Zucconi G (1997) The Pioneering Experimental Studies on Sleep Deprivation. Sleep 20:570–576

Blundell JE, Halford JCG (1998) Serotonin and appetite regulation. CNS Drugs 9(6):473–495

Borjigin J, Li X, Snyder SH (1999) The pineal gland and melatonin: molecular and pharmacologic regulation. Annu Rev Pharmacol Toxicol 39(1):53–65

Ben-Jonathan N, Liby K, McFarland M, Zinger M (2002) Prolactin as an autocrine/paracrine growth factor in human cancer. Trends Endocrinol Metab 13(6): 245–250

Berson D (2003) Strange vision: ganglion cells as circadian photoreceptors. Trends Neurosci 26(6):314–320

Basheer R, Strecker RE, Thakkar MM, McCarley RW (2004) Adenosine and sleep-wake regulation. Prog Neurobiol 73(6):379–396

Bryant PA, Trinder J, Curtis N (2004) Sick and tired: does sleep have a vital role in the immune system? Nat Rev Immunol 4:457–467

Berridge CW (2008) Noradrenergic modulation of arousal. Brain Res Rev 58:1–17

Born J, Wagner U (2009) Sleep, hormones, and memory. Obstet Gynecol Clin North Am 36:809–829

Bourjeily G (2009) Sleep disorders in pregnancy. Obstetric Med 2(3):100–106

Buckingham JC (2009) Glucocorticoids: exemplars of multi-tasking. Br J Pharmacol 147(S1):258–268

Beccuti G, Pannain S (2011) Sleep and obesity. Curr Opin Clin Nut Metab Care 14(4):402–412

Besedovsky L, Lange T, Born J (2012) Sleep and immune function. Pflugers Arch Eur J Physiol 463:121–137

Burke PR, Rios LF, Mendonça ET, Bittencourt AG, Tufik S, de Mello MT, Poyares D (2012) Shift work disorders: implications and proposed management, trabalho em turnos: consequências E propostas de gerenciamento. Sleep Sci 5(3):98–103

Bailes HJ, Lucas RJ (2013) Human melanopsin forms a pigment maximally sensitive to blue light (Λ Max ≈ 479 Nm) supporting activation of Gq/11 and Gi/O signalling cascades. Proc Royal Soc b: Biol Sci 280(1759):20122987–20122987

Benke KK, Benke KE (2013) Uncertainty in health risks from artificial lighting due to disruption of circadian rhythm and melatonin secretion: a review. Hum Ecol Risk Assess: an Int J 19(4):916–929

Boag S (2017) On dreams and motivation: comparison of freud's and hobson's views. Front Psychol 7:6–6

Blume C, Garbazza C, Spitschan M (2019) Effects of light on human circadian rhythms. Sleep Mood Somnologie 23(3):147–156

Binks H, Vincent GE, Gupta C, Irwin C, Khalesi S (2020) Effects of diet on sleep: a narrative review. Nutrients 12(4):936–936

Cardinali DP, Pévet P (1998) Basic aspects of melatonin action. Sleep Med Rev 2(3):175–190

Czeisler CA, Wright KP (1999) Influence of light on circadian rhythmicity in humans. Lung Biol Health Dis 133:149–180

Casez O, Dananchet Y, Besson G (2005) Migraine and somnambulism. Neurology 65(8):1334–1335

Claustrat B, Brun J, Chazot G (2005) The basic physiology and pathophysiology of melatonin. Sleep Med Rev 9(1):11–24

Colten HR, Altevogt BM (2006) Extent and health consequences of chronic sleep loss and sleep disorders. Sleep disorders and sleep deprivation: an unmet public health problem, vol 33063. National Academies Press, US

Christiansen JJ, Djurhuus CB, Gravholt CH, Iversen P, Christiansen JS, Schmitz O, Weeke J, Jørgensen JOL, Møller N (2007) Effects of cortisol on carbohydrate, lipid, and protein metabolism: studies of acute cortisol withdrawal in adrenocortical failure. J Clin Endocrinol Metab 92(9):3553–3559

Cappuccio FP, Taggart FM, Kandala NB, Currie A, Peile E, Stranges S, Miller MA (2008) Meta-analysis of short sleep duration and obesity in children and adults. Sleep 31(5):619–626

Carskadon MA (2011) Sleep in adolescents: the perfect storm. Pediatr Clin North Am 58(3):637–647

Cajochen C, Frey S, Anders D, Späti J, Bues M, Pross A, Mager R, Wirz-Justice A, Stefani O (2011) Evening exposure to a light-emitting diodes (LED)-backlit computer screen affects circadian physiology and cognitive performance. J Appl Physiol 110(5):1432–1438

Cannavò S, Marini F, Curtò L, Torre ML, de Gregorio C, Salamone I, Alibrandi A, Trimarchi F (2011) High prevalence of coronary calcifications and increased risk for coronary heart disease in adults with growth hormone deficiency. J Endocrinol Invest 34(1):32–37

Copinschi G, Caufriez A (2013) Sleep and hormonal changes in aging. Endocrinol Metab Clin North Am 42(2):371–389

Cowen PJ, Browning M (2015) What has serotonin to do with depression? World Psychiatry 14(2):158–160

Cao Y, Taylor AW, Pan X, Adams R, Appleton S, Shi Z (2016) Dinner fat intake and sleep duration and self-reported sleep parameters over five years: findings from the jiangsu nutrition study of chinese adults. Nutrition 32(9):970–974

Castrillon EE, Ou KL, Wang K, Zhang J, Zhou X, Svensson P (2016) Sleep bruxism: an updated review of an old problem. Acta Odontol Scand 74(5):328–334

Centers for Disease Control and Prevention (2017) How Much Sleep Do I Need? https://www.cdc.gov/sleep/about_sleep/how_much_sleep.html

Chen Y, Tan F, Wei L, Li X, Lyu Z, Feng X, Wen Y, Guo L, He J, Dai M, Li N (2018) Sleep duration and the risk of cancer: a systematic review and meta-analysis including dose-response relationship. BMC Cancer 18:1–13

Carter P, Ye L, Richards K, Vallabhaneni V (2019) Sleep and memory: the promise of precision medicine. Sleep Med Clin 14(3):371–378

Chopra A, Patel RS, Baliga N, Narahari A, Das P (2020) Sleepwalking and sleep-related eating associated with atypical antipsychotic medications: case series and systematic review of literature. Gen Hosp Psychiatry 65:74–81

Christensen M (2020) Modifiable lifestyle factors: exercise, sleep, stress, and relationships. Springer International Publishing, Integrative and Functional Medical Nutrition Therapy

Davidson JR, Moldofsky H, Lue FA (1991) Growth hormone and cortisol secretion in relation to sleep and wakefulness. J Psychiatry Neurosci: JPN 16(2):96–102

Dijk DJ, Edgar DM (1999) Circadian and homeostatic control of wakefulness and sleep. Lung Biol Health Dis 133:111–147

Dhand R, Sohal H (2007) Good sleep, bad sleep! the role of daytime naps in healthy adults. Curr Opin Int Med 6(1):91–94

Deak MC, Stickgold R (2010) Sleep and cognition. Wiley Interdisc Rev: Cogn Sci 1(4):491–500

Dijk D-J, Duffy JF, Silva EJ, Shanahan TL, Boivin DB, Czeisler CA (2012) Amplitude reduction and phase shifts of melatonin, cortisol and other circadian rhythms after a gradual advance of sleep and light exposure in humans. PLoS ONE 7(2):e30037–e30037

Drummond MJ, Dickinson JM, Fry CS, Walker DK, Gundermann DM, Reidy PT, Timmerman KL, Markofski MM, Paddon-Jones D, Rasmussen BB (2012) Bed rest impairs skeletal muscle amino acid transporter expression, mtorc1 signalling, and protein synthesis in response to essential amino acids in older adults. Am J Physiol-Endocrinol Metab 302(9):E1113–E1122

Dresler M, Spoormaker VI, Beitinger P, Czisch M, Kimura M, Steiger A, Holsboer F (2014) Neuroscience-driven discovery and development of sleep therapeutics. Pharmacol Ther 141:300–334

Dunlap JC, Loros JJ (2017) Making time: conservation of biological clocks from fungi to animals. In. American society of microbiology. pp 515–534

Daniele TMdC, de Bruin PFC, Rios ERV, de Bruin VMS (2017) Effects of exercise on depressive behavior and striatal levels of norepinephrine, serotonin and their metabolites in sleep-deprived mice. Behav Brain Res 332:16–22

Dolezal BA, Neufeld EV, Boland DM, Martin JL, Cooper CB (2017) Interrelationship between sleep and exercise: a systematic review. Advan Prev Med 2017:1–14

de Macêdo TCF, Ferreira GH, de Almondes KM, Kirov R, Mota-Rolim SA (2019) My dream, my rules: can lucid dreaming treat nightmares? Front Psychol 10:2618–2618

Doherty R, Madigan S, Warrington G, Ellis J (2019) Sleep and nutrition interactions: implications for athletes. Nutrients 11(4):822–822

Ellis JG, Gehrman P, Espie CA, Riemann D, Perlis ML (2012) Acute insomnia: current conceptualizations and future directions. Sleep Med Rev 16(1):5–14

Elder GJ, Wetherell MA, Barclay NL, Ellis JG (2014) The cortisol awakening response—applications and implications for sleep medicine. Sleep Med Rev 18(3):215–224

España RA, Schmeichel BE, Berridge CW (2016) Norepinephrine at the nexus of arousal, motivation and relapse. Brain Res 1641:207–216

Feinberg I (1974) Changes in sleep cycle patterns with age. J Psychiatr Res 10(3–4):283–306

Frazer T, Gavin JR, Daughaday WH, Hillman RE, Weldon VV (1982) Growth hormone-dependent growth failure. J Pediatr 101(1):12–15

Fredholm BB, Bättig K, Holmén J, Nehlig A, Zvartau EE (1999) Actions of caffeine in the brain with special reference to factors that contribute to its widespread use. Pharmacol Rev 51(1):83–133

Fink G (2000) Encyclopedia of stress. Academic Press

Fukuda K, Ishihara K (2001) Age-related changes of sleeping pattern during adolescence. Psychiatry Clin Neurosci 55(3):231–232

Franklin MS, Zyphur MJ (2005) The role of dreams in the evolution of the human mind. Evol Psychol 3(1):59–78

Faraut B, Boudjeltia KZ, Vanhamme L, Kerkhofs M (2012) Immune, inflammatory and cardiovascular consequences of sleep restriction and recovery. Sleep Med Rev 16:137–149

Fullagar HHK, Skorski S, Duffield R, Hammes D, Coutts AJ, Meyer T (2015) Sleep and athletic performance: the effects of sleep loss on exercise performance, and physiological and cognitive responses to exercise. Sports Med 45:161–186

Favero G, Franceschetti L, Buffoli B, Moghadasian MH, Reiter RJ, Rodella LF, Rezzani R (2017) Melatonin: protection against age-related cardiac pathology. Ageing Res Rev 35:336–349

Foster R, Kreitzman L (2017) Circadian rhythms: a very short introduction. Oxford University Press

Fredholm BB, Yang J, Wang Y (2017) Low, but not high, dose caffeine is a readily available probe for adenosine actions. Mol Aspects Med 55:20–25

Gooley JJ, Lu J, Chou TC, Scammell TE, Saper CB (2001) Melanopsin in cells of origin of the retinohypothalamic tract. Nat Neurosci 4(12):1165–1165

Gais S, Born J (2004) Low acetylcholine during slow-wave sleep is critical for declarative memory consolidation. Proc Natl Acad Sci USA 101(7):2140–2144

Gooley JJ, Chamberlain K, Smith KA, Khalsa SBS, Rajaratnam SMW, Van Reen E, Zeitzer JM, Czeisler CA, Lockley SW (2011) Exposure to room light before bedtime suppresses melatonin onset and shortens melatonin duration in humans. J Clin Endocrinol Metab 96(3):463–472

Gangwisch JE (2014) A review of evidence for the link between sleep duration and hypertension. Am J Hypertens 27(10):1235–1242

Godin I, Montplaisir J, Nielsen T (2015) Dreaming and nightmares in REM sleep behavior disorder. Dreaming 25(4):257–273

Grandner MA, Seixas A, Shetty S, Shenoy S (2016) Sleep duration and diabetes risk: population trends and potential mechanisms. Curr DiabRep 16:1–14

Ghafarzadeh J, Sadeghniiat-Haghighi K, Sadeghpour O, Akbarpour S, Amini-Behbahani F (2019) Investigating the prevalence of sleep disorder and the impact of sweet almond on the quality of sleep in students of Tehran, Iran. Iran J Public Health 48(6):1149–1154

Harvey S, Hull KL (1997) Growth hormone: a paracrine growth factor? Endocrine 7:267–279

Hublin C, Kaprio J, Partinen M, Koskenvuo M (1999) Nightmares: familial aggregation and association with psychiatric disorders in a nationwide twin cohort. Am J Med Genetics—Neuropsychiatric Genetics 88(4):329–336

Hauri PJ, Silber MH, Boeve BF (2007) The treatment of parasomnias with hypnosis: a 5-year follow-up study. J Clin Sleep Med 3(4):369–373

Hagenauer MH, Perryman JI, Lee TM, Carskadon MA (2009) Adolescent changes in the homeostatic and circadian regulation of sleep. Dev Neurosci 31(4):276–284

Hasler BP, Germain A (2009) Correlates and treatments of nightmares in adults. Sleep Med Clin 4:507–517

Huang Z-L, Zhang Z, Qu W-M (2014) Roles of adenosine and its receptors in sleep–wake regulation. In: International review of neurobiology, vol 119. Elsevier, pp 349–371.

Ireland JL, Culpin V (2006) The relationship between sleeping problems and aggression, anger, and impulsivity in a population of juvenile and young offenders. J Adolesc Health 38(6):649–655

Imeri L, Opp MR (2009) How (and why) the immune system makes us sleep. Nat Rev Neurosci 10:199–210

Izci Balserak B, Lee KA (2017) Sleep and sleep disorders associated with pregnancy. In. Elsevier, pp 1525–1539

Ikegami K, Refetoff S, Van Cauter E, Yoshimura T (2019) Interconnection between circadian clocks and thyroid function. Nat Rev Endocrinol 15(10):590–600

Ja C-S, Tapia-Ayuga CE (2020) Blue light emission spectra of popular mobile devices: the extent of user protection against melatonin suppression by built-in screen technology and light filtering software systems. Chronobiol Int 1–7.

Joëls M, Fernandez G, Roozendaal B (2011) Stress and emotional memory: a matter of timing. Trends Cogn Sci 15(6):280–288

Kerkhofs M, Van Cauter E, Van Onderbergen A, Caufriez A, Thorner MO, Copinschi G (1993) Sleep-promoting effects of growth hormone-releasing hormone in normal men. Am J Physiol—Endocrinol Metab 264(4):27–4

Kern W, Dodt C, Born J, Fehm HL (1996) Changes in cortisol and growth hormone secretion during nocturnal sleep in the course of aging. J Gerontol—Ser A Biol Sci Med Sci 51(1):3–9

Karasek M (2004) Melatonin, human aging, and age-related diseases. Exp Gerontol 39(11–12):1723–1729

Killgore WDS, Kahn-Greene ET, Lipizzi EL, Newman RA, Kamimori GH, Balkin TJ (2008) Sleep deprivation reduces perceived emotional intelligence and constructive thinking skills. Sleep Med 9(5):517–526

Kang J-H, Chen S-C (2009) Effects of an irregular bedtime schedule on sleep quality, daytime sleepiness, and fatigue among university students in Taiwan. BMC Public Health 9(1):248–248

Kierlin L, Littner MR (2011) Parasomnias and antidepressant therapy: a review of the literature. Front Psychiatry 2:1–8

Krueger JM, Majde JA, Rector DM (2011) Cytokines in immune function and sleep regulation. In: Handbook of clinical neurology, vol 98. Elsevier, pp 229–240

Kay M, Choe EK, Shepherd J, Greenstein B, Watson N, Consolvo S, Kientz JA (2012) Lullaby: a capture and access system for understanding the sleep environment. New York, New York, USA. ACM Press, pp 226–235

Kubiszewski V, Fontaine R, Rusch E, Hazouard E (2014) Association between electronic media use and sleep habits: an eight-day follow-up study. Int J Adolesc Youth 19(3):395–407

Kelley P, Lockley SW, Foster RG, Kelley J (2015) Synchronizing education to adolescent biology: 'let teens sleep, start school later.' Learn, Media Technol 40(2):210–226

Kim KW, Kang SH, Yoon IY, Lee SD, Ju G, Han JW, Kim TH, Lee CS, Kim T (2017a) Prevalence and clinical characteristics of insomnia and its subtypes in the korean elderly. Arch Gerontol Geriatr 68:68–75

Kim HD, Hong KB, Noh DO, Suh HJ (2017b) Sleep-inducing effect of lettuce (lactuca sativa) varieties on pentobarbital-induced sleep. Food Sci Biotechnol 26(3):807–814

Lange T, Mölle M (1997) Effects of sleep and circadian rhythm on human circulating immune cells. Article J Immunol 158(9):4454–4464

Laberge L, Tremblay RE, Vitaro F, Montplaisir J (2000) Development of parasomnias childhood to early adolescence. Pediatrics 106(1):67–74

Lambert GW, Reid C, Kaye DM, Jennings GL, Esler MD (2002) Effect of sunlight and season on serotonin turnover in the brain. Lancet 360(9348):1840–1842

Lorton D, Lubahn CL, Estus C, Millar BA, Carter JL, Wood CA, Bellinger DL (2006) Bidirectional communication between the brain and the immune system: implications for physiological sleep and disorders with disrupted sleep. NeuroImmunoModulation 13(5–6):357–374

Lange T, Dimitrov S, Born J (2010) Effects of sleep and circadian rhythm on the human immune system. Ann N Y Acad Sci 1193(1):48–59

Lee EK, Douglass AB (2010) Sleep in psychiatric disorders: where are we now? Can J Psychiat 55(7):403–412

Lin J-S, Anaclet C, Sergeeva OA, Haas HL (2011) The waking brain: an update. Cell Mol Life Sci 68(15):2499–2512

Lemola S, Schwarz B, Siffert A (2012) Interparental conflict and early adolescents' aggression: is irregular sleep a vulnerability factor? J Adolesc 35(1):97–105

Larcher S, Benhamou PY, Pépin JL, Borel AL (2015) Sleep habits and diabetes. Diabetes Metab 41:263–271

LaGrotte C, Fernandez-Mendoza J, Calhoun SL, Liao D, Bixler EO, Vgontzas AN (2016) The relative association of obstructive sleep apnea, obesity and excessive daytime sleepiness with incident depression: a longitudinal population-based study. Int J Obesity 40(9):1397–1404

Levenson JC, Shensa A, Sidani JE, Colditz JB, Primack BA (2016) The association between social media use and sleep disturbance among young adults. Prev Med 85:36–41

Li W, Ma L, Yang G, Gan WB (2017) REM sleep selectively prunes and maintains new synapses in development and learning. Nat Neurosci 20(3):427–437

Li J, Vitiello MV, Gooneratne NS (2018) Sleep in normal aging. Sleep Med Clin 13:1–11

Lazarus M, Oishi Y, Bjorness TE, Greene RW (2019) Gating and the need for sleep: dissociable effects of adenosine A1 and A2a receptors. Front Neurosci 13:1–12

Liu H, Chen A (2019) Roles of sleep deprivation in cardiovascular dysfunctions. Life Sci 219:231–237

Liu YU, Ying Y, Li Y, Eyo UB, Chen T, Zheng J, Umpierre AD, Zhu J, Bosco DB, Dong H, Wu LJ (2019) Neuronal network activity controls microglial process surveillance in awake mice via norepinephrine signalling. Nat Neurosci 22(11):1771–1781

Marriott BM (1994) Stress and monoamine neurons in the brain. In: Food components to enhance performance: an evaluation of potential performance-enhancing food components for operational rations. National Academies Press, US

Machado ERS, Varella VBR, Andrade MMM (1998) The influence of study schedules and work on the sleep-wake cycle of college students. Biol Rhythm Res 29(5):578–584

Morin LP (1999) Serotonin and the regulation of mammalian circadian rhythmicity. Ann Med 31(1):12–33

Mitchell HA, Weinshenker D (2010) Good night and good luck: norepinephrine in sleep pharmacology. Biochem Pharmacol 79:801–809

Mustafa SJ, Morrison RR, Teng B, Pelleg A (2009) Adenosine receptors and the heart: role in regulation of coronary blood flow and cardiac electrophysiology. In: Adenosine receptors in health and disease. Springer, pp 161–188

Marshall L, Helgadóttir H, Mölle M, Born J (2006) Boosting slow oscillations during sleep potentiates memory. Nature 444(7119):610–613

McEwen BS (2008) Central effects of stress hormones in health and disease: understanding the protective and damaging effects of stress and stress mediators. Eur J Pharmacol 583(2–3):174–185

McNamara P, Johnson P, McLaren D, Harris E, Beauharnais C, Auerbach S (2010) REM and NREM sleep mentation. In: International review of neurobiology, vol 92. Elsevier, pp 69–86

Malhotra RK, Avidan AY (2012) Parasomnias and their mimics. Neurol Clin 30(4):1067–1094

Marder M (2012) Flavonoids as gabaa receptor ligands: the whole story? J Exp Pharmacol 4:9–9

Mousavi F, Tavabi A, Iran-Pour E, Tabatabaei R, Golestan B (2012) Prevalence and associated factors of insomnia syndrome in the elderly residing in kahrizak nursing home, Tehran, Iran. Iran J Public Health 41(1):96–106

Morris CJ, Aeschbach D, Scheer FAJL (2012) Circadian system, sleep and endocrinology. Mol Cell Endocrinol 349:91–104

Meneses A, Liy-Salmeron G (2012) Serotonin and emotion, learning and memory. Rev Neurosci 23(5–6):543–553

Mezick EJ, Matthews KA, Hall MH, Richard Jennings J, Kamarck TW (2014) Sleep duration and cardiovascular responses to stress in undergraduate men. Psychophysiology 51(1):88–96

Meneses A (2015) Serotonin, neural markers, and memory. Front Pharmacol 6:1–22

McLellan TM, Caldwell JA, Lieberman HR (2016) A review of caffeine's effects on cognitive, physical and occupational performance. Neurosci Biobehav Rev 71:294–312

Melo G, Duarte J, Pauletto P, Porporatti AL, Stuginski-Barbosa J, Winocur E, Flores-Mir C, De Luca CG (2019) Bruxism: an umbrella review of systematic reviews. J Oral Rehabil 46(7):666–690

Nielsen TA, Paquette T, Solomonova E, Lara-Carrasco J, Popova A, Levrier K (2010) REM sleep characteristics of nightmare sufferers before and after REM sleep deprivation. Sleep Med 11(2):172–179

O'Donnell CP, King ED, Schwartz AR, Smith PL, Robotham JL (1994) Effect of sleep deprivation on responses to airway obstruction in the sleeping dog. J Appl Physiol 77(4):1811–1818

Ohayon MM, Priest RG (1999) Night terrors, sleepwalking, and confusional arousals in the general population: their frequency and relationship to other sleep and mental disorders. J Clin Psychiatry 60(4):268–276

Ohayon MM (2002) Epidemiology of insomnia: what we know and what we still need to learn. Sleep Med Rev 6:97–111

Olivier B (2004) Serotonin and aggression. Ann N Y Acad Sci 1036(1):382–392

Pagel JF, Helfter P (2003) Drug induced nightmares?an etiology based review. Human Psychopharmacol: Clin Exp 18(1):59–67

Penzel T, Kantelhardt JW, Lo CC, Voigt K, Vogelmeier C (2003) Dynamics of heart rate and sleep stages in normals and patients with sleep apnea. Neuropsychopharmacology 28(1):48–53

Power AE (2004) Slow-wave sleep, acetylcholine, and memory consolidation. Proc Natl Acad Sci USA 101:1795–1796

Pandi-Perumal SR, Zisapel N, Srinivasan V, Cardinali DP (2005) Melatonin and sleep in aging population. Exp Gerontol 40:911–925

Pandi-Perumal SR, Srinivasan V, Maestroni GJM, Cardinali DP, Poeggeler B, Hardeland R (2006) Melatonin: nature's most versatile biological signal? FEBS J 273(13):2813–2838

Poryazova R, Waldvogel D, Bassetti CL (2007) Sleepwalking in patients with parkinson disease. Arch Neurol 64(10):1524–1527

Pressman MR (2007) Disorders of arousal from sleep and violent behavior: the role of physical contact and proximity. Sleep 30(8):1039–1047

Perry JC, D'Almeida V, Souza FG, Schoorlemmer GHM, Colombari E, Tufik S (2007) Consequences of subchronic and chronic exposure to intermittent hypoxia and sleep deprivation on cardiovascular risk factors in rats. Respir Physiol Neurobiol 156(3):250–258

Palagini L, Rosenlicht N (2011) Sleep, dreaming, and mental health: a review of historical and neurobiological perspectives. Sleep Med Rev 15:179–186

Porkka-Heiskanen T, Kalinchuk AV (2011) Adenosine, energy metabolism and sleep homeostasis. Sleep Med Rev 15(2):123–135

Pressman MR (2011) Common misconceptions about sleepwalking and other parasomnias. Sleep Med Clin 6:xiii–xvii

Perogamvros I, Ray DW, Trainer PJ (2012) Regulation of cortisol bioavailability—effects on hormone measurement and action. Nat Rev Endocrinol 8(12):717–727

Peuhkuri K, Sihvola N, Korpela R (2012a) Dietary factors and fluctuating levels of melatonin. Food Nutr Res 56(1):17252–17252

Peuhkuri K, Sihvola N, Korpela R (2012b) Diet promotes sleep duration and quality. Nutr Res 32(5):309–319

Perogamvros L, Dang-Vu TT, Desseilles M, Schwartz S (2013) Sleep and dreaming are for important matters. Front Psychol 4:474

Paterson JL, Dorrian J, Ferguson SA, Jay SM, Dawson D (2013) What happens to mood, performance and sleep in a laboratory study with no sleep deprivation? Sleep Biol Rhythms 11(3):200–209

Pechanova O, Paulis L, Simko F (2014) Peripheral and central effects of melatonin on blood pressure regulation. Int J Mol Sci 15(10):17920–17937

Patel D, Steinberg J, Patel P (2018) Insomnia in the elderly: a review. J Clin Sleep Med 14(06):1017–1024

Porras-Segovia A, Pérez-Rodríguez MM, López-Esteban P, Courtet P, Barrigón MML, López-Castromán J, Cervilla JA, Baca-García E (2019) Contribution of sleep deprivation to suicidal behaviour: a systematic review. Sleep Med Rev 44:37–47

Rosenthal NE, Joseph-Vanderpool JR, Levendosky AA, Johnston SH, Allen R, Kelly KA, Souetre E, Schultz PM, Starz KE (1990) Phase-shifting effects of bright morning light as treatment for delayed sleep phase syndrome. Sleep 13(4):354–361

Reiter RJ (1991) Pineal melatonin: cell biology of its synthesis and of its physiological interactions. Endocr Rev 12(2):151–180

Rosen T, Eden S, Larson G, Wilhelmsen L, Bengtsson BA (1993) Cardiovascular risk factors in adult patients with growth hormone deficiency. Acta Endocrinol 129(3):195–200

Roky R, Obal F Jr, Valatx JL, Bredow S, Fang J, Pagano LP, Krueger JM (1995) Prolactin and rapid eye movement sleep regulation. Sleep 18(7):536–542

Roth T, Roehrs T, Pies R (2007) Insomnia: pathophysiology and implications for treatment. Sleep Med Rev 11(1):71–79

Rajagopalan N (2011) Obstructive sleep apnea: not just a sleep disorder. J Postgrad Med 57(2):168–175

Rothman SM, Mattson MP (2012) Sleep disturbances in alzheimer's and parkinson's diseases. NeuroMol Med 14:194–204

Rama AN, Zachariah R (2013) Normal human sleep. In. Elsevier, pp 16–23

Rasch B, Born J (2013) About sleep's role in memory. Physiol Rev 93(2):681–766

Rivera-Oliver M, Díaz-Ríos M (2014) Using caffeine and other adenosine receptor antagonists and agonists as therapeutic tools against neurodegenerative diseases: a review. Life Sci 101(1–2):1–9

Roller L, Gowan J (2014) Insomnia. Aust J Pharm 95 (1127):66–72

Riemann D, Krone LB, Wulff K, Nissen C (2020) Sleep, insomnia, and depression. Neuropsychopharmacology 45:74–89

Roesler C (2020) Jungian theory of dreaming and contemporary dream research—findings from the research project 'structural dream analysis.' J Anal Psychol 65(1):44–62

Samel A, Wegmann HM, Vejvoda M (1995) Jet lag and sleepiness in aircrew. J Sleep Res 4:30–36

Spiegel K, Luthringer R, Follenius M, Schaltenbrand N, Macher JP, Muzet A, Brandenberger G (1995) Temporal relationship between prolactin secretion and slow-wave electroencephalic activity during sleep. Sleep 18(7):543–548

Shalet SM, Toogood A, Rahim A, Brennan BMD (1998) The diagnosis of growth hormone deficiency in children and adults. Endocr Rev 19(2):203–223

Scacchi M, Pincelli AI, Cavagnini F (1999) Growth hormone in obesity. Int J Obes 23:260–271

Simonneaux V, Ribelayga C (2003) Generation of the melatonin endocrine message in mammals: a review of the complex regulation of melatonin synthesis by norepinephrine, peptides, and other pineal transmitters. Pharmacol Rev 55:325–395

Stepanski EJ, Wyatt JK (2003) Use of sleep hygiene in the treatment of insomnia. Sleep Med Rev 7(3): 215–225

Schredl M, Schmitt J, Hein G, Schmoll T, Eller S, Haaf J (2006) Nightmares and oxygen desaturations: is sleep apnea related to heightened nightmare frequency? Sleep Breathing 10(4):203–209

Scott JPR, McNaughton LR, Polman RCJ (2006) Effects of sleep deprivation and exercise on cognitive, motor performance and mood. Physiol Behav 87(2):396–408

Szewczuk LM, Tarrant MK, Sample V, Drury WJ, Zhang J, Cole PA (2008) Analysis of serotonin N-acetyltransferase regulation in vitro and in live cells using protein semisynthesis. Biochemistry 47(39):10407–10419

Schredl M (2009) Dreams in patients with sleep disorders. Sleep Med Rev 13:215–221

Schwartz J, Roth T (2009) Neurophysiology of sleep and wakefulness: basic science and clinical implications. Curr Neuropharmacol 6(4):367–378

Sterpenich V, Albouy G, Darsaud A, Schmidt C, Vandewalle G, Dang Vu TT, Desseilles M, Phillips C, Degueldre C, Balteau E, Collette F, Luxen A, Maquet P (2009) Sleep promotes the neural reorganization of remote emotional memory. J Neurosci 29(16):5143–5152

Srinivasan V, Singh J, Pandi-Perumal SR, Brown GM, Spence DW, Cardinali DP (2010) Jet lag, circadian rhythm sleep disturbances, and depression: the role of melatonin and its analogs. Advan Ther 27(11):796–813

Sandman N, Valli K, Kronholm E, Ollila HM, Revonsuo A, Laatikainen T, Paunio T (2013) Nightmares: prevalence among the finnish general adult population and war veterans during 1972–2007. Sleep 36(7):1041–1050

Singh A, Chaudhary R, Sonker A, Pandey HC (2016) Importance of donor history of restless leg syndrome and pica to asses iron deficiency. Transfus Apheres Sci 54(2):259–261

Stachowicz M, Lebiedzińska A (2016) The effect of diet components on the level of cortisol. Eur Food Res Technol 242:2001–2009

Stallman HM, Kohler M (2016) Prevalence of sleepwalking: a systematic review and meta-analysis. PLoS ONE 11(11):e0164769–e0164769

St-Onge MP, Mikic A, Pietrolungo CE (2016) Effects of diet on sleep quality. Advan Nutr 7:938–949

Simpson NS, Gibbs EL, Matheson GO (2017) Optimizing sleep to maximize performance: implications and recommendations for elite athletes. Scand J Med Sci Sports 27(3):266–274

Szaulińska K, Poradowska E, Wierzbicka A, Wichniak A (2017) Air travel is not only going on holiday—jet lag of airline employees, case narrative and brief review of literature | podróze lotnicze to nie tylko wyjazdy na wakacje—jet lag u pracowników linii lotniczych. Postepy Psychiatrii i Neurologii 26(1):44–54

Suzen S (2018) Melatonin and its antiaging activity: new approaches and strategies for age-related disorders. In: Molecular basis and emerging strategies for anti-aging interventions. Springer, Singapore, pp 217–235

Salehi B, Venditti A, Sharifi-Rad M, Kręgiel D, Sharifi-Rad J, Durazzo A, Lucarini M, Santini A, Souto EB, Novellino E, Antolak H, Azzini E, Setzer WN, Martins N (2019) The therapeutic potential of apigenin. Int J Mol Sci 20:1305

Scott H, Woods HC (2019) Understanding links between social media use, sleep and mental health: recent progress and current challenges. Curr Sleep Med Rep 5(3):141–149

Stepicheva NA, Weiss J, Shang P, Yazdankhah M, Ghosh S, Bhutto IA, Hose S, Zigler JS, Sinha D (2019) Melatonin as the possible link between age-related retinal regeneration and the disrupted circadian rhythm in elderly. In: Advances in experimental medicine and biology, vol 1185. Springer, pp 45–49

Sundaresan S, Migden MR, Silapunt S (2019) Treatment of leg veins for restless leg syndrome: a retrospective review. Cureus 11(4):4368–4368

Taylor A (1993) Night terrors. J Contemp Psychother 23(2):121–125

Turner R, Jones T (2003) Techniques for imaging neuroscience. Br Med Bull 65(1):3–20

Taheri S, Lin L, Austin D, Young T, Mignot E (2004) Short sleep duration is associated with reduced leptin, elevated ghrelin, and increased body mass index. PLoS Med 1(3):210–217

Ting L, Malhotra A (2005) Disorders of sleep: an overview. Primary Care—Clin off Practice 32:305–318

The GKH, Verkes RJ, Fekkes D, Bleijenberg G, van der Meer JWM, Buitelaar JK (2014) Tryptophan depletion in chronic fatigue syndrome, a pilot cross-over study. BMC Res Notes 7(1):650–650

Thun E, Bjorvatn B, Flo E, Harris A, Pallesen S (2015) Sleep, circadian rhythms, and athletic performance. Sleep Med Rev 23:1–9

Tobaldini E, Costantino G, Solbiati M, Cogliati C, Kara T, Nobili L, Montano N (2017) Sleep, sleep deprivation, autonomic nervous system and cardiovascular diseases. Neurosci Biobehav Rev 74:321–329

Ursin R (2002) Serotonin and sleep. Sleep Med Rev 6(1):55–67

Underwood E (2013) Sleep: the brain's housekeeper? Science 342:301

Van Cauter E, Plat L (1996) Physiology of growth hormone secretion during sleep. J Pediatr 128:32–37

Van Cauter E, Leproult R, Kupfer DJ (1996) Effects of gender and age on the levels and circadian rhythmicity of plasma cortisol. J Clin Endocrinol Metab 81(7):2468–2473

Van Cauter E, Leproult R, Plat L (2000) Age-related changes in slow wave sleep and REM sleep and relationship with growth hormone and cortisol levels in healthy men. J Am Med Assoc 284(7):861–868

Vanderveen J, Armstrong L, Butterfield G, Chenoweth W, Dwyer J, Fernstrom J, Kanarek R, Levander O, Sternberg E (2001) Caffeine for the sustainment of mental task performance. Caffeine for the Sustainment of Mental Task Performance, Washington, DC

van Stegeren AH (2008) The role of the noradrenergic system in emotional memory. Acta Physiol (oxf) 127(3):532–541

Weitzman ED, Nogeire C, Perlow M, Fukushima D, Sassin JON, McGregor P, Gallagher TF, Hellman L (1974) Effects of a prolonged 3-hour sleep-wake cycle on sleep stages, plasma cortisol, growth hormone and body temperature in man*. J Clin Endocrinol Metab 38(6):1018–1030

Weibel L, Follenius M, Spiegel K, Gronfier C, Brandenberger G (1997) Growth hormone secretion in night workers. Chronobiol Int 14(1):49–60

Walker MP, Stickgold R (2004) Sleep-dependent learning and memory consolidation. Neuron 44:121–133

Wilhelm I, Born J, Kudielka BM, Schlotz W, Wüst S (2007) Is the cortisol awakening rise a response to awakening? Psychoneuroendocrinology 32(4):358–366

Watson CJ, Baghdoyan HA, Lydic R (2010) Neuropharmacology of sleep and wakefulness. Sleep Med Clin 5:513–528

Wamsley EJ, Stickgold R (2011) Memory, sleep, and dreaming: experiencing consolidation. Sleep Med Clin 6:97–108

Watson NF, Harden KP, Buchwald D, Vitiello MV, Pack AI, Weigle DS, Goldberg J (2012) Sleep duration and body mass index in twins: a gene-environment interaction. Sleep 35(5):597–603

Wahl S, Engelhardt M, Schaupp P, Lappe C, Ivanov IV (2019) The inner clock—blue light sets the human rhythm. J Biophotonics 12(12):1–14

Xie L, Kang H, Xu Q, Chen MJ, Liao Y, Thiyagarajan M, O'Donnell J, Christensen DJ, Nicholson C, Iliff JJ, Takano T, Deane R, Nedergaard M (2013) Sleep drives metabolite clearance from the adult Brain. Science 342(6156):373–377

Young SN (2007) How to increase serotonin in the human brain without drugs. J Psychiatry Neurosci 32:394–399

Yazdi Z, Haghighi KS, Zohal MA, Elmizadeh K (2012) Validity and reliability of the iranian version of the insomnia severity index. Malays J Med Sci 19(4):31–36

Yamada RG, Ueda HR (2020) Molecular mechanisms of REM sleep. Front Neurosci 13:1402–1402

Zimmermann RC, McDougle CJ, Schumacher M, Olcese J, Mason JW, Heninger GR, Price LH (1993) Effects of acute tryptophan depletion on nocturnal melatonin secretion in humans. J Clin Endocrinol Metab 76(5):1160–1164

Zadra A, Pilon M, Montplaisir J (2008) Polysomnographic diagnosis of sleepwalking: effects of sleep deprivation. Ann Neurol 63(4):513–519

Zadra A, Desautels A, Petit D, Montplaisir J (2013) Somnambulism: clinical aspects and pathophysiological hypotheses. Lancet Neurol 12(3):285–294

Zeng Y, Yang J, Du J, Pu X, Yang X, Yang S, Yang T (2014) Strategies of functional foods promote sleep in human being. Curr Signal Transduct Ther 9(3):148–155

Zhang Y, Liu J, Yao J, Ji G, Qian L, Wang J, Zhang G, Tian J, Nie Y, Zhang YE, Gold MS, Liu Y (2014) Obesity: pathophysiology and intervention. Nutrients 6(11):5153–5183

Zhai L, Zhang H, Zhang D (2015) Sleep duration and depression among adults: a meta-analysis of prospective studies. Depression Anxiety 32:664–670

Zielinski MR, McKenna JT, McCarley RW (2016) Functions and mechanisms of sleep. AIMS Neurosci 3(1):67

Index

A
Adenosine, 167, 168, 170, 171
Antioxidant, vii, 3–5, 62, 65, 66, 76–84, 91–97, 99–101, 103, 105–109, 122, 123, 125, 132, 133, 135, 139, 140, 142
Anxiety, 4, 93, 94, 96, 110, 132, 143, 144, 146, 156, 158, 167, 172, 173, 180, 182, 185, 186

B
Bioactive, 16, 20, 21, 33, 62, 64, 65, 67, 68, 75, 77, 80, 82–85, 92–94, 97, 105, 108–110, 123, 139, 140
Biodiversity, 61, 66, 68–70, 143
Bioinspiration, 9–11, 22, 26
Biomedical, 16, 19, 20, 61, 67, 69, 144
Biomimetic, 2, 9–12, 14, 16–18, 22, 24
Biosynthetic, 36, 47, 66
Brain, 5, 6, 35, 36, 45, 67, 76, 95, 96, 101, 118, 134–137, 141, 144–147, 155–164, 167–175, 177, 180–183

D
Diabetes, vii, 2–4, 6, 62, 65, 67, 68, 76–78, 81, 82, 84, 91, 92, 96, 97, 99, 101, 103, 104, 107, 108, 122, 123, 129, 132, 134–141, 143, 145–148, 156, 173, 178, 179, 184
Diseases, 61–63, 65, 66, 68, 69
Drug-delivery, 16, 17
Drug design, 31, 32

E
Emotional, 155–163, 178, 180–182, 185
Exercise, 2, 3, 24, 132, 134, 139, 170, 180, 182, 186, 187

F
Free radicals, 1–3, 77, 84, 142
Functional food, vii, 3, 75–78, 83, 85, 92, 117, 123

H
Halal, 115–125
Hormone, 5–7, 34, 35, 37, 38, 80, 109, 132, 136, 137, 140, 159, 160, 167–170, 172–174, 176, 178, 180, 184, 185

I
Immune system, 3, 76, 134, 137–139, 143, 145, 156, 167, 173, 175, 176, 178, 180
Insomnia, 5, 6, 93, 94, 137, 146, 170, 171, 173, 177–179, 183–187

L
Life style, 134, 148

M
Melatonin, 5, 6, 80, 167–174, 176, 184–187

N
Nanotechnology, 17
Natural product, 31, 33, 61, 66, 68, 96
Nature, vii, 1–3, 7, 9–11, 13, 19, 31, 33, 36, 40, 49, 55, 77, 83, 103, 116, 129, 135, 136, 143, 146, 149, 157, 158
Nutrition, 3, 14, 69, 99, 116–119, 121, 129, 132, 134, 138, 157, 180, 181, 187
Nutritional, 75–77, 79–81, 84

O

Oxidative stress, 3, 4, 81, 95–97, 100, 101, 105, 108, 122, 129, 133, 134, 136, 139, 140, 145, 148, 149, 156

P

Probiotic, 79, 138
Psychoemotional, 155–164
Psychophysiological, 155, 160, 162–164

R

Radicals, vii, viii, 121–123

S

Synthetic, 16, 18–21, 31, 33, 34, 36, 37, 40, 44, 47–49, 51, 67, 68, 70, 84
System, 132–134, 137–139, 143–146

T

Technology, vii, 2, 9–15, 21, 23, 24, 26, 116, 125, 134
Tryptophan, 167, 168, 170, 186, 187